A *Jerry Baker* Health Book

Kitchen Counter Cures

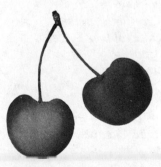

www.jerrybaker.com

A *Jerry Baker* Health Book

Kitchen Counter Cures

**117 Foods that Fight
Cancer, Diabetes, Heart Disease, Arthritis,
Osteoporosis, Memory Loss, Bad Digestion
and Hundreds of Other Health Problems!**

NOTICE

All efforts have been made to ensure accuracy. This is a reference volume only, not a medical manual. Although the information presented may help you make informed decisions about your health, it is not intended as a substitute for prescribed medical treatment. If you have a medical problem, please seek competent medical help immediately. Jerry Baker assumes no responsibility or liability for any injuries, damages, or losses incurred during the use of or as a result of following this information.

Published by American Master Products, Inc. / Jerry Baker
Kim Adam Gasior, Publisher

A Jerry Baker Health Book and A Blackberry Cottage Production
Ellen Michaud, editorial consultant, Blackberry Cottage Productions
Nest Publishing Resources, design
Carol Keough, editor
Wayne Michaud, illustrator
Patty Sinnott, copyeditor

Printed in the United States of America

Illustrations, copyright © 2001 by Wayne Michaud

Publisher's Cataloging-in-Publication

Cicero, Karen,
    Jerry Baker's giant book of kitchen counter cures:
    117 foods that fight cancer, diabetes, heart disease, arthritis,
    osteoporosis, memory loss, and hundreds of other health
    problems / Karen Cicero and Colleen Pierre;
    [edited by Jerry Baker]. —1st ed,
        p.   cm.
        ISBN: 978-0-922433-41-4

        1. Functional foods.   2. Nutrition.   3. Diet therapy.
    I. Pierre, Colleen.   II. Baker, Jerry.   III. Title.
    IV. Title: Giant book of kitchen counter cures.

RA784.C53 2001   613.2
                        QBI01-200875

                    28 26 25 27   hardcover

was all of 10 years old when I first went to live with my Grandma Putt. Back then, I wasn't just a little rough around the edges; I was a regular human pumice stone—a real rough-and-tumble little hellion!

But it didn't take long for me to realize that I wasn't such a tough nut to crack. Grandma Putt took me under her wing and taught me all about nature, instilling in me a lifelong passion for plants and all things natural. She recounted tales of her Native American heritage, which I've often passed along to you. And she taught me about the healing power of food, showing me time and time again that it's possible for food to taste good *and* be good for you.

These lessons are the ones that bring back my favorite memories of getting underfoot in Grandma Putt's kitchen. Every time I give my grandson horseradish on crackers for his stuffy nose, I remember how Grandma would make them for me, quietly explaining how the vapors would unclog my nose so I could breathe easy again. And every time the smell of freshly baked, whole wheat bread wafts through the air, I remember the way she looked there in her kitchen—hands beige with flour, apron tied in a perfect bow, kneading the dough back and forth, back and forth, until it was warm and resilient and ready for the oven.

Lately, I find myself thinking a lot about those good old days.

Maybe it's just old age creeping up on me. But I think it has more to do with living in a different time, where hard work and homespun tonics have given way to get-rich-quick schemes and an assortment of newfangled pills in pretty colors. Let's face it, folks—there doesn't seem to be a whole lot of room for old-time country wisdom within this technological revolution.

In fact, I was worried that it was going the way of the dinosaurs until I met Colleen and Karen, the authors of this book. They're two amazingly bright young women with the same homegrown values I always admired in Grandma Putt. And come to think of it, if I didn't know any better, I'd swear we were related! They're feisty. They're clever. And boy, oh boy, do these women *love* to eat!

Colleen is a registered dietitian and nutrition editor at *Child* magazine, and Karen is the food and nutrition director of *Child* magazine. Together they're teaching a new generation what Grandma Putt taught me so long ago—that good-tasting foods are good for you, too!

For instance, do you like chocolate? (I know, it's a silly question.) Well, don't feel guilty anymore for sneaking a bite of Snickers! In moderation, chocolate not only bolsters your mood and increases your life span (no wonder women live longer than men!), but those little kisses from heaven can also prevent heart disease.

Or how about cheese? A lot of folks have cut it out of their diets because of the fat content. That's too bad, because cheese that's lower in fat fights colon cancer.

And where's the beef? Probably not on the dinner table, given the recent hoopla about all that fat and cholesterol. But did you know that a lean cut of beef battles cancer, diabetes, and heart disease—all the while bolstering your energy and strengthening your immune system in the process?

I never would've guessed! Would you? Well, that's why I asked Colleen and Karen to write this book. They crammed it full of your favorite foods, added the latest discoveries from a bunch of very smart researchers, slipped in a bunch of recipes that show you how to get these foods to the table so even your picky Aunt Elmira will eat them, and then showed you how to use them to feel better and live longer.

So not only will you learn what each food battles and bolsters, but you'll also learn how red wine can help heal a cut, how brussels sprouts can prevent strokes, and how onions can relieve burns. You'll be a regular Florence Nightingale in the kitchen!

And those scrumptious, mouthwatering recipes! From old favorites such as apple-cranberry pork chops to new delights such as apricot waffles and a mesquite-flavored onion bloom—I tell you, this book is *bursting* with easy-to-make recipes that are sure to tempt your tummy and keep your family out of the doctor's office.

With *Kitchen Counter Cures*, Colleen and Karen have gone back to the basics, but with a twist. They've taken homespun values and old-time country wisdom and combined them with up-to-date research, proving that everything old really does become new again.

It's the kind of legacy that Grandma Putt would be proud of.

Jerry Baker

Table of Contents

COME ON IN! . . . xv

HEALTH FINDER . . . xviii

APPLES: THE CORE OF HEALTHY EATING PLANS . . . 1
An Apple a Day Keeps Stroke at Bay,
Fiber with A-Peel
Quick Fix: Diarrhea

APRICOTS: BRIMMING WITH CANCER FIGHTERS . . . 5
The Anticancer cocktail, Ticker Shock,
Gutsy Little Fighters
Quick Fix: Itchy Yeast Infections

ARTICHOKES: GLOBES OF GOODNESS . . . 11
Quick Fix: Poor Digestion

ASPARAGUS: KING OF FOLATE . . . 16
Rich in Essential Vitamins

AVOCADOS: PLENTY OF HEALTHY FAT . . . 20
Fight Fat with Fat,
Spread Yourself Thin
Quick Fix: Dastardly Dull Hair

BANANAS: THE BEST OF THE BUNCH . . . 28
Hearty Under Pressure

BARLEY: HEALTHY, HEARTY PEARLS . . . 33
Heart-to-Heart Talk,
Quick Fix: Constipation

BASIL: MEET THE GOOD HEALTH HERB . . . 37
New Herb on the Block
Quick Fix: Hangover

BEANS: A LEAN CUISINE . . . 41
Fight Cancer and Cholesterol,
Provide Stamina, Fill You Up
Quick Fix: Memory

BEEF: NO COMPLAINTS IF YOU BUY LEAN . . . 47
The Cut Counts,
Meat Your Vitamins

BEETS: HEALTHY VALENTINES FOR YOUR HEART . . . 55
Beet a Path to the Bathroom

BELL PEPPERS: RING IN HEALTH BENEFITS . . . 59
Sight Savers, Open Your Eyes, The
Pepper Palette

BLACKBERRIES: NUTRITIOUS BERRIED TREASURE . . . 63
Help for Allergy Sufferers

BLUEBERRIES: THEY'LL KEEP YOU IN THE PINK . . . 68
The Brainiest Berry
Quick Fix: Urinary Tract Infections
Quick Fix: Stomachache

BOK CHOY: ONE SECRET TO GOOD HEALTH . . . 72
Pressure Release Valve, Bone Builder
Quick Fix: Cuts, Hangnails

BROCCOLI: IT'S WORTH STALKING . . . 76
The Broccoli Bunch

BROCCOLI SPROUTS: THE HO, HO, HO HEALTH GIANT . . . 81
From Ho-Hum to Gung-Ho

BROWN RICE: THE WHOLE GRAIN FOR HEALTH GAIN . . . 86
Don't Frown on Brown, The Rice Bowl
Quick Fix: Heart Attack Risk

BRUSSELS SPROUTS: A CAPITAL IDEA . . . 91
DNA Protection, A Heart Helper, Too
Quick Fix: Stroke Risk

CABBAGE: POWER KRAUT . . . 96
Head of the Class, Comparing
Cabbages

CANOLA OIL: THE HEALTHIEST FAT . . . 101
Not All Oils Are Created Equal, Do You
Need an Oil Change?

CANTALOUPE: YOU CAN'T GET ENOUGH . . . 107
Cantaloupe Creations, The Real Skinny

CARROTS: BET ON BETA-CAROTENE . . . 112
The Smoking Gun,
Fantastic Foods or Bitter
Pills?

CAULIFLOWER: ANTICANCER FLOWER POWER . . . 117
The Bunch with the Biggest Punch
Quick Fix: Colds

CELERY: STALKING THE DIET CLAIMS . . . 123
Negative Calories

CEREAL: IT CARRIES CHOLESTEROL AWAY . . . 127
Feeling Your Oats, How Sweet It Isn't,
Name that Cereal
Quick Fix: Itchy Hives

CHEESE: GRATE FOR BONES . . . 132
Calcium Bargains
and Busts
Quick Fix: Muscle Cramps

CHERRIES: HEALTH IS JUST A BOWL FULL AWAY . . . 139
Newly Found Nutrients, Cherries
Equal Apples
Quick Fix: Gout

CHICKEN: HELPS YOU BE A FEATHERWEIGHT . . . 143
Give Your Heart a Leg Up
Quick Fix: Upper Respiratory Infection

CHILES: THEY'RE HOT FOR COLDS . . . 148
Feel Better Fast, Warm Your Heart
Quick Fix: Stuffy Nose

CHIVES: THE SINGLE-CALORIE SEASONING . . . 152
Bring Your Foods Alive with Chives

CHOCOLATE: A GIFT-WRAPPED ASSORTMENT OF HEALTH BENEFITS . . . 155
Health By Chocolate, A Kiss Can Make It Better

CINNAMON: OLD SPICE WITH A NEW TWIST . . . 160
Junk that Gunk, Ban the Bloat

CORN: A BITE FOR SORE EYES . . . 164
Now Ear This, Cancel Cataracts

CRANBERRIES: CONCENTRATED POWER THAT PROTECTS . . . 168
A Slender Alternative, The Daily Dilemma
Quick Fix: Allergy Sneezes

CUCUMBERS: THEY'RE WAY COOL . . . 173
Low-Calorie Crunch
Quick Fix: Puffy Eyes

CURRY POWDER: THE SPICE OF LIFE . . . 177
Kick Cancer, Defy Diabetes
Quick Fix: Heartburn

EGGS: INCREDIBLE! EDIBLE! AND GOOD FOR YOU! . . . 181
Let's Get Cracking, Grandma's Perfect Food
Quick Fix: Low Blood Sugar

FENNEL: SEEDS OF DESTRUCTION . . . 188
Ancient Seeds, Modern Medicine
Quick Fix: Icky Breath

FIGS: AN ANCIENT HEALTH FOOD . . . 193
Go Fig-ure!

FISH: GET HOOKED ON IT . . . 196
Don't Cell Yourself Short, Angling for the Fattiest Fish
Quick Fix: Irregular Periods

FLAXSEEDS: NUTTY NUGGETS ... 202
The Facts About Flax, Using Flax to the Max

GARLIC: THE CLOVE THAT LOATHES CANCER ... 207
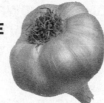
Cuts Cancer Risk, The ABCs of Peeling
Quick Fix: Athlete's Foot

GINGER: IT MAKES GOOD HEALTH A SNAP! ... 211
Ginger is Peachy, Weighty Matters
Quick Fix: The Queasies

GRAPEFRUIT: SOUR ON CANCER ... 215
Antioxidants at Your Service, Forever Fiber

GRAPES: A BUNCH OF HEALTH BENEFITS ... 219
Indulge in a Purple Passion, Late-Breaking News
Quick Fix: Morning Sickness

GREEN BEANS: HEALTH WITH NO STRINGS ATTACHED ... 223
The Bounty in Beans
Quick Fix: That Big Appetite!

GREENS: THEY'RE GLORIOUS! ... 227
Bravo to Beta-Carotene, Cooking the Green Way

HORSERADISH: THE CANCER-FIGHTING CONDIMENT ... 231
A Heart Helper and a Healer, A Toxin Neutralizer
Quick Fix: Stuffy Nose

KALE: YOUR EYES WILL SEE THE GLORY ... 235
A Sight Saver, A Cancer Fighter, A Heart Helper

KIWIFRUIT: THE DOWN UNDER DISEASE FIGHTER ... 240
A Far Sight Better

LENTILS: SMALL PACKAGES, BIG BENEFITS ... 245
Folate Finds, Fiber Factory
Quick Fix: Constipation

LETTUCE: GO FOR THE GREEN! ... 249
Play Your Cards Right, Lettuce Make a Rhyme

MANGOES: A TROPICAL FOLK REMEDY ... 255
Flesh It Out, Mango Mania
Quick Fix: Tummy Ache

MARGARINE: TAKE CONTROL OF CHOLESTEROL ... 261
Sizing Up the Spreads, Say Good-Bye to Stick Margarine

MILK: NATURE'S NEARLY PERFECT FOOD . . . 266
Weight, Weight, Don't Tell Me, Dueling Moo Juice
Quick Fix: Premenstrual Syndrome

MINT: IT HELPS KEEP YOU IN MINT CONDITION . . . 272
Cancer Crusader, Stomach Soother
Quick Fix: Fatigue

MUSHROOMS: FANTAS-TIC FUNGI . . . 277
Exotica Running Wild, Mushroom Mania

NECTARINES: NECTAR OF THE GODS . . . 282
Better Beta, Shooting the Gap, Eyes Bright!

NUTS: A HEART-SMART SNACK . . . 286
Heart Health in a Nutshell, Sometimes You Feel Like a Nut

OKRA: SOUTHERN-STYLE WELLNESS . . . 292
Saves Your DNA

OLIVE OIL: A BIG FAT DIFFERENCE . . . 295
Head Off Heart Disease, Relieve the Pressure
Quick Fix: Dry, Brittle Nails

OLIVES: RIPE FOR HEALTH . . . 300
Good Fat, Bad Fat
Quick Fix: Motion Sickness

ONIONS: POWER-PACKED BULBS . . . 306
Cancer Crackdown, Diabetes Deterrent
Quick Fix: Burns

ORANGES: BENEFITS BEYOND THE C . . . 311
Seasons in the Sun

PAPAYA: A TROPICAL TREASURE . . . 316
A Bonus Beta, Tropical Depression
Quick Fix: Hiccups

PARSLEY: A KISS OF HEALTH . . . 321
Safe to Smooch
Quick Fix: Garlic Breath

PASTA: USE YOUR NOODLE . . . 325
A Side of Energy, Does Pasta Make You Fat?
Quick Fix: PMS

PEACHES: THEY'RE KEEN FOR YOUR HEALTH . . . 332
What's All the Fuzz About?
Quick Fix: Sinusitis

PEANUT BUTTER: KEEPS YOU YOUNG AT HEART . . . 336
Weight a Minute, Crush Cholesterol and Cancer

PEARS: HEALTHY TO THE CORE . . . 341
Fiber Fill-Up, Dynamic Duo

PEAS: PROTEIN IN A POD . . . 347
It's Not Easy Being Green
Quick Fix: High Cholesterol

PINEAPPLE: YOUR HAWAIIAN HEALTH CONNECTION . . . 353
Tropical Relief, Outrigger Enzymes
Quick Fix: Callus

POMEGRANATES: THEY'RE SWEET TO YOUR HEART . . . 358
Of Mice and Men

PORK: FORK IT OVER . . . 363
Hogging All the Vitamins

POTATOES: SIMPLY SMASHING SPUDS . . . 368
Mood Smoother
Quick Fix: High Blood Pressure

PRUNES: THEY'RE PLUM GOOD CONSTIPATION FIGHTERS . . . 372
Quick Fix: The Blues

PUMPKIN: GIVE THANKS FOR ITS POTENT NUTRIENTS . . . 376
Power Veggie

QUINOA: IT'S KEEN MA! . . . 382
A Wagonload of Nutrients

RADISHES: CANCER-FIGHTING CRUNCH . . . 387
Radishes Rule, Stay-Slim Secrets

RAISINS: HEALTH THROUGH THE GRAPEVINE . . . 391
Blazin' Raisins
Quick Fix: Fatigue

RASPBERRIES: TAKE YOUR PICK OF HEALTH BENEFITS . . . 395
Cancer Enemy #1
Quick Fix: Lazy Gut

ROSEMARY: SAVOR THE FLAVOR . . . 400
Body and Soul
Quick Fix: Dizziness

SEEDS: POWER PACKETS . . . 404
Sunflower Seeds Shine, Sesame Seeds Build Bones

SHELLFISH: HEALTH ON THE HALF SHELL . . . 409
Lean, Mean Protein Machines, Swim or Sink with Zinc
Quick Fix: The Cold That Just Won't Go Away

SOY: A JOY FOR YOUR HEART . . . 415
Ticker Talk

SPINACH: SIGHT-SAVIN' GOODNESS . . . 424
Eye-Deal for Your Peepers,
A Memorable Veggie

SQUASH: ACORN-UCOPIA OF HEALTH . . . 429
The Color of Health, Pots of Potassium
Quick Fix: Sunburn

STRAWBERRIES: ANTIOXIDANTS BY THE PINT . . . 434
Berr-ific Antioxidants!

SWEET POTATOES: SUPERSTAR SPUDS . . . 438
A Veggie All-Star, Pass Up the Pills
Quick Fix: Nighttime Leg Cramps

TEA: A PARTY FOR YOUR BODY . . . 443
Half the Risk of a Heart Attack!
Quick Fix: Infections

TOMATOES: A MAN'S BEST FRIEND . . . 448
Prostate Protection, A Large
Pepperoni, Please

TURKEY: A NUTRITIONAL POWERHOUSE . . . 453
Talkin' Turkey,
New Ways to
Gobble It
Up

WATERMELON: THE SUMMERTIME HEALTH SAVER . . . 457
The Natural Sports "Drink,"
Heart Smart
Quick Fix: Queasy Moms

WHEATBERRIES: BERRY GOOD FOR YOU . . . 462
Whole for Heart and Diabetes, The
Whole Weight Problem
Quick Fix: Constipation

WHEAT GERM: HARVEST THE GOODNESS . . . 468
Wheat Basics, Fortified Folate,
Synergy for Bones

WHOLE WHEAT BREAD: THE REAL STAFF OF LIFE . . . 473
A Grain of Truth, Beats Diabetes

WINE: PARADOXICAL HEART HEALTH . . . 478
Two Magic Ingredients, Bonus Bennies,
More Is Less
Quick Fix: Cuts

YOGURT: THE BENEFITS OF HAVING CULTURE . . . 484
Beneficial Bugs,
The Scoop on Frozen Yogurt
Quick Fix: Canker Sores
Quick Fix: Body Fat

SUPER-CHARGED FOODS. . . 490

INDEX. . . 495

Come On In!

Sit down somewhere comfy, put up your feet, and have a cup of tea while we introduce ourselves. Actually, not much introduction is necessary since we're probably very much like you.

We work full-time jobs, never have enough time to do the marketing, and don't have anyone except a visiting friend or an occasional mom to help us out in the kitchen. In other words, we do all the work.

We also have husbands and kids who put their noses up at a lot of what's good for them. In fact, that's why we agreed to do this book. With all the responsibilities women have today, we knew that you needed a solid nutrition book that discusses scientific topics in plain English, that gives you practical advice, and that provides recipes that you don't have to be Martha Stewart to make.

This is that book. But it's also a book that you can trust.

To give you a little background, Colleen has been a registered dietitian for 20 years and still continues to counsel patients in her Baltimore office. Karen has been writing about nutrition in major magazines for more than a decade. She has interviewed literally hundreds of researchers over the years. We met at a nutrition conference, became fast friends, and worked on the nutrition pages of a couple of magazines together before writing this book.

Yet despite our combined years of experience, neither one of us was really prepared for the startling information that researchers gave us. We found a chicken soup recipe that's been proved in the lab to help fight colds, a cartful of foods that might save your eyesight, and yogurts that soothe your stomach. We were blown away countless times—and believe us when we say it, we're not easily impressed!

In all, the researchers we talked to nominated 117 foods that have the ability to keep us healthy and cure a whole lot of ailments. If you skipped ahead to the good stuff before you read this introduction (as we've sometimes done), you already know that we divided this book into 97 chapters—one chapter dedicated to each healthy food or food group.

Of course, you can't eat 117 foods every day. But you can fit them in over the course of a couple of weeks. To help you plan ways to incorporate these wonderful foods into your life, check out page 490 for seasonal menus based on the recipes in this book.

Research shows that people who eat the widest variety of foods are more likely to meet their nutrient requirements and remain healthy than those who get stuck in a food rut. That's because there's an incredible amount of synergy in nutrition. Nutrients work together—foods pair up—to keep your heart healthy, your blood pressure normal, your bones strong, and your memory sharp.

Even some foods that scientists

thought had no redeeming value—such as cucumbers and chocolate—turn out to have compounds beyond the good old vitamins and minerals. Many may hold the key to longer lives, cancer cures, or smoother skin—and every food in this book has at least some of those compounds.

Excited yet? Well, come on then! Join us as we explore the 117 foods in the supermarket that'll turn your kitchen into a healthy, healing place. Learn about all their benefits and, most of all, how to incorporate them into your family's meals—even if you feed the pickiest eaters. Dive right into our first chapter: apples. You know that old saying about an apple a day keeping the doctor away? As you'll soon find out, it's right on the money.

Karen

Karen Ciccro

COLLEEN

Colleen Pierre, M.S. RD.

HEALTHFINDER

Scattered throughout the following pages are more than 100 healing recipes that we've developed to keep you and your family in perfect health. Below is a sampling of those recipes, organized according to the diseases and conditions most likely to threaten your health.

If you'd like to keep any one of those ills at bay, just skim down the left-hand column until you reach a particular disease or condition in which you're interested, and look over the amazing recipes listed under it. Then think about including those recipes in your diet on a regular basis. Just keep in mind that no one food or recipe will ever prevent or relieve a condition on its own. But a healthy, balanced diet that includes the recipes in this book most certainly will. Bon Appetit!

Cancer
Amazing Apricot Waffles . . . 10
Artichoke Appetizer with Fresh Gazpacho Dip . . . 15
Hearty Purple Cow . . . 222
Pasta Chiller . . . 390

Depression
Grilled Salmon Primavera . . . 201
Tuna Tucks . . . 234

Diabetes
Aunt Shirley's Three-Bean Salad . . . 46
Chunky French Applesauce . . . 4
Mesquite Onion Bloom . . . 310
Wheatberry Breakfast . . . 466

Heart Disease and High Cholesterol
Blackberry-Peach Crisp . . . 67
Flax Prairie Bread . . . 206
Healthy Hot Pockets . . . 90
Mom's Garlic Pasta . . . 210

High Blood Pressure
Banana Breakfast Danish . . . 32
Bok Choy and Rice Noodles . . . 75
Ginger Butternut Soup . . . 433

Stroke
Baked Brussels Sprouts . . . 95
Colleen's Famous Gingerbread . . . 214
Cookout Citrus Splash . . . 218

Apples:

The Core of Healthy Eating Plans

BATTLES:
- cancer
- diabetes
- heart disease
- high cholesterol
- stroke

BOLSTERS:
- regularity

Colleen grew up with a Golden Delicious apple tree in her backyard, so she understands the apple's reputation for temptation. That's why she thinks Eve may have seduced Adam with an apple—to be sure he got some health food. (Women are, after all, the medical gatekeepers in most families.) Perhaps Eve knew instinctively that luscious, juicy apples were the perfect counterpoint to all those burgers and fries he was eating!

AN APPLE A DAY KEEPS STROKE AT BAY

If the first couple had lived in Finland, they might have been part of a recent study showing that men and women who munched an apple every day had a lower risk of embolic stroke (the kind caused by a tiny blood clot blocking an artery in the brain) than those who were halfhearted in their pursuit of the Isaac Newton special. The

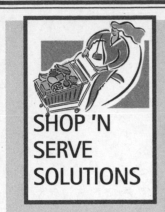

SHOP 'N SERVE SOLUTIONS

More than 2,500 varieties of apples are grown in the United States (good job, Johnny Appleseed!), but just 8 make up 80 percent of what we buy and eat.

Apples are at their juicy best when fresh-picked in the fall, but modern, controlled-atmosphere storage techniques keep us supplied with crispy, crunchy apples all year long.

WHEN SELECTING APPLES:

■ Look for those that are firm to hard. Apples are one of the few fruits that Colleen will let her husband, Ted, give the "thumb" test. If a gentle squeeze produces a dent, the apple is too soft.

■ Choose small ones. Little apples are usually better than big ones.

■ Pick pretty ones. Apples should have nice color for their type, tight skins, and no bruises or cuts.

WHEN STORING:

Apples are already fully ripe when you buy them, so take them home and put them right in the fridge, where they'll keep for up to six weeks. At room temperature, they'll get mushy–*fast.*

WHEN YOU'RE READY TO USE:

Scrub your apples well just before eating them, to remove pesticides and wax.

PREPARING AN APPLE A DAY

Enjoy these yummy ways to eat your apple a day:

◆ **Slice it.** Add the slices to winter salads for extra crunch and flavor.

◆ **Cook it.** Core a large Rome Beauty. Fill the center with a mixture of yellow raisins, chopped pecans, ground cinnamon, and brown sugar. Microwave until the apple is tender, about 5 minutes.

researchers expected apples' high quercetin content to be the key to stroke protection—but not so. Exactly why the apples were so powerful isn't clear. (Stay tuned. Scientists are hunting for yet another secret ingredient. Just have another apple while you're waiting!)

THE REAL SKINNY ON APPLES

Adam and Eve were likely short on knives and peelers, so they undoubtedly ate their apples with the skin on—and that's good. Apple skins are brimming with quercetin, a much-studied plant chemical that accounts for other health benefits. Quercetin fights heart disease by preventing cholesterol from transforming itself into the muck that plasters itself to your artery walls, narrowing them and setting you up for a heart attack.

And quercetin fights cancer, too, possibly by deactivating carcinogens, or causing them to just give up and die. One apple with skin delivers as much quercetin as $\frac{1}{2}$ cup of tea or $\frac{2}{3}$ cup of raw onion. So don't fight temptation. Give in!

FIBER WITH A-PEEL

In addition to loads of other nutrients, apples are bursting with fiber. In fact, one medium apple with skin delivers 20 percent of your daily fiber quota. The best news of all is that apples pony up both the insoluble and soluble forms of fiber.

Insoluble fiber keeps your bowels in good

Quick Fix:

Diarrhea

Suffering with diarrhea? Calm your tummy with the BRAT diet: bananas, rice, applesauce, and toast. Try it for a day or so, and your diarrhea will hit the skids. Just don't forget that you need plenty of water, as well. A bout with diarrhea could dehydrate a rain forest!

NUTRITION IN A NUTSHELL

Apple (1 medium)

Calories: 81

Fat: 0 g

Saturated fat: 0 g

Cholesterol: 0 mg

Sodium: 0 mg

Total carbohydrates: 21 g

Dietary fiber: 4 g

Protein: 3 g

Vitamin A: 1% of Daily Value

Vitamin C: 9%

Calcium: 1%

Iron: 1%

working order. Part of that insoluble fiber is pectin, a substance that can help calm diarrhea. What's more, pectin, in combination with the fruit sugars in apples, slows nutrient absorption, which helps people with diabetes keep their blood sugar under control. Soluble fiber works to lower blood cholesterol—by as much as 16 percent in one study! So indulge yourself.

Chunky French Applesauce

One great way to salvage the double-fiber appeal of apples that have lost their crunch is to simmer chunks—with the skin still on—to make this sweet-spicy sauce. It makes a great topping for waffles or pancakes, or a super side dish with lean ham or chicken.

4 Red Delicious apples, washed, cored, and cut into bite-size chunks
⅓ cup seedless raisins
¼ cup coarsely chopped walnuts
½ teaspoon ground cinnamon
⅛ teaspoon ground nutmeg
½ cup water

Place the apples, raisins, walnuts, cinnamon, nutmeg, and water in a heavy saucepan. Bring to a boil. Cover, reduce the heat to low, and simmer until the apples are fork-tender, stirring occasionally. Serve warm or cold.

Yield: Four servings.

Nutritional data per serving: Calories, 167; protein, 2 g; carbohydrates, 32 g; fiber, 5 g; fat, 5 g; saturated fat, less than 1 g; cholesterol, 0 mg; sodium, 2 mg; vitamin C, 9% of Daily Value; vitamin E, 4%; manganese, 20%; potassium, 8%.

Apricots:
Brimming with Cancer Fighters

BATTLES:

■ cancer
■ heart disease
■ high blood pressure
■ high cholesterol
■ stroke
■ yeast infections

BOLSTERS:

■ immune function

Just the other day, Karen's grandmother asked her which vegetables are rich in beta-carotene. Grandma had recently heard a report about the nutrient on the news, and she wanted to know if her produce drawer was stocked with the right stuff.

Glad to be of help and to show that she really had learned something in school, Karen rattled off the names of the most beta-carotene–rich veggies: carrots, pumpkins, and sweet potatoes. But Karen also pointed out that a food needn't be a vegetable in order to be brimming with

NUTRITION IN A NUTSHELL

Fresh apricots (3)

Calories: 48

Fat: 0 g

Saturated fat: 0 g

Cholesterol: 0 mg

Sodium: 1 mg

Total carbohydrates: 11 g

Dietary fiber: 2 g

Protein: 1 g

Vitamin A: 52% of Daily Value

Vitamin C: 17%

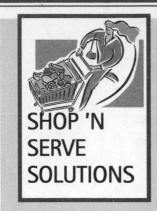

SHOP 'N SERVE SOLUTIONS

Depending on when you'd like to buy fresh apricots, they may be as difficult to find as a comfy pair of sandals. More than 95 percent of the U.S. crop comes from California and is available only between mid-May and late June. In August, your supermarket may carry apricots from Oregon and Washington, while Chilean imports usually appear in the supermarket from late November to April.

WHEN SELECTING FRESH APRICOTS:

■ Look for smooth skins.

■ Look for fruits that are soft, if you want to use them immediately, or somewhat firm, if you'd like to keep them for a few days.

■ Avoid apricots that have a greenish hue or are hard, because they may never fully ripen.

WHEN STORING:

■ Place ripe apricots in a plastic bag and refrigerate them. Eat them within three to seven days.

■ Place partially ripe apricots in a brown paper bag. Store them at room temperature, away from direct sunlight, until they're ready to eat, usually within a day or two. Then transfer them to the fridge.

Canned apricots. Can't get your hands on fresh apricots? A fine alternative is the canned version (more than 80 percent of U.S. apricots are canned), which you can substitute for fresh fare in most recipes.

beta-carotene. In fact, she told her grandmother, apricots, lovely yellow-orange fruits, were recently named to the *University of California–Berkeley Wellness Letter*'s list of top 10 beta-carotene sources. Turns out, just three apricots supply more than half of

Dried apricots. Weight watchers, be warned: Ounce for ounce, the dried fruit has three times the beta-carotene but five times the calories of its fresh counterpart.

FUTURE FAVORITES

Once you introduce apricots to your kitchen, you'll find plenty of ways to use them. Here are a few of Karen's favorites:

◆ **Mix them up.** Fold ¹/₂ cup of diced fresh, canned, or dried apricots into your batter for muffins or pancakes. They'll create quite a stir in your family!

◆ **Put your salad on the best-dressed list.** In a blender, combine 2 fresh pitted apricots with 2 tablespoons of white wine vinegar and 1 tablespoon of sugar. Slowly add ¹/₄ cup of canola oil. Continue blending until thick and smooth. Stir in 2 tablespoons of chopped fresh basil. Pour the dressing over a salad made of dark green lettuce, carrots, cucumbers, raisins, and feta cheese, and toss to coat. Or use the dressing as a marinade for chicken.

◆ **Break out the tortilla chips.** Dunk them in this easy-to-make apricot salsa: In a medium bowl, combine 2 tablespoons of lemon juice, 2 tablespoons of canola oil, ¹/₈ teaspoon of coarsely ground black pepper, 6 diced fresh apricots, ¹/₂ cup of diced red onion, and ¹/₃ cup of diced red bell pepper.

◆ **Make a snack pack.** Instead of raiding the vending machine when you're hungry at work, pull out a homemade trail mix from your purse or desk drawer. In a plastic bag, mix ¹/₄ cup each of dried apricots, mini pretzels, peanuts, raisins, and whole grain cereal, such as Wheat Chex or Cheerios. Crunch away!

the vitamin A you need daily. (Your body converts beta-carotene to vitamin A.)

While beta-carotene supplements may have limited—if any—benefits, getting plenty of the nutrient through foods makes amazing things happen. What's the difference? Beta-carotene boasts hundreds of lesser-known cousins that are present in foods, but not added to supplements. Scientists speculate that beta-carotene and its cousins—collectively called carotenoids—work together to stave off illnesses.

THE ANTICANCER COCKTAIL

It's not a drink, silly. It's just beta-carotene and the other carotenoids doing their job. Members of the carotenoid family attack cancer in different ways.

For instance, beta-carotene gobbles up free radicals, substances that cause cell damage, from fluids located inside and outside the body's fats. Lycopene, another carotenoid found in apricots, may arrest the growth of tumor cells. Still other carotenoids may stimulate an enzyme in your immune system that breaks down carcinogens, cancer-causing substances.

"A diet rich in beta-carotene from plenty of fruits and vegetables may reduce the risk of breast cancer recurrence by one-third," says Cheryl Rock, Ph.D., R.D., associate professor of family and preventive medicine at the University of California-San Diego.

Bring on the apricots for healthy men and women, too. A National Cancer Institute review of 156 studies found that a diet packed with fruits and veggies cuts the risk of most cancers—including bladder, cervical, lung, and stomach—by about half.

Quick Fix:

Itchy Yeast Infections

Bothered by yeast infections? Snack on some apricots. Their beta-carotene may bolster your immune system enough to ward off the infection. A study at Albert Einstein College of Medicine in New York City found that the vaginal cells of women with yeast infections had significantly lower levels of beta-carotene than did cells taken from healthy women.

TICKER SHOCK

Beta-carotene and company don't just fight cancer. They also stave off the leading killer of men and women in the United States—heart disease. How exactly? Beta-carotene and lycopene fight a process that makes bad low-density lipoprotein (LDL) cholesterol even worse, sticking more plaque to artery walls. A study of more than 85,000 nurses showed that a diet rich in beta-carotene reduced the risk of heart disease by a whopping 22 percent!

COOL UNDER PRESSURE

Besides boasting beta-carotene, apricots—particularly the dried variety—pack potassium, a nutrient that helps lower blood pressure and reduce the risk of stroke. In a Harvard University study of more than 40,000 men, those who got the most potassium had about 40 percent less chance of suffering a stroke as those who consumed the least.

So how much potassium does a $3\frac{1}{2}$-ounce serving of dried apricots offer? Close to 1,400 milligrams—three times the amount found in a banana!

Amazing Apricot Waffles

Dust off your waffle iron! Your family will love this waffle recipe that we got from pastry chef Diane Wagner.

1 can (15 ounces) apricot halves

1 cup all-purpose flour

1 cup whole wheat flour

3 tablespoons sugar

½ teaspoon salt

1½ teaspoons baking powder

¼ teaspoon baking soda

1¾ cups buttermilk

2 tablespoons butter, melted

1 egg yolk

3 egg whites

1 cup low-fat vanilla yogurt

⅓ cup maple syrup

Drain the apricots. In a blender or food processor, puree 3 apricot halves until smooth. Set aside. Finely chop the remaining apricots. Set aside. In a medium bowl, combine the flours, sugar, salt, baking powder, and baking soda. Set aside.

In a small bowl, mix the buttermilk, butter, egg yolk, and apricot puree until smooth. Pour the wet ingredients over the flour mixture and blend just until smooth. In another medium bowl, beat the egg whites until stiff, but not dry. Fold into the batter. Gently mix in the chopped apricots. Cook with a waffle iron. Spoon 2 tablespoons of the yogurt and drizzle some of the maple syrup over each waffle.

Yield: Four 2-waffle servings.

Nutritional data per serving: Calories, 254; protein, 9 g; carbohydrates, 45 g; fiber, 3 g; fat, 5 g; saturated fat, 3 g; cholesterol, 39 mg; sodium, 393 mg; calcium, 16% of Daily Value; iron, 13%.

Artichokes:
Globes of Goodness

BATTLES:
- cancer
- diarrhea
- heart disease
- high cholesterol

BOLSTERS:
- digestion
- regularity
- weight control

Yes, it's true: Artichokes are funny-looking. And for a long time, they presented a mystery too deep for us to tackle. Fortunately, Colleen has a couple of adventurous daughters who clued us in on how to take artichokes apart and have some delicious fun.

So why not follow our lead and learn to love artichokes, too? You'll discover that, in addition to being delicious, artichokes have some amazing health benefits.

HEART-SMART

To start with, you'll adore what artichokes do for your heart. First, they appear to help keep your blood supply flowing freely because they're packed with luteolin, one of the naturally occurring plant substances in the flavonoid family that acts as an antioxidant in your body. At least in lab dishes, concentrated luteolin taken from artichokes prevents the oxidation of bad low-density lipoprotein (LDL) cholesterol, the process that makes cholesterol gummy and lazy and very eager to find a resting place on your artery walls.

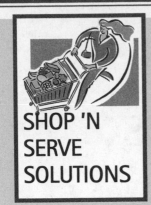

SHOP 'N SERVE SOLUTIONS

A few fresh artichokes are available year-round, but you'll find tons of them in your supermarket from March through May. Fall and winter globes may have a whitish or blistered look due to a little frostbite. But don't worry—they'll turn green when you cook them. In fact, these are often the tastiest 'chokes.

Artichokes come in three sizes. Babies weigh just 2 to 3 ounces each. They're great for appetizers, casseroles, or sautés. Medium 'chokes weigh in at 8 to 10 ounces each. They're great for dipping, stuffing, or as a light entrée. Large artichokes weigh about 1 pound each, big enough for a shared appetizer for two or more people.

WHEN STORING ARTICHOKES:

Sprinkle your artichokes with a little water, place them in an airtight plastic bag, and then chill them in the fridge. They'll keep for about a week.

COOKING MADE EASY

Start by slicing off the stem so that the artichoke can sit firmly on its bottom. Then cut off one-quarter to one-third of the top. Cook by one of the following three methods:

■ **Boil:** Stand trimmed artichokes in a deep saucepan with 3 inches of boiling water. Add lemon juice or seasonings, if desired. Cover and boil gently for 25 to 40 minutes, depending on size, or until a petal near the center pulls out easily. Stand the artichokes upside down to drain.

■ **Steam:** Place prepared artichokes on a rack above boiling water. Cover and steam for 25 to 40 minutes, or until done.

■ **Microwave:** Place prepared artichokes in a deep microwaveable cup or bowl. Add water, cover, and microwave on high until done. For one artichoke, use $\frac{1}{2}$ cup of water and microwave for 5 to 8 minutes; for two artichokes, 1 cup of water, 7 to 11 minutes.

And that makes arteries narrower and ripe for clogging.

Second, one medium artichoke provides about 15 percent of your daily folate requirement. Folate is a B vitamin that helps control blood levels of homocysteine, which, when out of control, can trigger a heart attack.

And third, artichokes are full of cynarin, which has been shown to lower cholesterol production. The idea here is that if you make less cholesterol, there's less for your body to deal with.

SKIN CITY

Cynarin may have benefits for your skin, too. In an Italian study, researchers found that cynarin (this time extracted from the herb echinacea) helped protect collagen, the conective tissue that holds your cells together, against sun damage. More research is needed, of course, and you may have to use it more like a sunscreen than an appetizer. Still, the possibilities are intriguing.

Meanwhile, Cleveland researchers have been pursuing the cancer prevention benefits of eating another artichoke ingredient, silymarin. At least in the lab, silymarin seems to forestall cancer development at several stages.

GET A MOVE ON

For better bowel function, you need a constant parade of fiber-rich fruits and vegetables in your diet.

NUTRITION IN A NUTSHELL

Boiled artichoke (1 medium)

Calories: 60

Fat: 0 g

Saturated fat: 0 g

Cholesterol: 0 mg

Sodium: 114 mg

Total carbohydrates: 13 g

Dietary fiber: 6 g

Protein: 4 g

Vitamin A: 4% of Daily Value

Vitamin C: 13%

Calcium: 5%

Iron: 9%

Quick Fix:

Poor Digestion

Suffering from digestive difficulties? Have an artichoke. It's a cholagogue, a vegetable that stimulates production of bile, which is an emulsifier that aids fat digestion.

And artichokes really wave the fiber flag, delivering about one-third of a day's supply in just one medium fat-free globe.

They'll help with weight control, too, if you dip them in lemon juice instead of drowning them in butter. Not only are artichokes low in calories (at just 60 each), but they also take a long time to eat, so your body gets a chance to register that you're full before you pack away too many calories!

GUTSY LITTLE FIGHTERS

It turns out that artichokes are prebiotics, too. In other words, they deliver just the right kind of carbohydrates to feed the good bacteria in your gut. Thus well fed, these bacteria then have the energy to multiply into a huge army that's strong enough to fight off a hostile bacterial invasion and the diarrhea that often comes with it.

ARTFUL ARTICHOKE SERVING

Now here's how to serve a cooked artichoke:

◆ **Dip it.** (It's the most fun appetizer.) Pull off the petals one at a time. Dip each into something healthy, such as the "Fresh Gazpacho Dip" on the opposite page. Put the petal in your mouth, holding on to the tip, and gently bite down. Now pull the petal out of your mouth, scraping off the tender flesh with your teeth. Throw away the skeleton, then pull off another petal.

◆ **Stuff it.** With a spoon, scrape the fuzzy center out of your cooked artichoke. Fill the 'choke with something cold, such as chicken or tuna salad, or something hot, such as warm crabmeat.

◆ **Slice it.** Again, de-fuzz the artichoke center, then remove some of the outer leaves for decoration. Thinly slice the artichoke and toss the slices into salad.

◆ **Hurry it.** In a rush? Fill the center of a canned artichoke heart with a jumbo ripe olive. Use it as a garnish for your dinner plate or salad.

Artichoke Appetizer with Fresh Gazpacho Dip

The only bad thing about eating artichokes is what you dip them in—usually butter. But change the dip, and you'll change the entire nutritional picture. So give this colorful dip a whirl. It comes from the California Artichoke Board, and it's packed with death-defying ingredients.

½ pound red, ripe tomatoes, chopped and seeded

1½ tablespoons tomato paste

2 teaspoons red wine vinegar

2 teaspoons fresh lime juice

1½ teaspoons extra virgin olive oil

2 teaspoons finely chopped shallots

¼ cup chopped sweet green pepper

2 teaspoons chopped fresh dill

¼ teaspoon freshly ground black pepper

⅛ teaspoon red pepper sauce

4 medium fresh artichokes, boiled

In a blender or food processor, whirl the tomatoes, tomato paste, vinegar, lime juice, and oil until blended. Transfer to a large mixing bowl. Stir in the shallots, sweet pepper, dill, black pepper, and pepper sauce. Cover and chill. To serve, place the gazpacho dip in a wide bowl. Pull the petals from the artichokes one at a time, dip into the gazpacho, and scrape off the tender part with your teeth.

Yield: Four servings.

Nutritional data per serving: Calories, 98; protein, 5 g; carbohydrates, 19 g; fiber, 8 g; fat, 2 g; saturated fat, less than 1 g; cholesterol, 0 mg; sodium, 126 mg; folate, 19% of Daily Value; vitamin A, 16%; vitamin C, 43%; copper, 18%; magnesium, 21%; potassium, 17%.

Asparagus:
King of Folate

BATTLES:
- birth defects
- heart disease

BOLSTERS:
- immune function

A sparagus is Colleen's favorite vegetable. Her husband, Ted, can't stand it, so he eats cauliflower instead. Hooray! That leaves more asparagus for her!

Colleen is happy not just because she thinks asparagus is tops in taste, but also because it's the king of vegetables in providing folate, the B vitamin now thought to play an important role in preventing heart attacks.

RICH IN ESSENTIAL VITAMINS

For many years, research was focused almost myopically on cholesterol as the culprit in heart disease. But that research uncovered only part of the problem. So nutrition detectives had to start looking for other clues.

What nutrition detectives found was that many heart attacks are triggered by

NUTRITION IN A NUTSHELL

Cooked asparagus (5 spears)

Calories: 18

Fat: 0 g

Saturated fat: 0 g

Cholesterol: 0 mg

Sodium: 8 mg

Total carbohydrates: 3 g

Dietary fiber: 1 g

Protein: 2 g

Folate: 27% of Daily Value

Vitamin A: 8%

Vitamin C: 9%

16

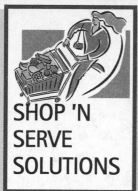

SHOP 'N SERVE SOLUTIONS

If you like your asparagus fresh, keep a lookout starting in January, when the first spears are hand-cut in California. Midwestern and eastern crops keep fresh asparagus coming through July.

WHEN SELECTING FRESH ASPARAGUS:

■ Size doesn't matter. Just choose spears of similar diameter so that they'll cook in the same amount of time.

■ Look for clean, round, mostly green stalks.

■ Look for tightly closed, purple tips.

■ Avoid shriveled spears or dry, brown, or "sprouting" tips. These are signs of old age and declining quality.

■ Avoid sandy spears. They're hard to clean, and the grit ends up in your teeth, ruining the pleasure of eating an otherwise elegant vegetable.

WHEN STORING:

■ Wrap the stalks in wet paper towels, or stand them in water. Then cover the asparagus with a plastic bag to prevent dehydration. Store them in the fridge.

■ Eat your asparagus as soon as possible, because every day you wait wastes some of the folate and vitamin C—and that fresh-from-the-field taste.

WHEN YOU'RE READY TO USE:

■ Wash the asparagus.

■ Snap off the tough part of each stem.

■ Then simply steam, boil, or grill just until crisp-tender.

Frozen asparagus. When fresh asparagus is out of season, you'll have to settle for frozen spears, which are still a good deal, both in taste and nutrition. In fact, there's nothing you can do with fresh asparagus that you can't do with the frozen kind.

DON'T MIX APPLES AND ASPARAGUS!

You probably know that putting an apple in a brown paper bag with "green" (unripe) fruits, such as peaches, speeds their ripening. That's because apples give off ethylene gas, the master synchronizer of chemical changes that cause fruits to turn soft and sweet, change color, and give off that tantalizing fragrance that makes you want to take a big, juicy bite. But separate apples from asparagus. Ethylene gas turns succulent stalks into tough, stringy spears.

high blood levels of the amino acid homocysteine. Coincidentally, they noticed that folks with high homocysteine levels also tended to have low blood levels of folate and folic acid, another form of the B vitamin. Clinical trials have shown that eating more folate-rich foods and folic acid supplements can lower blood levels of homocysteine. Now scientists are trying to prove that lowering homocysteine reduces heart disease risk.

Folate and folic acid are also critical for preventing certain birth defects. Just 1 cup of cooked asparagus provides two-thirds of the Daily Value for folate.

Asparagus is also a good source of vitamin C, part of the nutrition arsenal that keeps your immune system in fighting trim. Ten spears provide about 20 percent of the new higher daily recommendation for vitamin C of 75 milligrams for women and 90 milligrams for men.

Hazelnut Asparagus Salad

No vegetable is more elegant than asparagus. With flavor both distinctive and unique, it dazzles when prepared simply, as in this recipe.

2 pounds fresh asparagus, cut into 1½-inch pieces
3 teaspoons light soy sauce
2 teaspoons walnut oil
1 teaspoon honey
2 tablespoons chopped toasted hazelnuts (filberts)
Red leaf lettuce
Grape tomatoes (garnish)

Place the asparagus in a heavy saucepan with just enough water to cover. Bring the water to a boil, lower the heat, and cook the asparagus gently just until tender, 4 to 5 minutes. Pour off the hot water, then rinse the asparagus in cold water to stop cooking. Pat dry. Place in a glass or plastic refrigerator bowl. In a small bowl, combine the soy sauce, oil, honey, and hazelnuts. Pour over the asparagus. Cover and chill for 30 minutes. Serve on a bed of red leaf lettuce. Garnish with the tomatoes.

Yield: Six servings.

Nutritional data per serving: Calories, 61; protein, 3 g; carbohydrates, 6 g; fiber, 2 g; fat, 3 g; saturated fat, 0 g; cholesterol, 0 mg; sodium, 140 mg; folate, 45% of Daily Value; vitamin A, 13%; vitamin C, 15%; calcium, 3%; iron, 5%.

Avocados:
Plenty of Healthy Fat

BATTLES:
- cancer
- dry hair
- heart disease
- high cholesterol

BOLSTERS:
- weight control

Little can compare to the taste of a crispy tortilla chip dunked in a dish of creamy guacamole. Mmmmm! Unfortunately, in the last decade, as we counted fat grams ad nauseam, guacamole got a bad rep. Avocados suffered from the distinction of being one of the few fruits that are high in fat—up to 15 grams in one of medium size.

Fortunately, nutritionists have discovered that 80 percent of the fat in avocados is the type that offers health *benefits*. What's more, avocados exceed every fruit in certain plant compounds that scientists believe may help prevent cancer and heart disease.

In two words: *Guacamole returns!*

NUTRITION IN A NUTSHELL

California avocado (⅕ medium, or about ¼ cup)

Calories: 55

Fat: 5 g

Saturated fat: 1 g

Cholesterol: 0 mg

Sodium: 1 mg

Total carbohydrates: 3 g

Dietary fiber: 3 g

Protein: 1 g

Folate: 6% of Daily Value

A BUNCH OF BETA-SITOSTEROL

When you look at the vitamin and mineral content of avocados, it doesn't seem impressive. Sure, they have a little bit of folate, potassium, and vitamins B_6, C, and E, but the amounts are scrawny compared with those found in other fruits.

However, researchers at the University of California-Los Angeles recently dug deeper and found that avocados (at least the ones grown in California) boast 76 milligrams of beta-sitosterol in $3\frac{1}{2}$ ounces.

Beta *what?* Beta-sitosterol. It's a plant compound that can inhibit the absorption of cholesterol from your intestines, so you'll have a lower level in your bloodstream, reducing your risk of heart disease. What's more, animal studies have shown that beta-sitosterol inhibits the growth of cancerous tumors.

Ounce for ounce, avocados pack more than four times the beta-sitosterol of commonly eaten fruits such as oranges (17 milligrams), apples (11 milligrams), and strawberries (10 milligrams). They also contain at least twice the amount of beta-sitosterol found in other good sources such as corn, olives, and soybeans.

ANOTHER NEW NUTRIENT

And that's not all. Avocados also are loaded with glutathione, a plant compound that neutralizes free radicals, which are substances that cause cell damage. Studies suggest that glutathione helps prevent cancers of the mouth and pharynx, as well as heart disease.

Quick Fix:

Dastardly Dull Hair

To add shine to dull hair, try this: Mash a very ripe avocado and massage the pulp into your wet hair for about 5 minutes. Leave in for 10 minutes to an hour, then rinse. It may take several washes to remove it all, but you'll love the results.

Avocados offer about 28 milligrams of glutathione in 3½ ounces, while many other fruits, such as watermelon (7 milligrams), pears (5 milligrams), and bananas (4 milligrams), contribute considerably less.

FANTASTIC FAT

Yep, fantastic. Here's why: A diet rich in unsaturated fat, the main type in avocados, helps lower your level of low-density lipoprotein (LDL) cholesterol—the bad kind—while maintaining your level of high-density lipoprotein (HDL) cholesterol—the good kind. Dozens of studies have linked unsaturated fat to a reduced risk of ticker trouble, although most of them examined the amount of olive oil consumed rather than the amount of avocados.

To pinpoint the benefits of avocados specifically, researchers in Australia asked a group of women ages 37 to 58 to follow a high-carbohydrate, low-fat diet for three weeks and a diet rich in unsaturated fat from avocados for another three weeks. Depending on how much the women weighed, they ate ½ to 1½ avocados daily.

The impressive results: When the participants were on the avocado diet, their total cholesterol levels dropped by 8 percent on average, compared with just 4 percent when they followed the high-carb, low-fat plan. It gets better. The avocado diet didn't decrease the women's levels of good cholesterol, but the high-carb, low-fat plan lowered it by 14 percent!

FIGHT FAT WITH FAT

We know what you're thinking: "This sounds good, but if I start eating avocados and olive oil, my jeans won't fit." That's where you're wrong. If you substitute these foods for less healthy low-fat ones (such as fat-free cookies), you won't gain a pound. In fact, following a high-fat diet may even help you lose weight.

Here's the proof: An 18-month study at Brigham and Women's Hospital in Boston compared a diet rich in unsaturated

Spread Yourself Thin

You can drop a few pounds simply by substituting your usual topping on bagels, baked potatoes, sandwiches, and toast with lower-calorie fare. Check out how 1 ounce (about 2 tablespoons) of "One-Minute Avocado Spread" (see page 26) stacks up against the same amount of your typical condiments.

Topping	Calories	Healthy Fat (g)	Saturated Fat (g)
Avocado spread	53	4	1
Butter	215	8	15
Cream cheese	105	3	7
Mayonnaise	215	17	4

fat with a low-fat diet. Those on the high-fat plan were allowed about 45 grams of fat a day, mostly from foods such as avocados, nuts, and olive oil. The group on the low-fat diet received only 25 grams of fat a day.

After six months, both groups dropped the same amount of weight—about 13 pounds. But a year later, the low-fat group gained back about 7 pounds, while the high-fat folks put on just 2 pounds.

"The participants on the high-fat plan seemed to like the diet better, so they were far more likely to stick to it," says study leader Kathy McManus, R.D.

So it's your choice: steamed vegetables, fat-free salad dressings, and dry bagels—or veggies grilled in olive oil, plus avocados and nuts. Which sounds better to you?

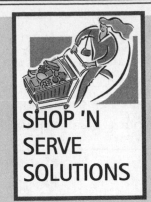

SHOP 'N SERVE SOLUTIONS

There are more than 100 varieties of avocados, but—mercifully—just two main types: California and Florida. You'll be able to find California avocados year-round, while the Sunshine State's avocados are usually available June through March.

Because they have distinctly different flavors, buy both types to determine which you prefer. In general, California avocados taste more buttery than their southern cousins do. That's probably because they have twice the fat and about one-third more calories. Everything else about the avocados—including their nutrient content—is identical.

No matter which type you try, determine how ripe the fruit is before you buy.

WHEN SELECTING AVOCADOS:

■ Look for a slightly soft avocado if you want to use it right away. To test it, squeeze it gently in the palm of your hand.

■ Look for a firm avocado if you're not planning to enjoy it until later in the week. Place it in a paper bag at room temperature. It will ripen within two to five days. (Tip: If you need that avocado in a hurry, place an apple in the bag, too. It will ripen even faster.)

SLICE THE SAFE WAY

When you're ready to use your avocado, you'll have to tackle seeding and peeling it. Relax. It looks a lot harder than it is. For safety's sake, we prefer to follow this technique recommended by the California Avocado Commission:

■ Cut the avocado lengthwise around the seed.

■ Rotate the halves to separate.

■ Remove the seed by sliding the tip of a spoon gently underneath it and lifting it out.

■ Peel the fruit by placing the cut-side down and removing the skin with a knife.

■ Alternatively, scoop out the avocado interior with a spoon.

■ Use the avocado immediately, or sprinkle it with lemon juice or white vinegar to prevent discoloration.

DICE TO SPICE

You can incorporate your beautiful green avocado into dozens of dishes besides guacamole. Here are a few:

◆ **Zing your salsa.** For an extra kick of nutrients and flavor, just stir chopped avocado into any commercial or homemade tomato salsa.

◆ **Stuff your sandwich.** Skip the mayo. Instead, flavor your wrap sandwiches—especially turkey—with avocado slices.

◆ **Perk up your pasta.** Tired of tomato sauce? Cook a pound of fettuccine (plain fettuccine is fine, but try the red pepper variety, too), and immediately toss with 2 tablespoons of olive oil, $\frac{1}{4}$ cup of white wine vinegar, $\frac{1}{2}$ cup of chopped fresh cilantro, $\frac{1}{2}$ cup of diced red bell pepper, $\frac{1}{2}$ cup of diced green or yellow bell pepper, 1 cup of diced sun-dried tomatoes, and, of course, 1 diced avocado.

One-Minute
Avocado Spread

Got a minute? That's barely all it takes to make this tempting topping for focaccia, crackers—even bagels.

1 medium avocado, seeded and peeled
2 tablespoons lemon juice
2 tablespoons chopped fresh basil

In a medium bowl, mash the avocado with a fork. Stir in the lemon juice and basil. Cover and chill for at least 1 hour to blend the flavors.

Yield: Six servings.

Nutritional data per serving: Calories, 53; protein, 1 g; carbohydrates, 2 g; fiber, 1 g; fat, 5 g; saturated fat, 1 g; cholesterol, 0 mg; sodium, 4 mg; folate, 5% of Daily Value.

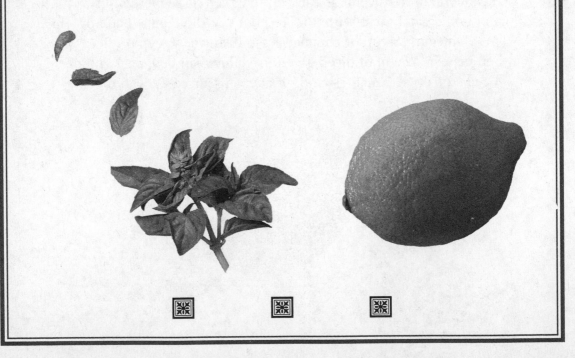

Mediterranean Salad

If you can't travel there, at least enjoy the fabulous flavors of the Mediterranean in your own dining room. Although you can use any salad greens, make this salad visually stunning with red radicchio lettuce.

½ **avocado, seeded and peeled**
4 **cups cleaned, chopped salad greens**
¼ **cup crumbled feta cheese**
8 **Kalamata olives**
½ **cup low-fat or fat-free balsamic vinaigrette, such as Old Cape Cod**

Slice the avocado into strips. In a large bowl, gently toss the avocado, salad greens, cheese, and olives with the vinaigrette until well coated.

Yield: Four servings.

Nutritional data per serving: Calories, 112; protein, 3 g; carbohydrates, 6 g; fiber, 2 g; fat, 9 g; saturated fat, 2 g; cholesterol, 8 mg; sodium, 408 mg; calcium, 8% of Daily Value; iron, 7%.

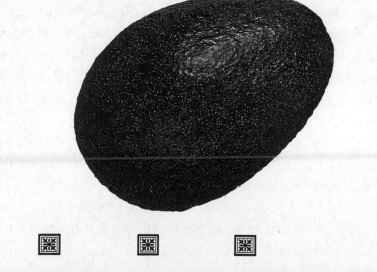

Bananas:

The Best of the Bunch

BATTLES:
- cancer
- heart disease
- high blood pressure
- kidney stones
- premenstrual syndrome
- stroke

BOLSTERS:
- energy

Colleen and her husband, Ted, have worked out the perfect system for getting their fill of perfect bananas.

Ted loves his bananas tinged with green and still very firm, and he can hardly wait to get them home from the grocery store to pop the peel. Colleen views bananas at this stage of ripening as crunchy and inedible. So she sets them out on the counter in a basket to tempt Ted. Then, when the first brown dot appears, Ted loses interest and Colleen's lights up. She loves her bananas creamy, sweet, and ripe. She rushes them into the fridge then, to stop the ripening process at this perfect place.

Worried about the skins turning black in the fridge? Get over it, Chiquita. The skins may turn dark, but the insides stay luscious longer when they're cold.

CARBO-LOADED

Bananas are Mother Nature's most perfect fast-food snack. They require no preparation (not even washing!) or refrigeration. They come prepackaged in a biodegradable wrapper and require no utensils for perfect enjoyment. What could be better than a banana?!

Babies love them (they're often a first food because they're so digestible), and athletes thrive on their quick, sustained carbohydrate energy. Gym rats toss them into their bags for the perfect preworkout boost. And women suffering from premenstrual syndrome can get a healthy serotonin surge by indulging in bananas.

HEARTY UNDER PRESSURE

Besides being just plain yummy, bananas help build a shield against heart disease. To start with, they're packed with potassium, which helps fend off high blood pressure—a big risk factor for heart disease and stroke. But you probably already knew that. (Getting more potassium may also help prevent kidney stones, especially if you eat a high-sodium diet.)

What may surprise you is that bananas are a powerful package of pyridoxine (also known as vitamin B_6), delivering one-third of your daily requirement in each medium-size finger.

In a study of 80,000 healthy professional women, those whose diets included the most vitamin B_6 and folate (another B vitamin) were the least likely to have a heart attack. In another study of almost 500 people at high risk for heart disease, increasing their intake of B_6, folate, and vitamin B_{12} helped control their blood homocysteine levels, another risk factor for heart attack. So whatever your risk level, havabanana.

NUTRITION IN A NUTSHELL

Banana (1 medium)

Calories: 109

Fat: 0 g

Saturated fat: 0 g

Cholesterol: 0 mg

Sodium: 1 mg

Total carbohydrates: 28 g

Dietary fiber: 3 g

Protein: 1 g

Vitamin A: 2% of Daily Value

Vitamin B_6: 34%

Vitamin C: 12%

Calcium: 1%

Iron: 2%

Potassium: 12%

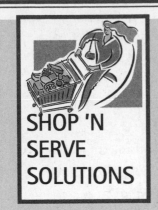

SHOP 'N SERVE SOLUTIONS

Bananas are available year-round.

WHEN SELECTING BANANAS:

■ Choosing the right banana is largely a matter of taste. Colleen finds that short, thick bananas seem to be the sweetest.

■ Avoid bananas with cuts or bruises.

■ After that, the degree of ripeness that you prefer is what counts.

WHEN STORING:

Store bananas at room temperature until they ripen to the stage that you prefer, then refrigerate them.

PREPARING YOUR BANANA BONANZA

Once you've found your perfect hand of bananas, enjoy them as a sweet treat or use them to add natural sweetness to other dishes. Here are a few ideas:

◆ **Stick 'em up.** Insert wooden sticks into peeled, overripe bananas. Dip the bananas in chocolate and freeze them for a tasty snack.

◆ **Whirl 'em up.** In a blender, whirl ripe bananas with yogurt or milk and vanilla for a cool milk shake.

◆ **Light 'em up.** Brighten a dull dinner with a candle salad. (Colleen learned this in Brownies when she was eight years old, and she still loves it!) On a salad plate, top a lettuce leaf with a pineapple ring. Cut a peeled banana in half crosswise. Stand a banana half in the pineapple ring, cut-end down. Top with a cherry on a toothpick to simulate a flame.

◆ **Cook 'em up.** Sauté banana slices, toss with brown sugar, and serve over your favorite broiled fish.

◆ **Sweeten up a sandwich.** Instead of jelly, use ripe banana slices on your peanut butter sandwich.

Reports about the beneficial effects of fiber in preventing bowel, colon, and colorectal cancers, change from Yes to No and back again day after day. The issues are complex, and fiber itself has so many parts. In one Hawaiian study, researchers looked at an array of fiber fractions, such as soluble and insoluble fiber, crude fiber, dietary fiber, and nonstarch polysaccharides. No wonder we're all confused!

In that study, only vegetable fiber worked. But one thing that the researchers learned along the way is that, fiber aside, eating certain plant foods, such as bananas, broccoli, carrots, and corn, had an inverse relationship to colorectal cancer risk. That means that the more study participants ate, the less likely they were to get that cancer. And in another study, bananas were ranked with oranges, peaches, and asparagus for ability to hamper the creation of new cancer cells. So while you're working on your five-a-day, say "Make mine banana."

Banana-Peanut "Pudding"

Here's a quickie dessert that delivers all the "comfort food" consistency of pudding, as well as all the calcium and potassium your body cries for to control blood pressure.

2 tablespoons crunchy peanut butter
1 cup fat-free plain yogurt
1 medium banana, quartered and sliced

In a microwaveable dish, melt the peanut butter in the microwave. Quickly stir in the yogurt. Add the banana and stir once more. Divide between two dessert dishes and serve.

Yield: Two servings.

Nutritional data per serving: Calories, 217; protein, 11 g; carbohydrates, 27 g; fiber, 2 g; fat, 8 g; saturated fat, 2 g; cholesterol, 2 mg; sodium, 172 mg; vitamin B_2 (riboflavin), 21% of Daily Value; vitamin B_6, 24%; calcium, 25%; potassium, 18%.

Banana Breakfast Danish

If you're focused on healthy eating, avoid the pastry cart. But when you long for the custardy taste of a cheese Danish pastry, satisfy your sweet tooth with this banana-sweetened treat. Its combination of fruit, dairy, whole grain bread, and heart-healthy walnuts makes it a complete breakfast all by itself (with a cup of steaming-hot coffee, of course!).

1 very ripe banana, peeled and mashed
¼ cup reduced-fat ricotta cheese
2 slices 100% stone-ground whole wheat bread
1 tablespoon finely chopped walnuts
½ teaspoon cinnamon sugar

In a medium bowl, stir the banana and cheese together until well blended. Spread half of the mixture on each slice of the bread. Sprinkle each with half of the nuts and cinnamon sugar. Toast in a toaster oven until the bottoms are crisp and the filling is custardlike.

Yield: One serving.

Nutritional data per serving: Calories, 386; protein, 13 g; carbohydrates, 55 g; fiber, 5 g; fat, 13 g; saturated fat, 8 g; cholesterol, 30 mg; sodium, 431 mg; vitamin B$_6$, 36% of Daily Value; calcium, 30%.

Barley:
Healthy, Hearty Pearls

BATTLES:
- diabetes
- heart disease
- high blood pressure
- high cholesterol

BOLSTERS:
- regularity

Whenever Karen goes out to dinner—even on the hottest days—she always asks about the soup du jour, secretly hoping that it's chicken, beef, or vegetable barley. Unfortunately, it hardly ever is. (In fact, it's usually cream of something.) But on the few occasions when the waiter mentions barley, Karen can't order a bowl fast enough.

HEART-TO-HEART TALK

So much nutrition information is couched in caveats. You've probably heard them all: "More research is needed," "These are preliminary findings," and so forth. Well, here's a *fact:* Barley is beneficial for your heart.

Researchers at Texas A&M University in College Station tested the effect of

NUTRITION IN A NUTSHELL

Cooked pearl barley (1 cup)

Calories: 193

Fat: 1 g

Saturated fat: 0 g

Cholesterol: 0 mg

Sodium: 5 mg

Total carbohydrates: 44 g

Dietary fiber: 6 g

Protein: 4 g

Folate: 7% of Daily Value

Vitamin B_3 (niacin): 16%

Iron: 11%

Magnesium: 9%

Phosphorus: 9%

Zinc: 8%

Quick Fix:

Constipation

If you're having trouble moving your bowels, you may not be getting the 20 to 35 grams of fiber you need daily. Just 1 cup of cooked barley can provide 6 to 14 grams of fiber. That's sure to get things moving in a hurry!

barley bran flour, barley oil capsules, or wheat flour on men and women with high cholesterol levels. All the participants followed a low-fat diet for about a month. The result: Those who used either kind of barley significantly lowered their cholesterol levels and their blood pressure.

So what's the magic ingredient in barley? Researchers think that several compounds in barley work together to keep your ticker trouble-free.

First, barley contains beta-glucan, a type of fiber that study after study has shown lowers cholesterol. (By the way, it's also what gives barley its creamy texture.) Beta-glucan traps some fat and cholesterol from the foods you eat and ushers them out of your body before they can be absorbed.

Plus, barley boasts tocotrienol, a substance that deactivates an enzyme that tells the liver to produce artery-clogging, bad low-density lipoprotein (LDL) cholesterol. Researchers also are testing a few other hard-to-pronounce substances in barley to see if they play a role. Stay tuned.

BLOOD SUGAR SURPRISE

Barley also helps fight heart problems through the back door—by controlling type 2 diabetes, which puts you at extra risk for a heart attack. Here are some of the latest research findings:

▶ At the University of California-Davis, researchers gave men meals made with regular pasta or pasta with barley flour. The guys who chowed down on the barley pasta didn't produce as much insulin (a hormone that plays a role in diabetes) as did those who ate the normal pasta.

▶ A Harvard University study on women suggests that eating whole grains such as barley lowers the risk of type 2 diabetes.

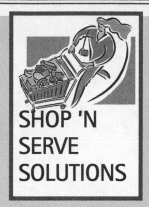

SHOP 'N SERVE SOLUTIONS

The next time you wander through the rice aisle at your supermarket, look for barley. This grain is sold in a variety of forms. No matter which you choose, barley is booming with vitamins, minerals, and flavor. Here's what's available:

■ **Pearl barley.** When barley is pearled, the husk is removed and the kernel is polished. This process strips barley of at least one-third of its fiber—although pearl barley still packs a sizable chunk.

■ **Hulled barley.** Here you get the whole grain. Hulled barley offers 14 grams of fiber—that's half of what you need for the entire day!—in just 1 cup, cooked.

■ **Quick-cooking barley.** This variety can be fully cooked in just 10 to 12 minutes, while pearl and hulled types generally take 45 and 95 minutes, respectively.

TRYING ON YOUR NEW STRAND OF PEARLS

Now that you've chosen your barley, here are some stylish serving suggestions:

◆ **Accent with apricots.** In a large saucepan, combine $1^{3}/_{4}$ cups of low-sodium chicken broth, 1 cup of orange juice, $^{1}/_{4}$ cup of white wine, 1 cup of pearl barley, $^{1}/_{4}$ cup of dried apricots, and $^{1}/_{4}$ cup of raisins. Bring to a boil. Cover, reduce the heat to low, and cook for 45 minutes, or until the barley is tender and the liquid is absorbed. Sprinkle with toasted nuts before serving.

◆ **Combine with chicken.** Sauté $^{1}/_{2}$ cup of sliced fresh mushrooms in 2 teaspoons of olive oil. Add 1 cup of pearl barley, 3 cups of low-sodium chicken or vegetable broth, $^{1}/_{4}$ teaspoon of dried rosemary, and 2 tablespoons of minced onion. Bring to a boil. Cover and cook for 45 minutes, or until the barley is tender and the liquid is absorbed.

◆ **Slurp supersoup.** If you're too busy to make your own, try Fantastic Foods Vegetable Barley Soup. Mmmmm!

Barley-Feta Toss

A few years ago, we got this recipe from the National Barley Foods Council, and it's been a favorite ever since.

1 cup pearl barley
3 cups water
1¼ teaspoons salt
⅓ cup olive oil
2 tablespoons fresh lemon juice
2 tablespoons red wine vinegar
½ teaspoon dried oregano
¼ cup finely chopped onion
¼ cup minced fresh parsley
2 medium tomatoes, diced
1 small green or red bell pepper, diced
½ cup crumbled feta cheese
Lettuce leaves, washed and chilled

In a large saucepan over high heat, bring the barley, water, and 1 teaspoon of the salt to a boil. Cover, reduce the heat to low, and cook for 45 minutes, or until the barley is tender and the liquid is absorbed. In a small bowl, combine the oil, lemon juice, vinegar, oregano, and the remaining ¼ teaspoon of salt. Pour over the cooked barley. Cool to room temperature. Gently stir in the onion, parsley, tomatoes, pepper, and cheese. Serve the salad chilled (Karen's favorite) or at room temperature on lettuce-lined plates.

Yield: Six servings.

Nutritional data per serving: Calories, 266; protein, 5 g; carbohydrates, 30 g; fiber, 6 g; fat, 15 g; saturated fat, 3 g; cholesterol, 8 mg; sodium, 558 mg; calcium, 10% of Daily Value; iron, 8%.

Basil:

Meet the Good-Health Herb

BATTLES:
- bloating
- colon cancer
- infections
- inflammation
- ulcers

BOLSTERS:
- bones

It's the fragrance of fresh basil that gets you. We grow it in our gardens for cooking, yes, but also for the aroma. Lawn mowing suddenly turns from work to wonder when you brush by the basil and its pungent perfume envelops you.

There are only four tastes, you know—sweet, sour, bitter, and salty. But basil, a member of the mint family, has been hailed since ancient times for the way its aromatic compounds turn basic food tastes into gourmet flavors with just a scissor snip.

Historically, basil has performed strictly as a cooking herb, not as a medicinal one. But now that's starting to change.

NUTRITION IN A NUTSHELL

Fresh basil (½ cup)

Calories: 6

Fat: 0 g

Saturated fat: 0 g

Cholesterol: 0 mg

Sodium: 0 mg

Total carbohydrates: 1 g

Dietary fiber: 1 g

Protein: 1 g

Vitamin A: 16% of Daily Value

Vitamin C: 4%

Calcium: 3%

Iron: 4%

Manganese: 15%

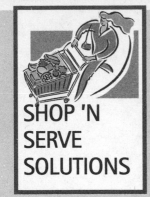

SHOP 'N SERVE SOLUTIONS

If you don't grow your own, you can find fresh basil in most health food stores and many large grocery stores.

WHEN SELECTING BASIL:

Look for sturdy, green leaves that aren't wilting or turning black.

WHEN STORING:

■ Store cut basil in the refrigerator. Colleen especially likes the Tupperware container with ventilation holes that allow basil to breathe.

■ Store basil bouquets in water either on your countertop or in the fridge. A bouquet—that's basil with the roots still attached—will stay alive for a week or two.

GO GOURMET

Once you start using basil, you'll go gourmet often. Here are some ideas to get you started:

◆ **Slip it into salads.** A handful of fresh basil tossed in with summer greens will have your guests asking, "Mmmmm, what's that?!"

◆ **Make luscious linguini.** For the best-dressed pasta when dining alfresco, stir together chopped fresh, ripe tomatoes, slivered fresh basil, some pressed garlic, and a little olive oil. Serve uncooked over hot pasta.

◆ **Store up summer.** If you end up with too much basil (is that possible?), you can pulverize it in the food processor with just enough olive oil to make a smooth paste. Use the paste instead of butter or mayonnaise on sandwiches for a dash of heart-healthy unsaturated fat. Or freeze it in ice-cube trays, then add it to soups, stews, and pasta dishes all year long.

◆ **Microwave memories.** Dry basil in the microwave. Wash the leaves and pat dry. Place a small handful at a time on a paper towel. Microwave on high for about 5 minutes, or until bone-dry and brittle. Crumble the leaves, then store them in an airtight container in a cool, dark place. Add to chicken dishes, pasta sauce, salads, and all Italian fare.

GROWING YOUR OWN

Basil is easy to grow in your garden, on your deck, or even in a deep flowerpot on your windowsill. All you need is a lot of sun and warmth and a little rain. In fact, basil is perfect for those hot spots that scorch most normal plants.

Sow the seeds when the weather turns warm, and let the soil dry out between waterings. After the plants have grown two sets of leaves, pinch off the top so that the plants will branch.

Two or three plants will provide more leaves than you can ever use.

Quick Fix:

Hangover

Overindulged just a tad last night, did we? Well, basil can at least help reduce the resulting bloating and flatulence. Make a tea by steeping 2 tablespoons of chopped fresh basil leaves or 2 teaspoons of dried leaves in 1 cup of just-boiled water for about 15 minutes. Strain and sip.

NEW HERB ON THE BLOCK

Researchers in India have been testing the oil from basil leaves on laboratory animals. According to their research, here's what basil can do:

▶ Dampen the ulcer-producing activity of aspirin and alcohol.
▶ Fight inflammation and swelling.
▶ Battle infection-causing bacteria.

Basil also may do the following:

▶ **Prevent colon cancer.** Basil contains eugenol, a compound that increases production of antioxidants, at least in the intestines of lab animals. The antioxidants help get rid of toxic substances that may cause cancer. So there's a hint that basil may be helpful in preventing colon cancer.

▶ **Help build bones.** Basil doles out small quantities of the minerals calcium, copper, magnesium, and manganese, all of which seem to be important for a sturdy skeleton.

Tomato-Basil Summer Salad

In the heat of summer, when your plants are loaded with the plumpest, most perfect tomatoes and roadside stands are spilling forth the lushest varieties, you'll want a salad that simply enhances their unbeatable flavor. Instead of lettuce, call on fresh basil to accentuate the positive.

1 large fully ripe, but firm, tomato
½ teaspoon balsamic vinegar
½ teaspoon olive oil
4 superthin shavings of Parmesan cheese (about 1 ounce total)
4 large fresh basil leaves
3 large green Cerignola olives or other olives as available (garnish)

Wash the tomato and pat dry. With a serrated knife, slice into four thick, juicy slabs. Arrange on a plate. Drizzle with the vinegar and then the oil. Top each tomato slice with a shaving of the cheese and a basil leaf. Garnish with the olives.

Yield: One serving.

Nutritional data per serving: Calories, 207; protein, 12 g; carbohydrates, 13 g; fiber, 3 g; fat, 13 g; saturated fat, 4 g; cholesterol, 22 mg; sodium, 612 mg; vitamin A, 33% of Daily Value; vitamin C, 49%; calcium, 36%.

Beans:

A Lean Cuisine

BATTLES:

- asthma
- birth defects
- cancer
- diabetes
- heart disease
- high cholesterol

BOLSTERS:

- energy
- memory
- weight control

When Karen was a kid, her family often made minestrone soup. While everyone else heartily dug in, Karen carefully navigated around the soup bowl, pushing aside the kidney beans until the bottom of the bowl was covered with them. Today, Karen's family still makes a mean minestrone, but now she eats the beans. Why? Because researcher after researcher has taught her that these luscious legumes are loaded with fiber and other nutrients that keep her body running in top shape.

NUTRITION IN A NUTSHELL

Cooked dried red kidney beans (½ cup)

Calories: 110

Fat: 0 g

Saturated fat: 0 g

Cholesterol: 0 mg

Sodium: 4 mg

Total carbohydrates: 20 g

Dietary fiber: 4 g

Protein: 8 g

Folate: 16% of Daily Value

Calcium: 5%

Iron: 14%

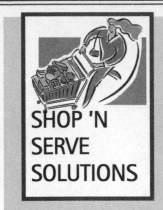

SHOP 'N SERVE SOLUTIONS

Many good cooks prefer using dried beans. But if you're a bean novice, start with canned beans. There's no doubt about it—they're bushels more convenient than dried. Here are some tips to get you off to a successful start using canned beans:

■ Try several brands. Flavors vary slightly from brand to brand, so experiment to see which you prefer.

■ Check for salt content. Look for brands that contain 350 milligrams of sodium or less per serving.

■ Rinse your beans. Tests by the nutrition advocacy group Center for Science in the Public Interest in Washington, D.C., have shown that you can eliminate one-quarter to one-third of the sodium in canned beans simply by rinsing them in cold water for about a minute.

THE ART OF COOKING BEANS

Now you're ready to try these bountiful, beautiful bean dishes:

◆ **Nab some nachos.** At a restaurant, the calories and fat in nachos add up quickly. At home, just dig into this low-fat recipe: Top baked tortilla chips with black beans, reduced-fat cheddar cheese, lettuce, chopped tomatoes, chopped sweet or hot peppers, and low-fat sour cream.

◆ **Make your hummus sing.** Sure, you can buy this spread, an ideal topping for crackers or a great alternative to mayo on breads.

FIGHT CANCER AND CHOLESTEROL

Just ½ cup of cooked beans kicks in 3 to 6 grams of fiber, both the insoluble type (a colon cancer fighter) and the soluble type (a cholesterol controller). A study at the University of Kentucky in

But it tastes so good when it's homemade. Try this: In a large bowl, mash one 15$\frac{1}{2}$-ounce can of garbanzo beans or 1$\frac{1}{2}$ cups of cooked dried garbanzos. Mix in 2 tablespoons of lemon juice, 1 tablespoon of olive oil, 1 teaspoon of minced garlic, 1 teaspoon of dried oregano leaves, and salt and ground black pepper to taste.

◆ **Give a hand to canned.** Open a can of beans, drain, rinse, and add to salads or soups (such as tomato or vegetable). Or heat them up, then mix with cooked brown rice. Or use them to make a pot of chili.

◆ **Whip up a snack.** Roasted garbanzo beans are a crunchy alternative to nuts. Just drain, rinse, and pat dry one 15$\frac{1}{2}$-ounce can of garbanzos. Put the beans on a jelly-roll pan. In a small bowl, combine 1 tablespoon of canola or olive oil and 1 teaspoon of chili powder. Drizzle the beans with the oil mixture. Bake at 400°F for 35 to 40 minutes, or until crisp.

Lexington found that eating 1 cup of canned beans in tomato sauce daily for three weeks lowered cholesterol in middle-aged men by about 10 percent. And lower cholesterol means less risk of heart disease.

PROTECT YOUR TICKER

First, beans are loaded with the B vitamin folate, which reduces blood levels of homocysteine, an amino acid implicated in heart disease. (And, yes, folate is the same vitamin that wards off birth defects.) Second, a recent study of 111 women suggests that bean eaters have more flexible arteries than legume loathers. Researchers at Cedars-Sinai Medical Center in Los Angeles are planning follow-up reports, but in the meantime, they recommend eating at least ½ cup of beans a day.

CONTROL BLOOD SUGAR

People with type 2 diabetes also may benefit from the soluble fiber in beans, because it slows the passage of carbohydrates from foods into the bloodstream. As a result, less insulin is needed to control blood sugar levels. By eating a diet rich in beans and

THE BEAN COUNTER

Size up the nutritional differences among your favorite beans. Nutritional values are based on ½ cup of cooked beans.

Bean	Calories	Fat (g)	Fiber (g)	Folate (% of Daily Value)	Calcium (% DV)
Black	114	0.5	4	32	2
Garbanzo (chickpea)	135	2	3	35	3
Great Northern	105	0.5	5	22	6
Lima	115	0.5	6	34	2
Navy	130	0.5	5	32	6
Pinto	118	0.5	6	36	4
Red kidney	110	0	4	16	5

other legumes, such as lentils, diabetics may be able to get away with using less medication to control their blood sugar levels. Just make sure you check with your doctor before altering your dosage.

INCREASE STAMINA

The poky release of carbohydrates into your bloodstream offers another perk: long-lasting energy. "Beans will sustain you longer than a food such as a potato, which quickly releases its carbohydrates," says nutritionist Kim Galeaz, R.D.

GET A FILL-UP

If that weren't enough, beans also fight the battle of the bulge. Studies at Pennsylvania State University in State College suggest that foods low in calories but high in volume and fiber (such as beans) help control your appetite, simply by taking up a lot of room in your tummy.

Quick Fix:

Tight Airways

Anybody with asthma knows the scary feeling that constricted airways cause. But now British scientists have found that people who have asthma are half as likely to develop constricted airways if they regularly eat foods rich in magnesium. One of the best? Black-eyed peas, which are actually a type of bean.

Quick Fix:

Memory

Keep losing your keys? Forgetting where you wrote an important telephone number? Studies have shown that deficiencies in iron and zinc can interfere with your concentration. Boost your brainpower by eating a serving of beans a few times a week—they're loaded with both minerals!

Aunt Shirley's Three-Bean Salad

When Karen told her grandmother that she was writing this book, Grandma asked her to include this dish, which is always a big hit at family gatherings. Oddly, the recipe isn't Grandma's, but one belonging to Karen's Aunt Shirley.

2 cans (15 ounces each) red kidney beans
2 cans (15 ounces each) yellow beans
2 cans (15 ounces each) green beans
1 small onion, chopped
1 sweet green or red pepper, chopped
⅔ cup white wine vinegar
½ cup sugar
⅓ cup olive oil

In a large colander, drain all the beans and then rinse under cold water for 1 minute. Transfer to a large bowl and add the onion and pepper. Set aside. In a saucepan over medium heat, cook the vinegar and sugar until the sugar melts. Remove from the heat and stir in the oil. Pour the oil mixture over the beans and toss until well combined. Refrigerate for 3 to 24 hours so the flavors can blend.

Yield: 12 servings.

Nutritional data per serving: Calories, 328; protein, 13 g; carbohydrates, 57 g; fiber, 9 g; fat, 7 g; saturated fat, 1 g; cholesterol, 0 mg; sodium, 193 mg; calcium, 7% of Daily Value; iron, 17%.

Beef:

No Complaints
If You Buy Lean

BATTLES:
- cancer
- heart disease

BOLSTERS:
- energy
- immune function

Beef? In a book about kitchen counter cures? We bet you can't believe your eyes. Truth is, at first, we weren't sure about including it, either. Then we mulled over all the research and realized that we couldn't leave it out.

While greasy hamburgers can send your cholesterol through the Golden Arches, some cuts of beef are comparable to chicken. Plus, beef is loaded with disease-fighting nutrients that are hard to come by even in a healthy diet. So you'd better sit down before you read on.

THE CUT COUNTS

Beef got a bad rep because, compared with other meats, it has a lot of saturated fat. Study after study has linked a diet high in saturated fat to heart disease. But not all cuts of beef are unacceptable. In fact, eight cuts of beef meet the USDA's standards for being considered lean. They are eye round, top round, round tip, top sirloin, bottom round, top loin, tenderloin, and flank steak.

A 3-ounce serving of most of these cuts contains 6 grams of

total fat and 2 grams of saturated fat. When you choose one of these lean cuts, your cholesterol level will respond the same way that it does to chicken.

LEAN BEEF MAY NOT RAISE CHOLESTEROL

In a recent study of 145 men and women with mild to moderately high cholesterol, researchers at three major medical centers compared the effects of lean white meat with those of lean red meat on the participants' cholesterol levels. For about nine months, half of the participants derived 80 percent of their meat from lean red meat. The other half of the group ate lean white meat. After a four-week break, the groups switched the type of meat they were eating. During the entire study, the participants were instructed to follow a healthy eating plan recommended by the American Heart Association.

The result: Whether the participants were eating red or white meat, they lowered their levels of bad low-density lipoprotein (LDL) cholesterol and improved their levels of good high-density lipoprotein (HDL) cholesterol. "A heart-healthy diet containing up to 6 ounces of lean red meat daily can positively impact blood cholesterol levels," says lead researcher Michael H. Davidson, M.D.

MEAT YOUR VITAMINS AND MINERALS

Okay, so now you know that eating lean beef won't attack your heart. But it has other perks, too. Beef supplies six vitamins and minerals that may be in short supply in your diet:

NUTRITION IN A NUTSHELL

Eye round (3 ounces, roasted)

Calories: 149

Fat: 5 g

Saturated fat: 2 g

Cholesterol: 59 mg

Sodium: 53 mg

Total carbohydrates: 0 g

Dietary fiber: 0 g

Protein: 25 g

Vitamin B_3 (niacin): 16% of Daily Value

Vitamin B_6: 16%

Vitamin B_{12}: 31%

Iron: 10%

Selenium: 33%

Zinc: 27%

▶ **Iron.** Consider iron the FedEx of nutrients: It delivers oxygen to cells where it is used to produce energy. Unfortunately, 7.8 million American women don't get enough iron, making it the top nutritional deficiency in the United States.

Without enough iron, you can become anemic, a condition that leaves you exhausted, irritable, and weak. Although most of the foods in your fridge contain iron, meat is your best bet because the iron from meat is absorbed six to nine times better than the iron from most nonmeat sources. For instance, to obtain the same amount of iron found in a 3-ounce serving of beef, you would have to eat at least 3 cups of spinach. And even then, you wouldn't be able to absorb it as well as the iron in beef.

▶ **Zinc.** Yes, indeed, that's the same nutrient found in those lozenges you take to zap colds. Nearly 75 percent of Americans don't meet the recommended zinc requirements. Not getting enough zinc may compromise the immune system or even cause memory loss.

A 3-ounce serving of beef supplies more than 25 percent of the Daily Value for zinc. (By comparison, chicken breast provides just 6 percent.) P.S. Too much zinc can be as bad for the immune system as too little, so you should hover around your daily requirement—15 milligrams for men and 12 milligrams for women.

▶ **Selenium.** A serving of beef supplies about one-third of your daily requirement for selenium. A powerful antioxidant, selenium may lower the risk of cancer (especially skin cancer), fight heart disease, and ward off infections.

▶ **B vitamins.** Beef boasts vitamin B_6 (a deficiency can cause

(Continued on page 52)

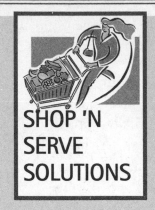

SHOP 'N SERVE SOLUTIONS

Unless your brother's a butcher, figuring out how to select the best-tasting and best-for-you beef can be a puzzle. So we'll walk you through it.

WHEN SELECTING BEEF:

■ Consider freshness first. Choose meat that has the most distant "sell-by" date on its label—a tip-off that it has been recently put on the shelf.

■ If you can't locate a "sell-by" date, look at the color of the fat and the meat. The fat should always be white; yellow fat is a sign of age. Unpackaged meat should look cherry red. Vacuum-packed meat should be dark purple. Notice brown or gray areas? That means the meat is on the old side—not necessarily spoiled, but not the freshest you can buy.

■ Select the leanest cuts. Look for beef that has only a little marbling or external fat. Remember, you can always ask your butcher to trim away excess fat.

■ Once you find the cut you like, check what grades are available. "Select" offers the least fat, followed by "choice" and then "prime."

BEWARE THE BURGER

What about ground beef? We recommend that you don't buy it very often. Even the leanest ground beef is still pretty high in fat.

Most supermarkets carry ground beef that ranges from 80 percent lean (that's 210 calories and 14 grams of fat for 3 ounces) to 93 percent lean (170 calories and 9 grams of fat). Occasionally, you'll see ground beef that is 96 percent lean.

Our call: If you must buy ground beef, choose the leanest you can find, and mix it with skinless ground turkey.

WHEN STORING BEEF:

■ Once you find the package of beef you want, tuck it inside a plastic bag so that any bacteria on the wrapper won't contaminate other foods in your shopping cart. Then head home right away—especially in the summer.

■ Store beef in the coldest part of your fridge—usually the meat drawer. Fresh beef is safe to eat until the "sell-by" date.

■ Alternately, you can freeze it. Roasts and steaks will keep for 6 to 12 months. Ground beef is fine in the freezer for 3 to 4 months.

WHEN YOU'RE READY TO USE:

Thaw beef properly. Always defrost meat in your refrigerator or in the microwave—never on the kitchen counter.

COOKING HINT

Time your cooking. Lean beef, as you'd imagine, isn't as forgiving of overcooking as fattier cuts are. So the trick is to broil or grill it long enough to avoid foodborne illness (dangerous bacteria such as *E. coli* can lurk in undercooked beef), but not so long that it tastes like shoe leather. Cook roasts and steaks to an internal temperature of 145°F (about medium-rare) and ground beef until a meat thermometer registers 160°F (about medium-well).

BEEF: IT'S WHAT'S FOR DINNER!

You probably have zillions of recipes for beef. But think about the following suggestions, because they use beef more as an accent than a main course:

◆ **Pump up your soup.** Toss a little leftover steak or roast into vegetable soup for the next day's lunch or dinner.

◆ **Mix up your meats.** Have a sandwich with a slice of roast beef and a slice of turkey. Or tuck a little bit of beef, a little bit of chicken, and a lot of vegetables into your tacos or fajitas.

◆ **Order surf and turf.** If you're dining out and dying for a steak, order surf and turf instead. That way, you'll get a better variety of food—a good-for-you lobster and a smaller piece of meat.

(Continued from page 49)

depression), vitamin B_{12} (not getting enough could lead to fatigue or even nerve damage), and vitamin B_3, or niacin (a severe deficiency can trigger disorientation and skin problems).

SLIMMING STEAK?

In addition to vitamins and minerals, beef contains a compound called conjugated linoleic acid (CLA). Studies on animals have found that CLA may inhibit tumors in the breasts, ovaries, lungs, and colon; decrease bad cholesterol levels; normalize reduced blood glucose levels; and—get this—decrease body fat.

We know this sounds like an infomercial, but this research is really happening. Scientists are now conducting human studies to see if the benefits hold true. In the meantime, keep your fingers crossed!

Beef Stir-Fry

You'll love this super, simple stir-fry recipe from the National Cattleman's Beef Association.

1 pound flank steak
2 tablespoons reduced-sodium soy sauce
4 teaspoons dark sesame oil, divided
1½ teaspoons sugar
1 teaspoon cornstarch
2 cloves garlic, crushed
1 tablespoon minced fresh ginger
¼ teaspoon crushed red pepper
1 small red bell pepper, cut into 1-inch pieces
1 can (15 ounces) whole baby corn, drained
¼ pound pea pods, cut into matchsticks

Cut the steak lengthwise in half and then crosswise into ⅛-inch-thick strips. In a medium bowl, combine the soy sauce, 2 teaspoons of the oil, the sugar, and cornstarch. Add the steak, tossing to coat, and set aside. Heat the remaining 2 teaspoons of oil in a large skillet over medium-high heat until hot. Add the garlic, ginger, and crushed red pepper, and cook for 30 seconds. Add the bell pepper and corn and stir-fry for 1½ minutes. Add the pea pods and stir-fry for 30 seconds. Remove the vegetables from the skillet. Add the steak (one-half at a time), and stir-fry for 1 to 2 minutes, or until the outside surface is no longer pink. Return the vegetables to the skillet and heat through.

Yield: Four servings.

Nutritional data per serving: Calories, 337; protein, 28 g; carbohydrates, 27 g; fiber, 3 g; fat, 14 g; saturated fat, 5 g; cholesterol, 57 mg; sodium, 668 mg; calcium, 3% of Daily Value; iron, 21%.

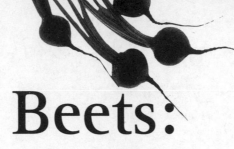

Beets:

Healthy Valentines for Your Heart

BATTLES:
- cancer
- diabetes
- heart disease

BOLSTERS:
- regularity

Way back when, one of Colleen's childhood playmates proudly gave her a handful of fresh beets that were grown in her own backyard garden. Colleen went running home, eager to have her mom cook them up for dinner. Unfortunately, their earthy taste was a bit much for Colleen. (New research says kids need 15 tastes of a new food before they consider it edible!) So she abandoned beets. That didn't seem like much of a problem, since nutritionists stuck beets on the back burner, anyway. After all, they offered only trivial amounts of the "big" vitamins such as A and C. (Who knew about phytochemicals then?)

Later, those high-protein, low-carbohydrate diet books started beet bashing. Somehow, their authors got the idea that beets were loaded with sweets that raise blood sugar and insulin and cause insulin resistance and even diabetes. Wrong.

Today, beets are starting to look better, now that the facts are finally sneaking out.

BEET HEART DISEASE

Beets are shaped like little hearts for a reason. Just 1 cup of fresh beets delivers one-third of your folate requirement for the day. That's the B vitamin noted for keeping homocysteine in check so that it can't trigger a heart attack. (Getting enough folate also dramatically reduces neural tube birth defects.)

BEET CANCER

Beta-cyanin is the phytochemical that gives beets their deep red color. It may also be a cancer fighter. Research done in Russia suggests that beet juice may help inhibit normal, healthy cells from mutating into cancer cells.

BEET DIABETES

Beets got a bad rap for raising blood sugar levels. Here's the issue: When you eat carbohydrates, they become blood sugar, also known as glucose. In your blood, glucose pairs up with insulin, which coaxes your cells to open up and let the glucose in, so that it can be used for fuel.

Some people's cells are reluctant to cooperate; that is, they're insulin-resistant. Insulin resistance has been linked to heart disease, high blood pressure, and diabetes. Some carbohydrate foods *slowly* raise blood sugar, making it

NUTRITION IN A NUTSHELL

Cooked fresh beets (1 cup)

Calories: 75

Fat: 0 g

Saturated fat: 0 g

Cholesterol: 0 mg

Sodium: 484 mg

Total carbohydrates: 17 g

Protein: 3 g

Dietary fiber: 3 g

Folate: 34% of Daily Value

Vitamin A: 1%

Vitamin C: 7%

Calcium: 3%

Iron: 7%

SAFE DYE

Need a healthy red food dye? Forget artificial food coloring, and use beet juice instead. Tests show that, unlike some synthetic dyes, beet juice is safe because it does not trigger liver cancer cell growth.

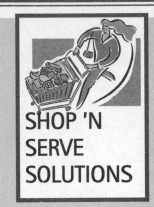

SHOP 'N SERVE SOLUTIONS

Fresh beets come in a range of sizes, from radish-size babies to 2$\frac{1}{2}$-inch-diameter giants. The babies are gourmet fare and may be expensive. The giants may be woody and tough. So shoot for the midsize beets, about 1$\frac{1}{2}$ inches in diameter. These young beets are perfect for most uses.

WHEN SELECTING BEETS:

■ Look for smooth, hard, round, deep red beets with thin taproots.

■ Any attached leaves should be small, fresh, and green.

WHEN STORING:

■ Before storing, trim any leaves to $\frac{1}{2}$ inch in length. If the leaves already have been clipped, be sure that there is at least $\frac{1}{2}$ inch of stem.

■ Leave about 2 inches of taproot, too, to prevent the beets from bleeding all over everything.

■ Store fresh beets in a plastic bag in the refrigerator, where they'll keep for up to three weeks.

WHEN YOU'RE READY TO USE:

■ Before cooking, scrub your beets well, but gently, trying not to break the skins. Leave the short stems and taproots on for color containment.

■ After cooking, peel, slice, and dice. Add vinegar or lemon juice to keep the crimson color.

easier for resistant cells to accept it. Other carbohydrates *rapidly* raise blood sugar, which aggravates the problem.

Beets were thought to be a rapid raiser. But it turns out that they're merely moderate. In fact, a full cup of cooked beets packs about the same amount of carbohydrates as a slice of whole wheat bread—and raises your blood sugar even more slowly. So eat your beets.

BEET A PATH TO THE BATHROOM

Beets are a good source of fiber, delivering about 3 grams in each cupful. Most Americans get only half the recommended 20 to 35 grams of fiber needed daily for good bowel function. And constipation makes you feel tired, cranky, and irritable. Who needs it? Have a glass of water, eat your beets, and get a move on!

Chilly Beet Soup

Okay, so in Russia, it's called borscht. But in the United States, this soup makes a great summer cooler. And you just have to smile when you see the shocking pink color! Then, when Old Man Winter turns your hometown into Siberia, heat up your soup for cozy comfort.

1 can (15 ounces) sliced beets, with juice
1 can (14¾ ounces) reduced-fat, reduced-sodium chicken broth
1 tablespoon dehydrated minced onion
1 tablespoon dried dillweed
1 teaspoon honey
2 tablespoons red wine vinegar
1 cup fat-free plain yogurt

In a blender, puree the beets and juice to a smooth consistency. Transfer to a medium bowl. Stir in the broth, onion, dillweed, honey, vinegar, and yogurt. Chill thoroughly, or heat gently until warm, but not boiling.

Yield: Four servings.

Nutritional data per serving: Calories, 88; protein, 7 g; carbohydrates, 14 g; fiber, 1 g; fat, 0 g; saturated fat, 0 g; cholesterol, 1 mg; sodium, 97 mg; folate, 8% of Daily Value; calcium, 14%; iron, 10%; potassium, 7%.

Bell Peppers:
Ring In Health Benefits

BATTLES:
- cancer
- colds
- heart disease

BOLSTERS:
- vision

In the summer, Karen fires up her blue Weber charcoal grill (okay, her husband does it) and cooks red bell peppers to perfection. She tosses them in salads, slips them into tortillas, and sometimes just eats them plain. Karen just can't get enough of them, because aside from their great taste, bell peppers have so much to offer. For one-third the calories of an orange, a red bell pepper packs twice as much vitamin C, a whopping 141 milligrams! A green one is on par with an orange, delivering about 66 milligrams of vitamin C. Amazing, no?

C NOTES

In your body, vitamin C acts as an antioxidant, gobbling up free radicals. These molecular troublemakers cause the cell damage that eventually leads to heart disease and cancer.

Based on promising research, the U.S. government recently raised the suggested daily intake of vitamin C from 60 milligrams to 75 milligrams for women and 90 milligrams for men. Smokers, the government suggested, should take in an additional 35 milligrams—for a total of 110 milligrams for women and 125

The Pepper Palette

Not sure which color bell pepper to buy? See why you should head for red. Nutritional values are based on 1 cup of chopped peppers.

Pepper	Vitamin C (mg)	Beta-carotene (units)	Lutein (mcg)
Red	191	2,379	6,800
Yellow	184	120	770
Green	89	198	700

milligrams for men who smoke. Nicotine apparently leads to both cell damage and depletion of vitamin C.

Vitamin C also may bolster your immune system, helping lessen the severity and duration of a cold. But, contrary to popular belief, there's not much evidence that even high amounts of vitamin C can stop sniffles altogether.

SIGHT SAVERS

Bell peppers, especially the red type, pack a powerful punch of lutein and zeaxanthin. These two key plant compounds may play a role in preventing age-related macular degeneration (ARMD).

Never heard of it before? The macula is a tiny spot in the center of your eye's retina that is responsible for sharp vision. It's what helps you read traffic signs and nutrition labels. ARMD, which is the most common cause of irreversible blindness in people over age 65, causes the macula to thin out and your vision to suffer.

OPEN YOUR EYES

Now here's where bell peppers come in: Lutein and zeaxanthin are common pigments found in the macula. Studies have shown that people who suffer from ARMD have fewer of these pigments than those who don't have the disease.

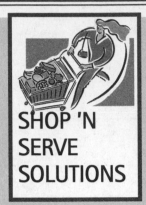

SHOP 'N SERVE SOLUTIONS

Summertime is pepper time. That's when you easily can find all colors of fresh bell peppers at a reasonable price.

WHEN SELECTING FRESH BELL PEPPERS:

■ Look for peppers that are firm and glossy, with unwrinkled skins.

■ Look for green stems.

■ Avoid peppers with soft or sunken areas.

■ Avoid those with cracks, slashes, or black spots.

WHEN STORING:

Store peppers in a plastic bag or container in the fridge. Green and yellow peppers generally last a week, while red peppers stay fresh for just three to four days.

WHEN YOU'RE READY TO USE:

■ Wash peppers just before eating or cooking them.

■ Scrub those that have a waxy coating.

Jarred and frozen peppers. If fresh bell peppers are too pricey for your pocketbook—in the winter, it takes Bill Gates's bank account to afford them—buy a jar of roasted red peppers for sandwiches and salads or frozen pepper strips for stir-fries. You'll save a bundle and still reap all the nutrition.

PETER PIPER'S PEPPERS

Here are ways to use peppers that even Peter Piper hadn't considered:

◆ **Brush up on bruschetta.** Instead of spreading Italian bread with the traditional tomato topping, cover it with roasted red bell peppers and fresh mozzarella cheese.

◆ **Pepper your dip.** In a blender, puree 1 cup of roasted red bell peppers, peeled and cut into strips. Add 1 cup of fat-free cheese and 2 cloves of garlic. Puree until smooth. Stir in 1 tablespoon of chopped fresh basil.

You can take supplements to boost your body's levels of lutein and zeaxanthin. However, most eye doctors recommend getting these compounds from foods because they may work synergistically with other nutrients not found in a pill.

So open your eyes to bell peppers, beets, kale, spinach, and other veggies that are rich in these compounds.

NUTRITION IN A NUTSHELL

Raw red bell pepper (1, approximately 3½ ounces)

Calories: 20

Fat: 0 g

Saturated fat: 0 g

Cholesterol: 0 mg

Sodium: 1 mg

Total carbohydrates: 5 g

Dietary fiber: 1 g

Protein: 1 g

Vitamin A: 8% of Daily Value

Vitamin C: 186%

Pasta Primavera Marinara

Cut the fat in your pasta sauce, while adding lots of fiber. Simply substitute veggies for ground beef.

3 cups prepared marinara sauce
Olive oil cooking spray
2 cloves garlic, minced
¾ cup broccoli florets
1 carrot, cut into 1½-inch-long matchsticks
1 red bell pepper, sliced into 1-inch pieces
1 pound large pasta shells or rotini
⅓ cup grated Parmesan cheese (garnish)

Fill a large pot with water for the pasta and place over high heat. Meanwhile, in a medium pot over medium-low heat, warm the marinara sauce, stirring occasionally. Coat a nonstick skillet with cooking spray, add the garlic, and sauté for 1 to 2 minutes. Add the broccoli, carrot, and pepper, and sauté until crisp-tender, tossing frequently.

When the water comes to a rapid boil, add the pasta. Cook according to package directions. Add the sautéed vegetables to the sauce, stirring well to combine. Reduce the heat to low. When the pasta has finished cooking, drain and transfer to a large bowl. Add the sauce to the pasta and stir until well mixed. Divide among six serving bowls. Garnish with the cheese.

Yield: Six servings.

Nutritional data per serving: Calories, 390; protein, 13 g; carbohydrates, 62 g; fiber, 6 g; fat, 7 g; saturated fat, 2 g; cholesterol, 3 mg; sodium, 743 mg; calcium, 10% of Daily Value; iron, 30%.

Blackberries:
Nutritious
Berried Treasure

BATTLES:
- allergies
- cancer
- heart disease
- high cholesterol

BOLSTERS:
- regularity
- weight control

For years, Karen would pick up raspberries and blueberries at the grocery store—and bypass blackberries. But at a restaurant in Virginia recently, she had an old-fashioned southern-style blackberry cobbler for dessert.

How did she like it? Let's just say you can always find these plump purple berries in Karen's shopping cart now. And the timing is perfect: New research suggests that blackberries contain just as many healthy compounds as—if not more than—their popular cousins do.

A TROVE OF NEW NUTRIENTS

Blackberries are brimming with two recently discovered compounds: catechin and epicatechin. Ounce for ounce, blackberries have about 50 percent more catechin and three times as much epicatechin as red raspberries do. Research has shown that these compounds can help do the following:

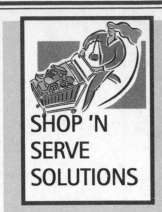

SHOP 'N SERVE SOLUTIONS

During some months, fresh blackberries are so pricey that you may have to stop by the ATM for extra cash. Preserve your investment by buying only the best.

WHEN SELECTING BLACKBERRIES:

■ Look for berries that are shiny and black, not dull or reddish.

■ Avoid berries that look a little wet, because moisture speeds decay.

■ Avoid those that appear to have been squeezed or flattened.

■ Avoid berries that are dripping juice—a telltale sign that they're past their peak.

WHEN STORING:

Once you find the cream of the crop, refrigerate your berries immediately. You'll have just two to three days to eat them before they start to spoil.

WHEN YOU'RE READY TO USE:

Just before eating them, place the berries in a shallow pan lined with paper towels and carefully wash them. Pat them dry with additional paper towels.

BERRY DELIGHTS

Now that you've found the best blackberries, see how they can add excitement to everyday dishes:

◆ **Perk up pancakes.** Instead of maple syrup, sprinkle your pancakes with fresh blackberries and top with a dollop of whipped cream.

◆ **Add pizzazz to pudding.** Stir blackberries into lemon or vanilla pudding that you make from an instant mix. Try the same with yogurt.

▶ **Prevent cancer.** Catechin and epicatechin neutralize free radicals, substances that damage cells' genetic material and provoke cancer-causing mutations in DNA. Although scientists aren't sure exactly how these two compounds work their magic, they speculate that they may inhibit an enzyme associated with the reproduction of free radicals.

▶ **Prevent heart disease.** What's more, a Japanese study has shown that catechins help lower cholesterol levels, especially levels of low-density lipoprotein (LDL) cholesterol—the bad kind. And reduced cholesterol levels lower your risk of heart disease.

The Berry Bowl

See how your favorite berries stack up in vitamins and minerals. Nutritional values for each are based on a 3½-ounce serving. (The equivalent in cups is listed next to each berry type.)

Berry	Calories	Fiber (g)	Folic Acid (mcg)	Vitamin C (mg)	Potassium (mg)
Blackberries (⅔ cup)	52	4	34	21	196
Blueberries (⅔ cup)	56	3	6	13	89
Raspberries (¾ cup)	49	4	26	25	152
Strawberries (⅔ cup)	30	2	18	57	166

HELP FOR ALLERGY SUFFERERS

In addition to catechins, blackberries also contain a compound called quercetin. In fact, they boast at least four times as much quercetin as raspberries do. (And raspberries pack plenty!) Like the catechins, quercetin also attacks the production of free radicals and helps prevent bad cholesterol from damaging blood vessels.

But quercetin also has a very surprising additional health benefit: It halts the production of histamine. That's the substance that makes allergy sufferers sneeze, wheeze, and generally feel miserable. Isn't it wonderful that blackberries ripen just as the hay fever season starts?

FILLING FIBER

While scientists are studying these newly discovered nutrients, we shouldn't forget about an old standby—fiber. Blackberries pack a whopping 7 grams of the good stuff in just a single cup—one-third of what you need for the entire day!

Fiber fills you up, so you feel satisfied on fewer calories. It also prevents constipation, helps reduce your risk of heart disease, and may lower your chance of developing colon cancer. Not too shabby, huh?

NUTRITION IN A NUTSHELL

Blackberries (1 cup)

Calories: 75

Fat: 1 g

Saturated fat: 0 g

Cholesterol: 0 mg

Sodium: 0 mg

Total carbohydrates: 18 g

Dietary fiber: 7 g

Protein: 1 g

Folate: 12% of Daily Value

Vitamin A: 5%

Vitamin C: 50%

Calcium: 5%

Blackberry-Peach Crisp

A few years ago, when Karen worked at a health magazine, representatives from the Oregon Raspberry and Blackberry Commission stopped by her office. They presented her with dozens of recipes—and a big bag of blackberries. That night, she made this dessert, and it's been a hit at family gatherings ever since.

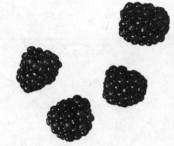

1 cup rolled oats
1 cup brown sugar
¾ cup flour
½ cup butter
4 cups fresh blackberries
2 cups sliced peaches

Preheat the oven to 350°F. In a large bowl, combine the oats, sugar, and ½ cup of the flour. Using a pastry blender or two knives, cut in the butter until the mixture is well blended and moist enough to form a ball. Place the blackberries in the bottom of an 8-inch-square baking dish. Toss with the remaining ¼ cup of flour. Add the peaches to the baking dish. Sprinkle the crumb mixture evenly over the fruit. Bake for 35 to 40 minutes, or until golden brown.

Yield: 12 servings.

Nutritional data per serving: Calories, 200; protein, 2 g; carbohydrates, 30 g; fiber, 3 g; fat, 8 g; saturated fat, 5 g; cholesterol, 20 mg; sodium, 83 mg; calcium, 3% of Daily Value; iron, 7%.

Blueberries:

They'll Keep You in the Pink

BATTLES:
- cancer
- heart disease
- urinary tract infections
- wrinkles

BOLSTERS:
- memory

You've heard it all your life: Crunch on carrots (for your eyes), finish your spinach (for your muscles), and pack a banana (for the potassium, of course). But we'll bet no one ever told you to eat a blueberry.

Well, sit down and hear this: If a blueberry comes within 10 feet of you—*eat it!* In a recent study at Tufts University in Boston, blueberries outranked more than 50 fruits and vegetables in amount of antioxidants—compounds that protect you against cancer, heart disease, and even wrinkles. Turns out, the health-promoting bounty comes from the very pigment that gives these berries such a cool color.

NUTRITION IN A NUTSHELL

Fresh blueberries (1 cup)

Calories: 81

Fat: 0 g

Saturated fat: 0 g

Cholesterol: 0 mg

Sodium: 9 mg

Total carbohydrates: 21 g

Dietary fiber: 4 g

Protein: 1 g

Vitamin C: 30% of Daily Value

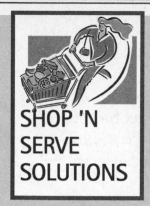

SHOP 'N SERVE SOLUTIONS

Ounce for ounce, wild blueberries pack double the antioxidants of their plumper cultivated cousins. So if you spot them at the supermarket, snatch them up. Wyman's, the largest wild-blueberry marketer, sells them fresh, frozen, and canned.

But if the only blueberries you can locate are the cultivated kind, don't pass them by. You've still found a blue-ribbon winner!

WHEN SELECTING FRESH BLUEBERRIES:

Look for berries that are dry, firm, and uniformly colored.

WHEN STORING:

■ Store your berries in the refrigerator. They'll last for at least a week—if you don't devour them immediately.

■ If you pick a boatload at a local farm, place them in a single layer on a baking sheet or tray and freeze them for a few hours. When you're sure they're frozen, transfer them to airtight containers and store them in the freezer until you need them. They'll keep for at least a year.

COLOR YOUR FOODS BLUE

You've bought the best. Now put your blueberries to the test in the kitchen. Try these tasty treats:

◆ **Make your salad chic.** Leave the iceberg lettuce at the supermarket because it offers very few nutrients. (Think of it as crunchy water!) Instead, buy dark greens, such as spinach or romaine lettuce. Then top your greens with fresh blueberries, feta cheese, and low-fat balsamic vinaigrette.

◆ **Give your desserts a blue hue.** Instead of topping your frozen yogurt with sprinkles, try blueberries. Or frost a cake and then coat it with blueberries. For a dessert that's supereasy, just fill a dish with blueberries and top them with a dollop of whipped cream.

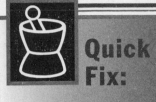

Quick Fix:

Urinary Tract Infections

Blueberries are bursting with tannins, compounds that boot out the bacteria responsible for urinary tract infections. Researchers at Rutgers University in Chatsworth, New Jersey, found that these tannins prevent the germs from attaching to the wall of your bladder, where they thrive. How many blueberries should you eat? Researchers aren't sure. But if you suffer from frequent urinary tract infections, you might want to think about tossing a handful in your mouth whenever you're in the kitchen!

Scientists call it anthocyanin. This pigment gobbles up free radicals, substances that cause cell damage in your body.

"If you'd eat just ½ cup of blueberries daily, you'd double the antioxidants you get for the entire day," says study leader Ronald Prior, Ph.D., who admits that he hardly ever ate blueberries— except in an occasional pancake—until he conducted this research. Now he has a half-pint-a-day habit.

THE BRAINIEST BERRY

Following up on Dr. Prior's work, other researchers at Tufts uncovered the first hint that blueberries may help reverse short-term memory loss. They divided older rats into four groups. One group received their usual diet, while the others got a supplement of blueberry, strawberry, or spinach extract. By far, the blueberry group outperformed all the others on memory tests.

Now scientists are working to isolate the memory-boosting compounds in blueberries and test them on humans. In the meantime, eat blueberries so that you'll remember . . . *to eat blueberries!*

Quick Fix:

Stomachache

Got a tummyache? Reach for a few tablespoons of dried blueberries. Recently, they've been reported to inhibit the ability of bacteria to stick to things in your body— which reduces the chance of a nasty infection in the lining of your stomach. Pass up fresh or frozen berries, though, because they may aggravate tummy troubles.

Blueberry Breeze

This drink is so invigorating that it'll seem like a breath of fresh air. Pair it with a whole wheat English muffin for a nutritionally balanced breakfast, or enjoy it as a midafternoon snack. It'll be love at first sip!

1 cup frozen blueberries
1 cup low-fat or skim milk
6 ounces low-fat lemon yogurt
1 teaspoon lemon extract
2 teaspoons honey or sugar (optional)

Pour the blueberries, milk, yogurt, lemon extract, and, if using, the honey or sugar into a blender. Cover and blend until smooth. If needed, add ice to reach the desired consistency.

Yield: Two servings.

Nutritional data per serving: Calories, 186; protein, 8 g; carbohydrates, 35 g; fiber, 2 g; fat, 2 g; saturated fat, 1 g; cholesterol, 10 mg; sodium, 117 mg; calcium, 29% of Daily Value.

Bok Choy:
One Secret to Good Health

BATTLES:
- cancer
- high blood pressure

BOLSTERS:
- bones
- wound healing

Colleen loves to stir-fry—it's such a great way to turn a little bit of meat or poultry into a big pile of food when she mixes in lots and lots of veggies. In fact, it's one of her secret weapons for changing the portions on her husband Ted's plate. And lately, she's started adding bok choy, a vegetable with a secret.

Think of bok choy as Chinese celery. It's about the same size as the hefty celery stalks that show up around Thanksgiving. But the ribs are stark white, and the flat, ruffled leaves are deep hunter green. Very striking. More likely, you'll remember it from Asian dishes you've eaten in restaurants. There, it appears as crosswise slices, in the style of romaine lettuce cut for Caesar salad. "Oh, that stuff," you're probably saying.

NUTRITION IN A NUTSHELL

Bok choy (1 cup)

Calories: 20

Fat: 0 g

Saturated fat: 0 g

Cholesterol: 0 mg

Sodium: 58 mg

Total carbohydrates: 3 g

Dietary fiber: 3 g

Protein: 3 g

Folate: 17% of Daily Value

Vitamin A: 87%

Vitamin C: 49%

Calcium: 16%

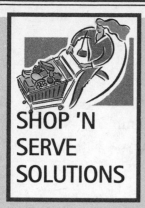

SHOP 'N SERVE SOLUTIONS

Although bok choy was once considered fairly exotic, today many supermarkets carry it in the produce aisle.

WHEN SELECTING BOK CHOY:

■ Look for stalks with sturdy, crisp white ribs with no cuts or bruises.

■ Look for leaves that are dark green. If they're turning pale green or yellow, they're getting old and losing their vitamins, so move on and look for a better bunch.

WHEN STORING:

Store bok choy in the vegetable crisper of your refrigerator, and use it within a few days. Cruciferous vegetables tend to fade fast and change flavor if kept too long.

WHEN YOU'RE READY TO USE:

Separate the ribs, wash them thoroughly, and pat dry.

EXOTIC ADVENTURES

Now you're ready for some exotic little adventures. Cut across the ribs and slip some slices of bok choy into everyday fare that's all in good taste. Try these serving suggestions:

◆ **Sensationalize salads.** Replace half the lettuce in your next salad with bok choy. The dark leaves create a lush backdrop for colorful veggies.

◆ **Add sizzle to stir-fries.** Bok choy adds bulk, fiber, vitamins, and minerals to stir-fries (see "Bok Choy and Rice Noodles" on page 75), but very few calories.

◆ **Simmer up soups.** Double the nutrition in canned soups. Stir in a cup or two of bok choy and simmer for 2 to 3 minutes.

CRUNCHY CRUCIFER

Bok choy is a very mild-mannered Asian member of the cabbage family known as crucifers. As a cruciferous vegetable, bok choy is related not just to cabbage, but also to broccoli, cauliflower, kale, kohlrabi, and the new baby in the family, broccolini.

Cruciferous vegetables have long been recognized as powerful cancer fighters. But that's not bok choy's big secret.

PRESSURE RELEASE VALVE

The word is out that eating plenty of fruits and vegetables (8 to 11 servings) each day, along with a couple of dairy foods, can lower blood pressure just as well as medication can. The reason? It's probably a combination of all the nutrients working together in ways we can't yet even imagine. But part of the answer is potassium, which in big doses, has been shown to lower blood pressure. And bok choy is packed with potassium—more, in fact, than your breakfast banana or glass of orange juice. But that's not bok choy's secret, either.

BONE BUILDER

Okay, it's time to let the cat out of the bag: Bok choy's secret is that it's loaded with calcium! Just 1 cup serves up as much of this bone builder as half a glass of milk, an unusually large quantity for a nondairy food.

And the especially cool part is that you can absorb bok choy's calcium, unlike the calcium in some other greens (like spinach), as easily as you can the calcium in milk. For that reason, bok choy is especially important for vegetarians who don't "do" dairy.

Along with the calcium, you also get some manganese and iron, which are needed for bones and blood.

Quick Fix:

Cuts, Hangnails, and Incisions

Bok choy is brimming with vitamin C. Just 1 cup provides half of what you need for the day. And although vitamin C won't cure your cold, it will help heal your wounds, from paper cuts and hangnails to surgical incisions.

Bok Choy and Rice Noodles

4 ounces thin rice noodles
1 tablespoon low-sodium soy sauce
2½ teaspoons fish sauce
2½ teaspoons sugar
1 tablespoon sesame seeds
1 tablespoon peanut oil
2 large cloves garlic, pressed or finely chopped
½ cup thinly sliced onion
½ cup baby carrots
2 cups thinly sliced bok choy
1 cup chopped sweet green, red, and yellow peppers, mixed
6 ounces cooked pork tenderloin, sliced and quartered

Cover the rice noodles with hot water, soak for 5 minutes, and drain. Set aside. In a small bowl, stir together the soy sauce, fish sauce, and sugar until the sugar dissolves. Set aside. In a wok over high heat, toast the sesame seeds until golden. Remove to a small bowl and set aside.

Heat the oil in the wok over high heat. Add the garlic, onion, and carrots, and cook for 3 minutes, stirring constantly. Add the bok choy, peppers, and pork, and cook for 3 minutes, stirring constantly. Add the noodles and sauce. Cook until the noodles are warm, stirring until the vegetables and noodles are well mixed. Divide between two large dinner plates. Sprinkle with the sesame seeds.

Yield: Two servings.

Nutritional data per serving: Calories, 543; protein, 33 g; carbohydrates, 68 g; fiber, 5 g; fat, 15 g; saturated fat, 3 g; cholesterol, 67 mg; sodium, 956 mg; folate, 26% of Daily Value; vitamin A, 225%; vitamin C, 167%; vitamin E, 12%; calcium, 14%; copper, 14%; iron, 22%; magnesium, 22%; manganese, 22%; zinc, 22%.

Broccoli:

It's Worth Stalking

BATTLES:
- cancer
- heart disease

BOLSTERS:
- bones
- vision

For years, our friend Ellen hated broccoli. It was understandable because broccoli, if overcooked or overly mature, can be hard to swallow—no matter how much cheese sauce you pour on it—and Ellen's mother always cooked broccoli until it was nothing but green slime with a few hard bumps.

Fortunately, when Ellen got married, her new sister-in-law introduced her to fresh broccoli. Now Ellen keeps a stash in the fridge at all times. She grates it over salads; serves it up freshly blanched, with dip; or just grabs it and crunches away when she's feeling tense.

It's a good thing she learned how great broccoli can taste, because broccoli is a real fighter against cancer and other major health problems.

NUTRITION IN A NUTSHELL

Broccoli (1 medium stalk)

Calories: 45

Fat: 0.5 g

Saturated fat: 0 g

Cholesterol: 0 mg

Sodium: 55 mg

Total carbohydrates: 8 g

Dietary fiber: 5 g

Protein: 5 g

Vitamin A: 15% of Daily Value

Vitamin C: 220%

Calcium: 6%

Iron: 6%

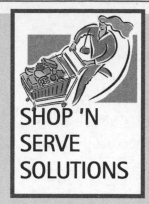

SHOP 'N SERVE SOLUTIONS

In the market for some fresh broccoli? Choose carefully!

WHEN SELECTING BROCCOLI:

■ Look for uniformly dark green or purplish blue-green florets. They're richer in vitamins A and C than paler florets.

■ Check out the color of the stalks and stems, too. They should be green and rich-looking.

■ Avoid broccoli with yellowing florets, because it's past its prime and won't taste good no matter how you prepare it.

■ No time to clean broccoli? Look for packaged washed florets, such as Mann's Broccoli Wokly (cute, huh?), in the produce section next to bagged salad mixes.

WHEN STORING:

■ Once you buy broccoli, baby it. Store it in a plastic bag in the crisper of your fridge to protect the veggie's vitamins. Ideally, you should use broccoli within a day or two. It'll keep for no longer than four to five days.

■ Don't wash broccoli before storing it, because that will speed up the growth of mold.

WHEN YOU'RE READY TO USE:

Right before you're ready to eat or cook your broccoli, wash it in cold water. Soak it for a few minutes if you're having trouble removing all the dirt.

POWER YOUR PASTA

Stir broccoli into your tomato sauce (see "Pasta Primavera Marinara" on page 62), or make a pasta topping with broccoli, garlic, olive oil, and a few tablespoons of the hot water you used to boil your pasta.

THE BROCCOLI BUNCH

Like the Brady Bunch, broccoli is comprised of at least six do-gooders: vitamin A, vitamin C, vitamin K, fiber, and the plant compounds lutein and sulforaphane. Scientists believe that many of these elements work *together* to provide broccoli's health benefits. Chief among the perks: preventing cancer. Specifically, here's what broccoli can do:

▶ **Prevent prostate problems.** A recent study at the Fred Hutchinson Cancer Research Center in Seattle found that eating three servings of vegetables daily can lower the risk of prostate cancer by an amazing 45 percent! "If some of those vegetables are the cruciferous kind like broccoli, men could drop their risk even further," says study coauthor Alan Kristal, Dr.P.H.

▶ **Waylay bladder cancer.** Another investigation of 50,000 men determined that those who ate a $1/2$-cup serving of broccoli just twice a week reduced their chance of developing bladder cancer—the fourth leading cancer—by half.

▶ **Confound colon cancer.** Research at the University of Utah Medical School in Salt Lake City suggests that broccoli also may cut the risk of colon cancer.

ADDITIONAL BENEFITS

Beyond the cancer front, studies have shown that broccoli may be just what the doctor ordered for these health problems:

▶ **Heart disease.** Researchers recently found that women who ate broccoli just once a week had half the risk of heart disease as those who didn't pile any on their plates.

▶ **Hip fractures.** The vitamin K in broccoli may help lower the chance of fracturing a hip when you get older, according to a study at Tufts University in Boston.

▶ **Cataracts.** In a Harvard University study of more than 36,000 men, scientists discovered that eating foods high in lutein—specifically, broccoli and spinach—may reduce the risk of developing cataracts.

BROCCOLI FOR LUNCH BUNCH

Now, you could load up on broccoli every day to ensure that you receive all its health benefits, but you probably don't have to. Researchers do say, however, that you should try to eat at least a ½-cup serving of cruciferous veggies daily. These include not only broccoli, but also bok choy, brussels sprouts, cabbage, cauliflower, and kale.

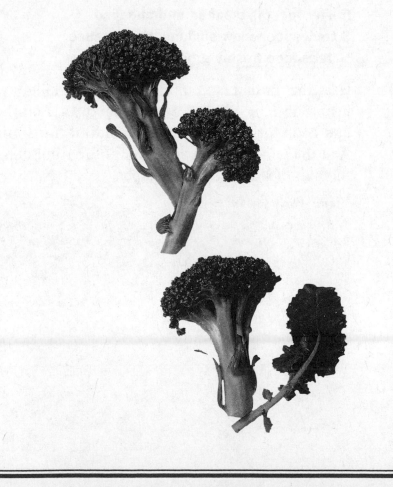

Simple Stir-Fried Broccoli

Sure, you can cook broccoli in gourmet recipes. But who has time for that every night? Instead, try this quick recipe, which will help you get your broccoli two or three times a week. The best part: One serving delivers almost all the vitamin C you need for the entire day!

1½ tablespoons canola oil
2 cloves garlic, minced
1 bag (1 pound) fresh broccoli florets or 1 bunch (1½ pounds) fresh broccoli, cleaned and chopped
3 tablespoons low-sodium stir-fry sauce
¼ teaspoon freshly ground black pepper

Heat the oil in a large nonstick wok or skillet over medium heat. Sauté the garlic for 1 to 2 minutes. Add the broccoli, and cook for 2 to 3 minutes, or until it turns bright green. Add the stir-fry sauce and stir-fry for 1 minute. Remove from the pan. Season with the pepper.

Yield: Four servings.

Nutritional data per serving: Calories, 85; protein, 5 g; carbohydrates, 7 g; fiber, 3 g; fat, 5 g; saturated fat, 0 g; cholesterol, 0 mg; calcium, 5% of Daily Value; iron, 7%.

Broccoli Sprouts:

The Ho, Ho, Ho, Health Giant

BATTLES:
■ cancer

BOLSTERS:
■ immune function

Mama always said: "An ounce of prevention is worth a pound of cure." And that's really the cancer-fighting strategy of Paul Talalay, M.D., the researcher at Johns Hopkins University in Baltimore who tapped into the chemoprotective power, first, of broccoli and then, of broccoli sprouts.

Why wait till you have a dread disease, such as breast cancer, he reasoned, to try to do something about it? Wouldn't it be better to fight cancer cells before they take hold? So Dr. Talalay went to work with test tubes and laboratory mice to figure out how to use real, live foods to turn on the body's natural defense mechanisms.

PREVENTION VERSUS CHEMOPROTECTION

Researchers have long known that people who eat the most cruciferous (cabbage family) vegetables have very low rates of certain cancers. But the "why" remained to be seen. So Dr. Talalay went hunting.

What he found was a natural chemical called sulforaphane

that hampered the growth of breast cancer cells in lab dishes. Digging further, he discovered that all cabbage family vegetables packed sulforaphane, but broccoli delivered the biggest dose. It was an interesting finding that started an amazing chain of events.

The goal of cancer *prevention* is to cut down on our exposure to carcinogens, cancer-causing agents such as cigarette smoke, air pollution, radiation, and alcohol, so that they can't attack our cells and make them sick. The hang-up here is that you need to know that a substance is a carcinogen in order to avoid it.

Dr. Talalay's strategy is to find foods that make the body's defenses stronger so that it can fight off carcinogens, both known and unknown. The cool thing about this approach, called *chemoprotection,* is that you don't have to know what you're fending off. It's like building a bigger fortress and a moat so that no matter which marauding invaders attack, you have everything covered.

So even though Dr. Talalay is working with breast cancer cells, the protection being stirred up by broccoli's sulforaphane should defend against other cancers, as well.

HO, HO, HO, LITTLE SPROUT

Cells produce a family of enzymes that neutralize carcinogens before they can attack your DNA and start cancer cells growing. When Dr. Talalay moved from test tubes to mice, he learned that sulforaphane was dynamite for increasing the activity of detoxification enzymes.

Among animals simultaneously infected with potent carcinogens and fed sulforaphane, he found the following:

NUTRITION IN A NUTSHELL

Broccoli sprouts (½ cup)

Calories: 5

Fat: 0 g

Saturated fat: 0 g

Cholesterol: 0 mg

Sodium: 1 mg

Total carbohydrates: 1 g

Dietary fiber: 0 g

Protein: 1 g

Vitamin C: 2% of Daily Value

Manganese: 2%

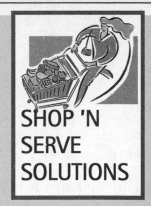

SHOP 'N SERVE SOLUTIONS

Broccoli sprouts are available in the produce section of your grocery store. Choose carefully!

WHEN SELECTING BROCCOLI SPROUTS:

■ Seek out perky-looking sprouts that are just bursting to get out of their container.

■ Pass up any that appear shriveled or weak.

Caution: Thoroughly wash any sprouts you buy, especially if you plan to eat them raw, since some sprouts are contaminated with *E. coli* bacteria. For safety and guaranteed sulforaphane levels, look for trademarked BroccoSprouts, which are grown from sterilized seeds, tested weekly for contamination, and then cleaned, packed, refrigerated, and subjected to surprise inspections.

FROM HO-HUM TO GUNG HO

When you're ready to add a spicy bite to ho-hum foods, try these top-notch ideas:

◆ **Make a statement.** Make a bold salad even bolder. Toss arugula, watercress, and spinach leaves with broccoli sprouts. Sweeten with light Catalina dressing.

◆ **Cause a stir.** Swirl a handful of broccoli sprouts into your favorite soup—from tomato to vegetable to classic chicken noodle.

◆ **Stack a sandwich.** On a hearty slice of seven-grain bread, stack romaine lettuce, turkey, sweet red and green pepper rings, a pile of broccoli sprouts, slivers of onion, and a slice of avocado. Attack with a knife and fork (because you'll never get your mouth around it!).

◆ **Wrap 'n roll.** Fill a tortilla with tuna salad, grated carrots, sliced celery, red leaf lettuce, and a handful of broccoli sprouts. Wrap the bottom of the tortilla over the middle, then roll up the rest. Or try our "Southwestern Sprout Wrap" on page 85.

► The number that developed tumors decreased by 60 percent.

► The number of tumors in each animal that developed tumors dropped by 80 percent.

► The size of the tumors was smaller by 75 percent.

► In addition, the tumors showed up later and grew more slowly.

Now tests are being done on women to see if sulforaphane stimulates human detoxification enzymes.

Dr. Talalay also learned that the amount of sulforaphane in some broccoli was 10 times higher than in others. In trying to grow his own standardized broccoli, he stumbled onto the fact that, ounce for ounce, three-day-old broccoli sprouts packed 20 to 50 times more sulforaphane than mature broccoli did. But the sprouts he bought varied as much as the broccoli did.

Consequently, he developed a standardized seed and a process for growing sprouts that, together, guarantee to deliver a high dose of sulforaphane. He calls his product BroccoSprouts. You can get them at your grocery store or grow your own. For a seed-sprouting kit, call Whole Alternatives at (800) 626-5357.

Southwestern Sprout Wrap

When Baltimore held its own version of the Race for the Cure for breast cancer, a local restaurateur wrapped and rolled 3,000 chemoprotective sandwiches similar to this version, which has been scaled down for at-home lunching.

2 tablespoons fat-free spicy bean dip
1 whole wheat tortilla
¹⁄₁₆ teaspoon cumin seeds
¹⁄₁₆ teaspoon ground coriander
4 slices jalapeño pepper
¼ cup sliced onion
¼ cup chopped ripe tomato
½ cup broccoli sprouts

Spread the bean dip down the middle third of the tortilla. Sprinkle with the cumin seeds and coriander. Top with the pepper, onion, tomato, and sprouts. Wrap the bottom third of the tortilla over the mixture, then roll sideways to complete the wrap.

Yield: One serving.

Nutritional data per serving: Calories, 135; protein, 7 g; carbohydrates, 31 g; fiber, 5 g; fat, 1 g; saturated fat, 0 g; cholesterol, 0 mg; sodium, 325 mg; vitamin C, 15% of Daily Value; iron, 10%; magnesium, 10%.

Brown Rice:

The Whole Grain for Health Gain

BATTLES:
- diabetes
- heart disease

Chances are, you love rice. Most of us eat about 25 pounds of it every year—unfortunately, it's mostly the white kind. It's too bad we choose white, though, because as our friend Ellen keeps telling us, brown rice overshadows its paler cousin in nearly every vitamin and mineral. (For a comparison of the two types, see "The Rice Bowl" on page 89.)

"Do you know that all rice actually starts out brown?" she'll ask, with an admonishing wag of her finger right under our noses. The grain is harvested in its hull, a hard, inedible covering that protects whole brown kernels. To make rice look shiny and white, manufacturers remove—

NUTRITION IN A NUTSHELL

Cooked brown rice (⅔ cup)

Calories: 170

Fat: 1.5 g

Saturated fat: 0 g

Cholesterol: 0 mg

Sodium: 10 mg

Total carbohydrates: 34 g

Dietary fiber: 2 g

Protein: 4 g

Vitamin B_3 (niacin): 8% of Daily Value

Copper: 4%

Iron: 2%

Magnesium: 15%

Zinc: 6%

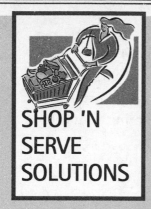

SHOP 'N SERVE SOLUTIONS

You'll find different types of brown rice at your local supermarket. Here are your choices:

■ **Instant brown rice.** For those days when you don't have a second to spare in the kitchen, try a package of instant brown rice. It'll be ready to eat in just 10 minutes—a far cry from the 30 to 45 minutes that traditional brown rice takes.

■ **Regular brown rice.** But if you're not racing to beat the clock, opt for regular brown rice, because it has a better flavor and consistency than the instant version. You also can speed the cooking process for regular rice by using a rice cooker or by soaking the rice in water for 2 to 3 hours beforehand.

If you choose regular rice, you'll need to decide on the length of grain you'd like:

■ **Medium grain** is considered the all-purpose length. (Instant rice, incidentally, almost always comes in a medium grain.)

■ **Short grain** works best in puddings and stuffings.

■ **Long grain** is ideal for pilafs, salads, and stir-fries.

AN INTERNATIONAL FLAVOR

You can use brown rice in virtually any dish that calls for its white cousin. It'll add a slightly nutty flavor and a heartier texture. Try these brown rice treats:

◆ **Send your palate to Peking.** Use whole grain brown rice in your favorite Chinese dishes, such as Moo Shu Chicken. Karen often asks Chinese restaurants to substitute this whole grain for the sticky white rice they usually deliver. Why not do the same?

◆ **Make a Thai score.** You'll think you're in Bangkok when you fix brown rice with a spicy seafood stir-fry.

◆ **Be an all-American.** What's as American as Mom's apple pie? How about chicken and brown rice soup?

Quick Fix:

Heart Attack Risk

A recent study found that eating two servings of whole grains daily can reduce the risk of dying from a heart attack by about 30 percent. "We're now trying to determine what exactly it is in the whole grains that seems to be protective—the fiber, the vitamins and minerals, the phytochemicals, or the entire package," says Lawrence Kushi, Sc.D., professor of human nutrition at Columbia University in New York City. In the meantime, feel free to chow down on brown rice and other whole grains!

or in techno terms, *refine*—the kernels' husk, bran, and germ. Yet, researchers have found that these are the parts that store a vast array of vitamins, minerals, and disease-fighting phytochemicals. Happily, these components, and the nutrients they contain, remain intact in brown rice.

DON'T FROWN ON BROWN

So what are all those nutrients going to do for you? Glad you asked. Here's what brown rice can do for you:

BROWN RICE MADE EASY

Nowadays, you can find rice in everything from breakfast bars to frozen dinner entrées. But isn't most of that rice of the—how shall we put it?—less colorful variety? Yes, but there are some delicious exceptions. These companies boast convenience foods with the brown stuff:

■ **Grainaissance** (www.grainaissance.com). Makes beverages and puddings with organic brown rice.

■ **Hain Kidz** (www.thehainfoodgroup.com). Sells those quintessential chocolate chip and marshmallow treats (hint: snap, crackle, and pop!) made with brown rice.

■ **Lundberg Family Farms** (www.lundberg.com). Markets brown rice cakes and instant side-dish mixes. (The roasted garlic pesto is tops!)

■ **Mon Cuisine** (www.moncuisine.com). Uses brown rice in its vegetarian frozen dinner entrées.

The Rice Bowl

Which is healthier—brown or white rice? We'll lay out the facts; you keep score. Nutritional values are based on ½ cup of cooked rice.

Rice	Fiber (g)	Vitamin E (mg)	Phosphorus (mg)
Brown	1.6	2	79
White	0.03	0	34

▶ **Prevent heart disease.** A recent study at Columbia University in New York City suggests that women who eat three daily servings of whole grains, such as brown rice, have a 27 percent lower risk of developing heart disease than those who eat only refined grains, such as white rice.

▶ **Cut the danger of diabetes.** While those researchers are working to isolate rice's magic, a group at Harvard University is examining why brown rice and other whole grains seem to protect you from type 2 diabetes. A study of more than 65,000 nurses revealed that those who ate large amounts of refined grains had twice the risk of developing diabetes as those who consumed mostly unrefined carbohydrates. "Your pancreas needs to quickly secrete a lot of insulin for your body to absorb refined carbohydrates," explains Walter Willett, M.D., chairperson of Harvard's nutrition department. "Over time, your pancreas may slow down insulin production, triggering diabetes."

So what's the bottom line? Ellen sums it up in two words: "Buy brown!"

Healthy Hot Pockets

Stuck in a sandwich rut? Whip up this veggie-packed, but filling, creation. Delicious for lunch, this dish delivers all the vitamin C and one-third of the fiber you need for the day.

1 tablespoon olive or canola oil
2 cloves garlic, minced
1 small red onion, chopped
2 red or green bell peppers, chopped
¼ pound baby carrots, sliced
½ cup sliced mushrooms
2 cups cooked instant brown rice
1 teaspoon Italian seasoning
Salt to taste
Ground black pepper to taste
4 whole wheat pita pockets

Heat the oil until hot in a large nonstick skillet or wok over medium-high heat. Add the garlic, onion, bell peppers, carrots, and mushrooms, and sauté for 4 to 6 minutes, or until tender, but not mushy. Reduce the heat to medium-low, and mix in the rice, Italian seasoning, salt, and black pepper. Sauté for 2 to 3 minutes, stirring frequently. Divide the rice mixture in fourths and stuff into the pita pockets.

Yield: Four servings.

Nutritional data per serving: Calories, 296; protein, 8 g; carbohydrates, 156 g; fiber, 8 g; fat, 6 g; saturated fat, 1 g; cholesterol, 0 mg; sodium, 252 mg; vitamin C, 100% of Daily Value.

Brussels Sprouts:

A Capital Idea

BATTLES:
- birth defects
- cancer
- heart disease
- stroke

BOLSTERS:
- bones
- immune function

Contrary to popular belief, brussels sprouts don't taste all that bad. Just season them with a little oil or butter and some bread crumbs, and they're good to go. Unfortunately, many of you probably don't share even a tiny bit of our enthusiasm. But if ever there was a maligned vegetable, it's brussels sprouts. And that's a shame, because brussels sprouts offer plenty of protection against big-time diseases—namely, cancer, osteoporosis, and heart trouble.

DNA PROTECTION

Consider brussels sprouts as security guards that help protect your DNA from cancer-causing villains. When researchers gave people 10½ ounces of cooked brussels

NUTRITION IN A NUTSHELL

Cooked brussels sprouts (½ cup)

Calories: 30

Fat: 0 g

Saturated fat: 0 g

Cholesterol: 0 mg

Sodium: 16 mg

Total carbohydrates: 7 g

Dietary fiber: 4 g

Protein: 2 q

Folate: 12% of Daily Value

Vitamin A: 11%

Vitamin C: 80%

Iron: 5%

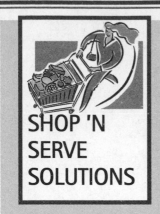

SHOP 'N SERVE SOLUTIONS

You'll find brussels sprouts in your super-market all year long, although they're most plentiful in November and December. If you've never bought brussels sprouts, don't worry—they're a cinch to select.

WHEN SELECTING BRUSSELS SPROUTS:

■ Examine their color and texture. Firm, bright green sprouts are the best.

■ Avoid those that look yellow, are wilted, or feel soft.

■ Choose sprouts that are sold loose rather than those packed in a tub, so that you can select same-size sprouts. They'll cook more evenly.

WHEN STORING:

Place brussels sprouts in a plastic bag in your refrigerator right away. They'll stay fresh for three to five days. At room temperature, they'll turn yellow fast.

WHEN YOU'RE READY TO USE:

■ Drop your sprouts in a pot of lukewarm water for about 10 minutes to make sure that there are no insects hidden in the leaves.

■ Trim the stem ends—but not quite flush with the bottoms, or the outer leaves will fall off during cooking.

■ Use a sharp knife to cut a shallow X in the base so that the core cooks as fast as the leaves.

COOKING LESSONS

You can steam, boil, or microwave your sprouts—each method will take about 6 to 10 minutes. Cook them until they're still slightly firm—like al dente pasta. You can test for doneness by poking the bases with the tip of a knife. The sprouts are ready when the bases are slightly tender.

sprouts daily for three weeks (really, this wasn't torture), they noted a 28 percent drop in DNA damage as measured by a compound excreted in the participants' urine.

Then they went a step further and examined the effect of the sprouts on cancer-fighting enzymes in the colon-rectal area. Their findings: The sprouts supersized levels of these enzymes, indicating that they may be able to prevent colon cancer.

Other studies suggest that brussels sprouts may stave off bladder and prostate cancers, too:

▶ Harvard University researchers studied nearly 48,000 men and found that those who consumed five servings of cruciferous veggies a week—namely, brussels sprouts, broccoli, cabbage, and cauliflower—were half as likely to develop bladder cancer as those who ate only one serving per week or less. It didn't matter how many other veggies the men consumed, overall.

▶ At the Fred Hutchinson Cancer Research Center in Seattle, researchers showed that men who consumed three or more servings of veggies daily—especially the cruciferous kind—could lower their risk of prostate cancer by nearly 50 percent.

A BONE-S FROM BRUSSELS

If you're feeling a little left out with all this talk about cancer in men, say no more.

Quick Fix:

Stroke Risk

If your doctor tells you that you're at high risk for a stroke (or if you have high blood pressure, which ups your odds), start incorporating cruciferous veggies—namely, brussels sprouts—into your diet. A recent study showed that eating at least five servings of fruits and veggies daily, especially citrus fruits and members of the cabbage family (we hate to nag you, but that means brussels sprouts), can lower your chance of stroke by about 30 percent.

Brussels sprouts may help protect women from osteoporosis—a bone disease that plagues more than three times as many women as men.

But brussels sprouts don't help in the way you might suspect. They don't supply calcium; instead, they offer vitamin K.

A Harvard University study suggests that women who consume at least 109 micrograms of vitamin K daily—that's less than the amount in a 3-ounce serving of brussels sprouts—can reduce their chance of a hip fracture by 30 percent.

A HEART HELPER, TOO

Brussels sprouts also supply other essential vitamins. Just ½ cup of cooked sprouts packs nearly all the vitamin C (great for your heart and immune system) that you need daily and about 12 percent of the daily requirement for folate (another heart helper that is also essential for reducing birth defects).

So eat up!

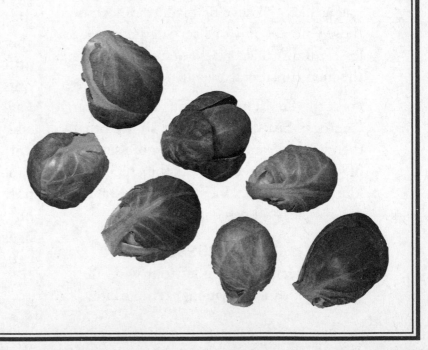

Baked Brussels Sprouts

Serve this delicious side dish with chicken, lean beef, or fish.

1 pound brussels sprouts
2 tablespoons olive oil
¼ cup bread crumbs
2 tablespoons grated Parmesan cheese
2 tablespoons pine nuts (pignoli), toasted

Preheat the oven to 350°F. Prepare the brussels sprouts for cooking as directed in "Shop 'n Serve Solutions" on page 92. In a large saucepan, boil the sprouts just until tender. Drain and toss with 1 tablespoon of the oil. Transfer to an oven-proof baking dish. In a small bowl, mix the bread crumbs, cheese, pine nuts, and the remaining 1 tablespoon of oil. Sprinkle over the sprouts. Bake for 5 to 7 minutes, or until the bread crumbs are light brown.

Yield: Four servings.

Nutritional data per serving: Calories, 156; protein, 6 g; carbohydrates, 15 g; fiber, 6 g; fat, 9 g; saturated fat, 2 g; cholesterol, 2 mg; sodium, 140 mg; calcium, 11%; iron, 12%.

Cabbage:
Power Kraut

BATTLES:
- cancer
- heart disease
- stroke

BOLSTERS:
- bones
- vision

Poor, poor cabbage. It's so misunderstood. Here's a vegetable that is chock-full of cancer fighters, heaping with heart menders, brimming with bone builders, and no one wants to cook it because they fear it'll smell—okay, really reek.

Well, here's a newsflash to all of you who can't stand the smell: *Cabbage offends your nose only because you're cooking it way too long!* So just take it out of the pot in a jiffy, and you'll get the good stuff without the bad aroma.

HEAD OF THE CLASS
Along with broccoli and kale, cabbage is a cruciferous vegetable. While broccoli has gotten all the glory, scientists have consistently found that cabbage is every bit as healthy as broccoli—if not more so!

NUTRITION IN A NUTSHELL

Red cabbage
(1 cup shredded)

Calories: 20

Fat: 0 g

Saturated fat: 0 g

Cholesterol: 0 mg

Sodium: 30 mg

Total carbohydrates: 8 g

Dietary fiber: 1 g

Protein: 4 g

Vitamin C: 70% of Daily Value

Calcium: 4%

Comparing Cabbages

All cabbages contribute plenty of vitamin C, but some varieties kick in more vitamin A and calcium than others do. See how 1-cup servings of different cabbages stack up against each other and against America's second favorite hot-dog topping, canned sauerkraut. The bottom line: They're all winners!

Cabbage	Calories	Folate (mcg)	Vitamin A (RE)	Vitamin C (mg)	Calcium (mg)
Bok choy	9	46	210	31	73
Green	18	30	9	22	32
Red	19	15	3	19	36
Savoy	19	56	70	21	24
Sauerkraut, canned	44	56	4	35	70

"Cabbage contains at least 11 of the 15 families of vegetable-related compounds found to prevent cancer," says Wendy Demark, Ph.D., R.D., researcher at the Duke University Comprehensive Cancer Center in Durham, North Carolina.

IT EARNS AN A FOR INDOLES

Foremost among those compounds are indoles, which scientists believe can destroy carcinogens before they trigger cancer or can stop the process in its tracks.

At Rockefeller University Hospital in New York City, researchers extracted a specific indole from cabbage and gave it to men and women for one to eight weeks. The compound lowered their levels of estrogen, a hormone thought to play a role in breast and prostate cancers.

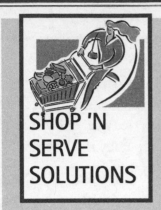

SHOP 'N SERVE SOLUTIONS

Sizing up fresh cabbage is a snap.

WHEN SELECTING CABBAGE:

■ Look for solid, well-trimmed heads. Each head should have no more than three or four outer leaves, which should be free of worm damage. (Worms can penetrate the interior.)

■ Look for crisp leaves and a dry stem.

■ Avoid heads with yellow leaves—a sign that the cabbage has been hanging around too long.

WHEN STORING:

■ Store cabbage in a plastic bag in the fridge so that it retains its vitamin C. Most kinds of cabbage will keep for about two weeks, but Savoy cabbage lasts just a week or so.

■ Wash your cabbage in cold water after you've chopped it.

■ Sprinkle the unused portion of the head with lemon juice to prevent browning, then cover with plastic wrap. Use the leftovers within a few days.

And scientists from the University of Illinois in Urbana found that indoles protected mice exposed to a carcinogen from developing breast and skin tumors.

Meanwhile, in a study of more than 47,000 men, researchers at Harvard University determined that those who ate just one ½-cup serving of cabbage or two ½-cup servings of broccoli once a week lowered their risk of bladder cancer by 44 percent, compared with those who ate less than one serving of either vegetable weekly.

5 WAYS TO CABBAGE HEAVEN

Here are some tips to help you get more delicious cabbage in your life:

◆ **Cook quick.** In general, most people cook cabbage way too long, which is the reason it gives off an unpleasant odor. Endless cooking also destroys the vitamin C in cabbage. So cook it quickly.

◆ **Wok it up.** In a large nonstick skillet or wok, heat 1 tablespoon of canola oil and $\frac{1}{4}$ cup of chopped scallions. Add 3 cups of shredded cabbage and 2 tablespoons of sesame seeds. Sauté over medium heat for about 8 to 10 minutes, or until the cabbage begins to wilt.

◆ **Thank frank.** Traditional hot dogs pack a wad of calories and fat, but they're oh-so-good with sauerkraut. Make this favorite healthier by using low-fat beef franks instead. Cook a few franks, slice into small pieces, and add to warmed kraut.

◆ **Pair it with pasta.** Slice cabbage into long, thin strips and stir the strips into your favorite pasta sauce. Serve with fettuccine.

◆ **Make cool slaw.** You don't have to make coleslaw with a creamy dressing. Instead, toss shredded cabbage with apple or pear wedges in a citrus vinaigrette, or make the "Five-Minute Asian Slaw" on page 100.

MORE GOOD GRADES

Cruciferous veggies, studies show, may also reduce your risk of heart disease, stroke, and cataracts.

And here's one more A+ for cabbage: Compared with other veggies in the crucifer family, some types of cabbage are high in calcium, boosting your bone density.

So, what do you say? Want to give cabbage another chance?

Five-Minute Asian Slaw

Karen's family loves creamy coleslaw, but last Fourth of July, Karen realized that she didn't have all the ingredients or the time to make it. So she whipped up this recipe and crossed her fingers that her guests would approve. The result: Let's just say there were no leftovers.

½ bag Mann's Broccoli Cole Slaw or 3 cups shredded cabbage and ¼ cup shredded carrots
2 tablespoons chopped peanuts
2 tablespoons sunflower seeds
½ cup low-fat sesame-ginger salad dressing

In a large bowl, combine the coleslaw, peanuts, and sunflower seeds, and toss with the dressing. Refrigerate for at least 1 hour to blend the flavors.

Yield: Six servings.

Nutritional data per serving: Calories, 72; protein, 2 g; carbohydrates, 6 g; fiber, 1 g; fat, 5 g; saturated fat, 1 g; cholesterol, 0 mg; sodium, 228 mg; calcium, 2% of Daily Value; iron, 4%.

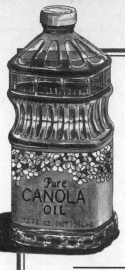

Canola Oil:

The Healthiest Fat

BATTLES:
- cancer
- heart disease
- high cholesterol
- rheumatoid arthritis
- stroke

BOLSTERS:
- immune function

Whenever we try to eat healthier, it often requires a sacrifice—ditching Danish pastries for granola, replacing Alfredo sauce with tomato sauce, or trading french fries for a baked potato. But switching your cooking oil from vegetable to canola isn't a hardship. In fact, it'll make your foods taste better!

THE CANOLA CONTRIBUTION

You probably think that olive oil is the only healthy fat. And why shouldn't you? It's the one that grabs all the headlines. While olive oil certainly qualifies as healthy, it contains twice as much saturated fat—and only half as much vitamin E—as canola oil.

What's more, canola oil is the only cooking oil rich in heart-healthy alpha-linolenic acids. These substances protect against heart disease by lowering levels of low-density lipoprotein (LDL) cholesterol (the bad kind) and triglycerides (another troublesome

NUTRITION IN A NUTSHELL

Canola oil (1 tablespoon)

Calories: 120

Fat: 14 g

Saturated fat: 1 g

Cholesterol: 0 mg

Sodium: 0 mg

Total carbohydrates: 0 g

Dietary fiber: 0 g

Protein: 0 g

Vitamin E: 31% of Daily Value

component of cholesterol), as well as by reducing the stickiness of blood cells.

And, yes, canola oil packs a lot of the healthy monounsaturated fat that has made olive oil famous.

A BIG IMPACT

Because canola oil battles heart disease from a variety of angles, it makes a big impact. Scientists studied 600 men and women in Lyons, France, who had recently suffered a heart attack. They put half of the participants on a Mediterranean-style diet that derived most of its fat from canola oil. The other half of the group followed an American diet.

Although both groups ate about the same amount of fat, those on the canola oil diet were 68 percent less likely to have a subsequent heart attack in the next four years than those on the American plan. The results were so dramatic that the researchers stopped the study early so that all the participants could enjoy canola oil's benefits!

NOT ALL OILS ARE CREATED EQUAL

After hearing about the promise of canola oil in the French study, researchers at the University of Maryland at Baltimore decided to take a closer look. They gave 10 men with normal cholesterol levels meals that contained 50 grams of fat. One day the men received bread and canola oil (not much of a meal); another day, bread and olive oil; and a third day, salmon (now we're talking!).

Before and after each meal, the researchers measured blood flow in the arteries. The canola oil and the salmon didn't cause any significant changes—which was good—but the olive oil actually decreased blood vessel function.

Do You Need an Oil Change?

Tablespoon for tablespoon, all oils have the exact same number of calories (120) and grams of fat (14). But they're far from nutritionally equal. Depending on the type of oil, the 14 grams of fat are split in different ways among saturated (bad), polyunsaturated (good), and monounsaturated (very good). Check out the percentage of each in your favorite oil.

Oil	Saturated Fat (%)	Polyunsaturated Fat (%)	Monounsaturated Fat (%)
Canola	7	32	61
Corn	13	58	29
Olive	15	10	75
Peanut	19	33	48
Safflower	10	76	14
Sunflower	12	72	16
Vegetable	14	64	22

What did the researchers make of this? "We were surprised," says Robert Vogel, M.D., chief of cardiology at the university. "We expected to see a benefit with *all* the oils." Dr. Vogel is now conducting the study with a large number of participants.

In the meantime, he suggests that you consider cooking with canola oil more often. Check with your doctor first if you're taking the blood thinner Coumadin (warfarin sodium), because canola oil contains quite a bit of vitamin K, which actually encourages blood clotting.

If you don't try canola oil for your ticker, do it for all its other health benefits. The alpha-linolenic acids in canola oil may help reduce the risk of stroke, protect against cancer, ease rheumatoid arthritis, and boost the immune system.

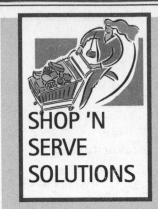

SHOP 'N SERVE SOLUTIONS

You'll spot several brands of canola oil at your supermarket. Consider buying the type that says "first press" or "expeller press" on the label, even though it's a little pricey.

Canola oil producers extract about 35 percent of the plant's oil by rolling or flaking the seeds. To get the remaining oil, some manufacturers soak the seeds in a chemical solvent. Traces of the solvent probably end up in your oil. No one knows for sure whether that will cause you any harm. But to be on the safe side, look for a bottle from the first press—before the solvent was added.

WHEN STORING:

Once you have your oil, store it in a cool, dark place or in your refrigerator. It should keep for up to one year.

CANOLA BASICS

Unlike olive oil, canola oil doesn't have a strong taste. So it's ideal for dishes that require fat without an overwhelming flavor. Try these two uses:

◆ **Whip up cookies.** You can substitute canola oil for the butter or margarine in your homemade cookie, cake, and brownie recipes and in boxed mixes. If the recipe requires less than $\frac{1}{4}$ cup of butter or margarine, use the same amount of canola oil. If it calls for $\frac{1}{4}$ cup or more, use about 20 percent less canola oil. For instance, substitute $3\frac{1}{2}$ tablespoons of canola oil for $\frac{1}{4}$ cup (4 tablespoons) of butter or margarine, or 7 tablespoons of oil for $\frac{1}{2}$ cup of shortening. And if the recipe calls for vegetable oil? Make it with the same amount of canola oil.

◆ **Create a stir.** Heat 2 tablespoons of canola oil in a nonstick wok or skillet, add onions and garlic (as much as you like!), and stir-fry your favorite veggies along with chicken, pork, or lean beef.

Berry-Good Muffins

Canola oil replaces the margarine without a hitch in this weekend breakfast favorite.

Canola oil cooking spray
1¾ cups oats
2 tablespoons brown sugar
1 cup all-purpose flour
½ cup sugar
1 tablespoon baking powder
1 cup skim or 1% milk
1 egg, lightly beaten
3 tablespoons canola oil
1 teaspoon vanilla extract
¾ cup fresh or frozen (unthawed) raspberries

Preheat the oven to 400°F. Coat 12 medium muffin-pan cups with cooking spray. In a small bowl, combine ¼ cup of the oats and the brown sugar. Set aside. In a large bowl, combine the remaining 1½ cups of oats with the flour, sugar, and baking powder until well mixed. In a small bowl, mix the milk, egg, oil, and vanilla extract. Add to the dry ingredients in the large bowl. Stir until moistened, but don't overmix. Lightly stir in the raspberries.

Divide the batter equally among the muffin cups. Sprinkle with the oats–brown sugar mixture. Bake for 20 to 25 minutes, or until golden brown. Cool in the muffin pan for 5 minutes. Remove and serve warm.

Yield: 12 muffins.

Nutritional data per serving: Calories, 171; protein, 4 g; carbohydrates, 28 g; fiber, 2 g; fat, 5 g; saturated fat, 1 g; cholesterol, 18 mg; sodium, 18 mg; calcium, 9% of Daily Value; iron, 8%.

Basil Balsamic Vinaigrette

Karen's basil plants thrived last year, so she had plenty of the herb left even after she had made lots of Colleen's "Family-Party Pesto" (see page 299). So instead of buying bottled dressing for a summer picnic, she tossed everyone's greens with this fresh-from-the-garden concoction. A healthy bonus: It has about 75 percent less sodium than most bottled dressings.

⅔ cup canola oil
⅓ cup balsamic vinegar
2 cloves garlic
¼ cup chopped fresh basil
¼ teaspoon salt

In a food processor, combine the oil, vinegar, garlic, basil, and salt until well blended.

Yield: 10 servings.

Nutritional data per serving: Calories, 135; protein, 0 g; carbohydrates, 2 g; fiber, 0 g; fat, 14 g; saturated fat, 1 g; cholesterol, 0 mg; sodium, 55 mg; iron, 1% of Daily Value.

Cantaloupe:
You Can't Get Enough!

BATTLES:

■ cancer

BOLSTERS:

■ bones
■ immune function
■ skin
■ vision

When a friend of ours visits family in California, the first thing she does after checking into her hotel is head for a restaurant and order a big bowl of fresh cantaloupe. Why? Because she knows that while California's hot, dry summers may be hard on the grass, they are just what the doctor ordered for growing the sweetest, juiciest cantaloupes—which is why 95 percent of the nation's cantaloupes come from California farms. The heat concentrates the naturally occurring sugars in the fruit, creating a sweetness that is signaled by that heady, musky aroma.

But cantaloupe is a lot more than just good eating. It's also one of the best natural sources of beta-carotene. Beta-carotene's

(Continued on page 110)

NUTRITION IN A NUTSHELL

Cantaloupe (¼, or about 1 cup cubed)

Calories: 48

Fat: 0 g

Saturated fat: 0 g

Cholesterol: 0 mg

Sodium: 12 mg

Total carbohydrates: 12 g

Dietary fiber: 1 g

Protein: 1 g

Vitamin A: 90% of Daily Value

Vitamin C: 65%

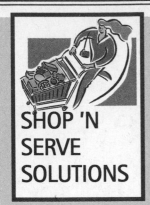

SHOP 'N SERVE SOLUTIONS

Cantaloupe connoisseurs know just how to find the sweetest, juiciest melons—and how to treat them with care. You can easily do the same. Here's how.

WHEN SELECTING CANTALOUPE:

■ Look for an evenly shaped melon, without dents, bruises, cuts, or discoloration.

■ Check out the color of the skin under the netting—it should be glowing golden.

■ Look for a melon that's smooth and well rounded at the stem end. Unlike other ripe melons, which have a bit of vine attached, mature cantaloupes dehisce, smoothly slipping free of the stem attachment.

■ Choose a melon that's heavy for its size—the sign of juiciness.

■ Make sure your melon is intoxicatingly fragrant.

WHEN STORING:

■ Refrigerate a ripe melon until you're ready to use it.

■ Leave a too-firm melon on your kitchen counter for a few days, until it begins to soften and its greenish color turns golden.

WATCH OUT FOR SALMONELLA

Before slicing your cantaloupe, wash your hands and then wash the outside of the melon with soap and hot running water. Cantaloupe can carry salmonella bacteria, and you'll drag those germs through the melon with the very first cut. Cut the melon in half and scrape out the seeds. Then clean up thoroughly. Wash your hands, cutting board, and utensils so that you don't transfer the germs to other fruits and vegetables.

Several salmonella outbreaks caused by cantaloupe triggered fever, cramps, and diarrhea in more than 400 people. Children, older folks, and people with compromised immune systems due to chemotherapy or AIDS are especially at risk.

CANTALOUPE CREATIONS

Once your cantaloupe has cleaned up its act, turn it into some luscious treats. Here's how:

◆ **Bowl it over.** Half a cantaloupe makes a great edible bowl. Load it up with blueberries, raspberries, and a little vanilla yogurt for a berry-nice breakfast. Or fill it with high-calcium cottage cheese and serve it with a piece of thinly sliced and rolled lean ham for lunch. For special events, carve a cantaloupe basket and fill it with honeydew and watermelon balls drizzled with honey and dusted lightly with cinnamon.

◆ **Cube some refreshment.** Nothing beats an ice-cold wedge of cantaloupe for instant refreshment after a long, hot run or your daily workout. So in your downtime, cut your cantaloupe into wedges, carve off the rind, and store the naked pieces in an airtight container in the fridge. They'll be ready when you are.

◆ **Turn over a new leaf.** Toss red leaf lettuce, thinly sliced red onion, fresh cilantro, sliced water chestnuts, and cantaloupe chunks with light Catalina dressing for a distinctive and summery side salad.

◆ **Skewer melon kebabs.** Use a large-size melon baller to make cantaloupe, honeydew, and watermelon balls. Thread the balls on bamboo skewers.

◆ **Don't chicken out.** Jazz up your pasta salad. Mix cooked chicken chunks, cantaloupe balls, low-fat mayo, and a few chopped cashews with your favorite cooked pasta shape for light luncheon fare.

◆ **Go slushy in the summer.** Freeze cantaloupe chunks, then whirl a cupful in your blender with $1/2$ cup of skim milk and $1/4$ teaspoon of mint flavoring for an instant slushy cooler. Or freeze cantaloupe balls to use as never-melt ice cubes for your drinks.

(Continued from page 107)

main job is to act as the raw material for creating vitamin A. Liver, fish liver oils, eggs, fortified milk, butter, and margarine deliver fully active, preformed vitamin A, which is stored in your liver. That sounds good, but too much straight vitamin A at one time can be toxic. Fortunately, however, vitamin A can also be created from carotenoids—mostly beta-carotene, which is *never* toxic, because your body can't store it the way it can straight vitamin A.

THE REAL SKINNY

One of vitamin A's top jobs is to take care of your body's surfaces, inside and out, which are lined with epithelial cells that protect your body against germ warfare.

Outside, vitamin A makes epithelial cells tough, to create skin. Inside, it makes them tender, to create the mucous membranes that line the nose, mouth, lungs, stomach, intestines, bladder, urethra, uterus, and vagina, forming a barrier against invading germs. Vitamin A also creates the mucus itself. This sticky fluid is essential. It prevents your stomach lining from being digested along with your food. And in your lungs, mucus traps debris and hauls it out of your airways before it can hurt your body.

Vitamin A is also vital for maintaining vision, building bones, and building healthy babies. Plus, researchers suspect that it beefs up sensors that notice cancer cells and warn your immune system to take action.

Chill-a-Melon Soup

Dining alfresco? Indulge in this refreshing cold soup to beat the summer heat.

1 medium ripe cantaloupe, peeled and cut into cubes (about 4 cups)
⅓ cup calcium-fortified orange juice
¼ cup fat-free plain yogurt
2 tablespoons honey
Juice of 1 lime
1 teaspoon grated lime peel
6 fresh strawberries (garnish)
6 mint leaves (garnish)

In a food processor, combine the cantaloupe, orange juice, yogurt, honey, lime juice, and lime peel until smooth. Cover and chill for about 2 hours or overnight. To serve, divide among six chilled bowls. Garnish each with 1 strawberry and 1 mint leaf.

Yield: Six servings.

Nutritional data per serving: Calories, 77; protein, 2 g; carbohydrates, 18 g; fiber, 1 g; fat, 0.5 g; saturated fat, 0 g; cholesterol, 1 mg; sodium, 10 mg; vitamin A, 69% of Daily Value; vitamin C, 66%; calcium, 6%.

Carrots:
Bet on Beta-carotene

BATTLES:
- cancer

BOLSTERS:
- bones
- immune function
- vision

Colleen practically grew up on horseback, and she loved the chomping, crunching sound of her favorite mount sharing her handful of carrots. But now she keeps those carrots all to herself. "Let 'em eat grass!" she says. Why the change in attitude? Carrots are loaded with beta-carotene, making them one of the leading vegetable contenders for the title of cancer-fighting champ.

Just one 7-incher packs four days' worth of beta-carotene. And when Colleen's too pooped to peel, she snags a bag of babies. A generous handful of these golden nuggets nets her three days' worth of beta-carotene.

Researchers have long known that people who eat the most beta-carotene–rich fruits and vegetables have the lowest risk of lung cancer. Now the research goes on, trying to pin down exactly why. Is it the beta? One of its relatives? Or is it the interplay of

NUTRITION IN A NUTSHELL

Raw baby carrots (10)

Calories: 38

Fat: Less than 1 g

Saturated fat: 0 g

Cholesterol: 0 mg

Sodium: 35 mg

Total carbohydrates: 8 g

Dietary fiber: 2 g

Protein: 1 g

Vitamin A: 300% of Daily Value

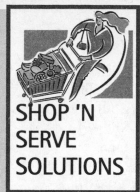

SHOP 'N SERVE SOLUTIONS

Most of the carrots we buy come to us packaged in plastic bags with tricky, fine orange lines that make the carrots look better and with black borders that hide the freshness clues the carrot tops can give us. Try to wiggle the bag around to get a better look inside.

WHEN SELECTING CARROTS:

■ Look for carrots that are bright orange, with no little root hairs growing out of them.

■ Choose those that have narrow shoulders, which signals a thinner core and sweeter carrot. If the shoulders are a little green, that's okay, although the green part is bitter and you might want to trim that off before eating.

WHEN STORING:

■ Keep carrots fresh by twisting off the tops. Otherwise, they'll just keep growing and sucking up their own sugars.

■ Keep them in the refrigerator so that they'll stay fresh and tasty till you put them in the pot.

■ Keep carrots away from apples in the fridge. Apples produce ethylene gas, which helps other fruits ripen but prompts carrots to produce isocoumarin, a bitter-tasting chemical that keeps bugs from biting carrots in the field and may stop you from biting them, too.

COLORFUL CARROT CONCOCTIONS

Here are some easy ways to add carrots to your diet:

◆ **Make liquid gold.** Puree cooked carrots and onions to use as a thickener for soups and sauces. It makes great fat-free "gravy" for Yankee pot roast, grilled pork tenderloin, or baked chicken, too.

◆ **Sliver for slaw.** To create the most colorful slaw, shred both green and red cabbage, then toss in long slivers of carrot.

KEEP 'EM CRISP!

Almost everyone thinks that vegetables are best eaten raw. But occasionally, everyone can be wrong. It turns out that the same plant materials that give carrots and other veggies their crispy, crunchy texture also imprison their sugars and carotenes. Light cooking, just to the crisp-tender stage, actually releases the beta-carotene in carrots, so you can absorb more of it. But don't overcook carrots. If you cook them too long—say, 20 minutes—all their food value ends up in the cooking water, and the carrots end up tasting terrible.

the entire nutrient mix in a beta-rich whole food that gets to wear the winner's crown?

THE SMOKING GUN

One recent study of nonsmokers gave the nod to vegetables—tomatoes, lettuce, and carrots—and suggested that eating more of these and other vegetables might lower lung cancer risk by 25 percent for nonsmokers. And an Italian study found that among people who never smoked, eating more fruits and carrots, along with reducing alcohol and saturated fat intake, might cut the risk of cancers of the mouth and pharynx.

And 16 years into the Nurses' Health Study, researchers have learned that eating more vegetables, especially carrots, might significantly lower lung cancer risk, even in women who smoke. Don't get us wrong: Eating better is no substitute for quitting smoking. But eating more carrots while you're quitting looks like a plus.

BETA FOR BONES

Carrots are tops among vegetables for delivering beta-carotene. And beta-carotene, more than any of its 500-plus carotenoid cousins, stands ready to convert to vitamin A as the need arises. So carrots should get called on a lot.

Bone building is a case in point. When children's bones are trying to grow, remodeling is in order. Just as you would tear down a part of your house to attach an addition, vitamin A tears down the finished ends of bones so that additional bone can be added. Remodeling goes on all the time in adults, too—not to make bones longer, but to make them stronger. Calcium, you see, is constantly being subtracted from and added to existing structures.

FANTASTIC FOODS OR BITTER PILLS?

Beta-carotene is a powerful antioxidant that may help deter cancer. So should you boost your protection by taking a hefty supplement? Not a good idea. A Finnish study found that lung cancer actually *increased* among 29,000 smokers taking high-dose beta-carotene supplements. And in a study of 22,000 American male doctors, researchers found that scarfing down 50-milligram supplements every other day had absolutely no effect, good or bad, on the men's risk of cancer, heart disease, or death for any reason.

So focus on plant foods instead of pills. Orange, yellow, and red fruits and vegetables, such as carrots, butternut squash, cantaloupe, and apricots, are packed with beta-carotene, so it's easy to get all you need from them. And they're also loaded with fiber, fluid, an array of carotenoids, and other newly discovered (and possibly *undiscovered*) elements that work together for better health.

HAVE YOU GONE JAUNDICED?

Probably not. It's true, you can take on an orange hue when you eat lots of carrots, because the same pigments that color the carrots can settle in your skin. But not to worry. The condition, called carotenemia, is harmless, and the color will start to fade the minute you cut back on carrots. However, if the whites of your eyes turn yellow, you could be jaundiced, and you need to check in with your doctor.

Sugar Baby Carrots

Glazed carrots as a side dish add glamour to simple broiled or grilled fish. But—gasp!—what about the butter? Some dishes just demand the taste of real butter. The secret is to add the tiniest bit right at the end of cooking, so that it's the first thing that touches your tongue. Here's how to make decadent carrots in 10 minutes or less.

1 cup baby carrots, cut lengthwise
1 tablespoon brownulated sugar (light brown sugar that pours)
1 teaspoon butter

Put the carrots in a small saucepan with just enough water to cover. Bring the water to a boil. Cover and simmer the carrots until crisp-tender, about 5 minutes. Drain the water and return the saucepan containing the carrots to the stove. While cooking over medium heat, sprinkle the sugar over the carrots and stir until dissolved. Add the butter and stir until melted and mixed. Serve immediately.

Yield: Two servings.

Nutritional data per serving: Calories, 59; protein, 1 g; carbohydrates, 10 g; fiber, 2 g; fat, 2 g; saturated fat, 1 g; cholesterol, 5 mg; sodium, 47 mg; vitamin A, 300% of Daily Value.

Cauliflower:

Anticancer Flower Power

BATTLES:
- birth defects
- cancer
- heart disease
- stroke

BOLSTERS:
- immune function

Have you ever noticed that whenever there's a vegetable tray at parties, cauliflower is, well, a wallflower? Guests gobble up the broccoli, snatch the red bell peppers, and leave the cauliflower behind. For this book, we asked a friend why she eats broccoli but not cauliflower. Her reason: Broccoli is supposed to be really good for you—while cauliflower is nothing special.

Well, our friend is half right. Broccoli is an incredible disease fighter, but cauliflower is every bit as good. Both are members of the family of cruciferous vegetables, a clan of anticancer crusaders that share a lot of the same traits.

THE BUNCH WITH THE BIGGEST PUNCH

You know that most vegetables contain cancer-fighting compounds with hard-to-pronounce names. But study after study suggests that the compounds in cruciferous veggies pack the heaviest punch. Let's look at some of the scientific studies:

▶ In studying prostate cancer, researchers at the Fred

Hutchinson Cancer Research Center in Seattle found that men who ate three or more servings of vegetables daily—especially the cruciferous kind—had about half the risk of developing prostate cancer as those who didn't "do" veggies.

▶ In researching bladder cancer, scientists at Harvard University couldn't link overall vegetable consumption with a lower chance of bladder cancer, but they did connect cruciferous veggies with it.

▶ The study's authors discovered that nonsmoking men who consumed five or more servings of cruciferous veggies per week had a 51 percent reduction in their risk of bladder cancer, compared with men who ate just one serving per week.

▶ New findings on breast cancer prevention show that cruciferous veggies aren't just good for guys. Researchers at the University of Buffalo think that cauliflower, broccoli, and the rest of the family may be able to lower a woman's risk of breast cancer, especially before she reaches menopause.

Exactly how these vegetables work their magic in preventing breast cancer is a little complicated, but we'll try to explain: Your body can break down the hormone estrogen in a number of ways. If your body produces estrogen by-products with little biological activity, the researchers found, your risk of breast cancer may drop by 40 percent. Cruciferous veggies make your estrogen by-products less active.

STROKE STOPPERS

The latest stroke research shows that cruciferous vegetables also lower your risk of having a stroke. In a study of more than

NUTRITION IN A NUTSHELL

Cooked cauliflower
(½ cup)

Calories: 14

Fat: 0 g

Saturated fat: 0 g

Cholesterol: 0 mg

Sodium: 9 mg

Total carbohydrates: 3 g

Dietary fiber: 1 g

Protein: 1 g

Folate: 7% of Daily Value

Vitamin C: 46%

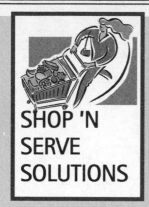

SHOP 'N SERVE SOLUTIONS

You can find cauliflower year-round, although its availability usually peaks in the spring and fall.

WHEN SELECTING CAULIFLOWER:

■ Choose heads that are firm, heavy, and white or creamy white.

■ Look for leaves that are fresh and green.

■ Avoid heads with brown spots.

WHEN STORING:

Once you bring your cauliflower home, store it in a plastic bag in the crisper of your fridge, where it'll keep for up to a week. Wash it when you're ready to use it.

CAULIFLOWER CREATIONS

Cauliflower tastes great both raw and cooked. To get more folate, we prefer to eat it raw at least sometimes. If you're cooking cauliflower, squeeze a little lemon juice into the water so that the cauliflower retains its white color.

Ready for some serving ideas? Here you go:

◆ **Dunk it.** Cauliflower's mild flavor is perfectly matched with hummus, that wonderful chickpea spread.

◆ **Mash it.** Mix chopped cauliflower florets into your family's mashed potatoes. They're the perfect camouflage—kids, big or small, won't know the cauliflower is there.

◆ **Bread it.** Toss cooked cauliflower in a little olive oil, sprinkle some bread crumbs on top, and bake until the crumbs are light brown.

◆ **Soup it.** Stir cooked cauliflower pieces into canned tomato soup for the ultimate prostate-cancer–fighting duo.

◆ **Top it.** Skip the pepperoni, and put cauliflower and broccoli florets on top of your pizza.

Quick Fix:

Colds

Plagued by a parade of colds? Maybe you're not getting enough vitamin C. But don't run out for a supplement; just eat more foods that are rich in the nutrient. Cauliflower, unexpectedly, is loaded with vitamin C.

75,000 women, researchers found that those who ate the most produce, especially cruciferous veggies, had a 30 percent lower chance of suffering a stroke than those who consumed the least amount of produce.

CAULIFLOWER CONTRIBUTIONS

In addition to being part of a family rich in cancer- and stroke-fighting compounds, cauliflower also offers big helpings of vitamin C and folate. Vitamin C helps protect your heart by gobbling up free radicals, compounds that play a role in the development of heart disease. Folate may also safeguard your heart by lowering your level of the amino acid homocysteine, which increases your risk of ticker trouble.

Plus, a diet rich in folate (and its synthetic version, folic acid) keeps unborn babies from developing neural tube birth defects, such as spina bifida.

But don't wait until you're pregnant to make sure that you get enough folate. These birth defects can occur early in a pregnancy—often before a woman knows that she's in the pink (or blue). Researchers, therefore, suggest that all women capable of having children, no matter if they're trying to or not, eat a diet rich in this B vitamin. Since cauliflower can lose a lot of its folate when it's boiled, eat it raw sometimes, too.

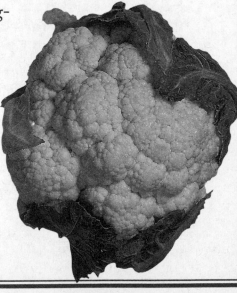

Broccoli-Cauliflower Wreath

The creative nutritionists at the University of Michigan's Comprehensive Cancer Center in Ann Arbor passed along this recipe just in time for a big party at Karen's house. It teams up two potent cancer fighters in a festive presentation. Plus, it's a cinch to make.

½ cup low-fat, low-sodium chicken broth
1 tablespoon chopped fresh parsley
1 tablespoon sliced green onion
1 teaspoon dried basil
½ teaspoon dried oregano
¼ teaspoon drled thyme
2 cups cauliflower florets
2 cups broccoli florets
¼ cup sliced red bell pepper strips

In a large microwaveable container, combine the broth, parsley, onion, basil, oregano, and thyme. Add the cauliflower and broccoli and cover with a lid or plastic wrap. Microwave on high until the vegetables are tender, about 5 minutes. On a large platter, arrange the cooked cauliflower and broccoli in a wreath shape. Use the pepper strips for a bow. Drizzle with any remaining hot herb broth.

Yield: Four servings.

Nutritional data per serving: Calories, 33; protein, 3 g; carbohydrates, 6 g; fiber, 3 g; fat, 1 g; saturated fat, 0 g; cholesterol, 1 mg; sodium, 42 mg; calcium, 4% of Daily Value; iron, 5%.

All-Occasion Vegetable Platter

Karen likes to make the veggie platters at her parties the center of attention—so that guests flock to them and not the potato chips that her husband puts out. How does she do it? By spelling short words with the produce. For instance, at Christmastime, she arranges the veggies so that they spell "Noel." For cookouts, she writes "Spring," "Summer," "Picnic," or even "Hot." On birthdays, she spells the guest of honor's first name. With a little imagination, the possibilities are endless. Here is a recipe that provides enough veggies to spell a five-letter word. You can add other veggies, such as radishes or grape tomatoes, if you need to spell something longer.

2 cups cauliflower florets
2 cups broccoli florets
10–15 sliced carrot sticks
10–15 sliced red bell pepper strips
10–15 sliced celery strips
Assorted low-fat dips

On a large colored platter, use each vegetable to create one letter of the word you'd like to spell. Around the edge of the platter, place dollops of several kinds of low-fat dips.

Yield: Eight servings.

Nutritional data per serving: Calories, 26; protein, 2 g; carbohydrates, 6 g; fiber, 2 g; fat, 0 g; saturated fat, 0 g; cholesterol, 0 mg; sodium, 29 mg; calcium, 3% of Daily Value; iron, 4%.

 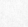

Celery:
Stalking the Diet Claims

BATTLES:
- high blood pressure

BOLSTERS:
- hydration
- weight control

Colleen loves to use thick chunks of celery as a bulking agent for her tuna salad. The recommended serving of tuna, about 3 ounces, just isn't enough to fill up her pita pocket. So she packs the mix with celery and stuffs in a folded large red lettuce leaf and a tomato slice, and—voilà!—she's gotten in three of her vegetable servings for the day. Besides feeling fuller, she loves that crispy celery crunch.

NEGATIVE CALORIES

As Colleen munches away, she contemplates celery rumors, good and bad. Every dieter has heard the "negative calorie" rumor, for example—you know, the one that you burn more calories by chewing celery than you get from digesting it. And it's almost true! An 8-inch celery stalk nets out about 6 (count 'em, 6) calories after chewing. Technically, that's not negative, but it's darn close. You'd have to nosh an entire farm field of celery to get into calorie trouble at that rate.

So you can pretty much eat celery at will and still drop the pounds. Substitute a celery rib for a couple of Oreos, and you'll save 100 calories. If your usual afternoon snack is a candy bar,

Quick Fix:

High Blood Pressure

Got high blood pressure? Eat some celery. Researchers have uncovered a naturally occurring chemical in celery, called phthalide, that actually helps lower blood pressure (at least in rats) by dilating blood vessels.

you'll save more than 200. And it helps that celery tastes so good, especially the sweet inner stalks. (Okay, it's not chocolate, but what do you want from a simple stem?) Celery is also fat- and cholesterol-free, and it consists mostly of water, so it will even help keep you hydrated.

SODIUM SCARE?

Celery also has a reputation for being high in sodium. If you have kidney disease and you're on dialysis, the sodium content in a couple of stalks of celery might be an issue. But that concern somehow has been picked up by folks with high blood pressure who've been advised to eat a low-sodium (2,000 milligrams) diet.

Yet a celery stalk serves up only 35 milligrams of sodium, less than a carrot, which has almost 40 milligrams! Add to that the recommendation of the Dietary Approaches to Stop Hypertension (DASH) diet to eat 8 to 11 fruits and vegetables daily to lower blood pressure, and celery takes its rightful place in the healthy foods parade! (For more about the DASH diet, see "Dash Away from High Blood Pressure" on page 269.)

NUTRITION IN A NUTSHELL

Celery (one 8-inch stalk)

Calories: 6

Fat: 0 g

Saturated fat: 0 g

Cholesterol: 0 mg

Sodium: 35 mg

Total carbohydrates: 2 g

Dietary fiber: Less than 1 g

Protein: Less than 1 g

Folate: 3% of Daily Value

Vitamin A: 1%

Vitamin C: 3%

Calcium: 2%

Iron: 1%

Potassium: 3%

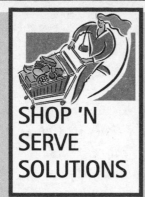

SHOP 'N SERVE SOLUTIONS

Celery is "in season" year-round. And stalking the best celery is a snap if you just use your eyes and nose.

WHEN SELECTING CELERY:

■ Look for a tight, shiny, well-shaped green bunch with bright green, fresh-looking leaves. Yellow leaves are a sure sign of old age.

■ Your celery should feel firm and crisp. Leave limp or yellow celery behind.

■ Avoid celery that looks abused, with cuts, bruises, or ragged stalks.

■ Then give it the "sniff" test. If it smells bitter, better leave it alone.

WHEN STORING:

Store your celery in its plastic bag in the vegetable drawer of your fridge, and pull off the stalks as you need them.

WHEN YOU'RE READY TO USE:

■ Wash the stalks thoroughly and trim off the ends.

■ If your celery has become limp, trim off the root end and the tops, then stand it in a glass of water for an hour or two. It'll stiffen right up.

ADD SOME NEGATIVE CALORIES

Celery's calories may be negative, but we're positive that you'll enjoy the flavor and texture this veggie gives to everyday foods. Try these ideas:

◆ **Spice up soups and stews.** Add chopped celery to soups and stews. For best flavor and firm texture, toss it in about 20 minutes before the dish has finished cooking.

◆ **Give a hand to canned.** Freshen canned soups by adding a few celery leaves.

◆ **Spoon-feed the kids.** Use the wide ends of large celery stalks as edible spoons for soup. The kids will love it!

Italian Braised Celery

If you're looking for a quick and zesty side dish to spice up a bland entrée such as chicken or pork tenderloin, this is it! Celery stars in a veggie mix kissed by classic Italian ingredients. We like braised celery served in a shallow soup bowl, topped with a baked chicken breast, and with a slice of crusty Italian bread on the side. Mama mia! *That's good eating!*

4 eight-inch stalks celery, cut into two-inch pieces
4 Italian plum tomatoes, sliced
2 cloves garlic, pressed or minced
½ cup water
1 cup frozen Italian green beans
½ cup chopped sweet green pepper
½ cup chopped sweet red pepper
½ cup chopped onion
¼ teaspoon anise seeds
Dash of ground cayenne pepper
1 teaspoon olive oil
¼ teaspoon dried oregano
½ teaspoon dried basil

Place the celery in a large skillet. Top with the tomatoes, garlic, and water. Bring to a boil. Cover, reduce the heat, and simmer for 10 minutes. Add the beans, sweet green and red peppers, onion, anise seeds, cayenne pepper, oil, oregano, and basil. Simmer, covered, for 10 minutes, or until the celery is tender.

Yield: 4 servings.

Nutritional data per serving (vegetables only): Calories, 133; protein, 5 g; carbohydrates, 26 g; fiber, 8 g; fat, 3 g; saturated fat, less than 0.5 g; cholesterol, 0 mg; sodium, 87 mg; vitamin A, 73% of Daily Value; vitamin C, 169%; calcium, 10%; iron, 13%; potassium, 24%.

Cereal:

It Carries Cholesterol Away

BATTLES:
- diabetes
- heart disease
- high blood pressure
- high cholesterol

BOLSTERS:
- insulin sensitivity
- regularity

What could be better on a frosty morning than a steaming bowl of hot, whole grain cereal to coax you into the day? And if it's oatmeal, your heart and all its blood vessels, from your big coronary arteries to your tiniest capillaries, will want to give you a great big hug—a hug you deserve for taking such tasty good care of yourself!

FEELING YOUR OATS

Oatmeal and oat bran cereals were the first individual foods ever permitted to bear an FDA-approved health claim on their packages. The reason? An impressive pile of

NUTRITION IN A NUTSHELL

Dry quick oats (½ cup)

Calories: 155

Fat: 3 g

Saturated fat: 0 g

Cholesterol: 0 mg

Sodium: 2 mg

Total carbohydrates: 27 g

Dietary fiber: 4 g

Protein: 6 g

Vitamin B_1 (thiamin): 20% of Daily Value

Magnesium: 15%

Manganese: 74%

research showed that adding oats to your diet lowers total and bad low-density lipoprotein (LDL) cholesterol without lowering good high-density lipoprotein (HDL) cholesterol. And that's just what a struggling heart needs.

Nationwide, hearts started beating louder, because the folks who benefit most from oats are those in greatest jeopardy. If cholesterol measures 229 or less, a drop of 2 to 3 percent is common. But at levels above 229, a whopping 4 to 7 percent drop rewards those who skip the lumberjack breakfast and, instead, start the day by eating enough oats to provide 3 grams of beta-glucan, the soluble fiber in oats. That amount is equivalent to ½ cup of dry (uncooked) oats.

Quick Fix:

Itchy Hives

To soothe the itchiness of hives, soak for 10 to 15 minutes in a bathtub full of warm water and some finely ground colloidal oatmeal. Colloidal oatmeal is an over-the-counter bath powder made by Aveeno that stays suspended in water. It won't clog your drain—and it will fix your itch.

DRAMATIC DRUG-FREE IMPROVEMENT

Now the story gets even better. In a recent study of a 500,000-member HMO group, 50 percent of patients on blood pressure medication were able to stop taking their medication after eating 5 grams of soluble fiber from oatmeal and oatmeal squares every day for four weeks. Another 20 percent were able to cut their medication in half. (Warning: Don't try this at home. Always consult with your doctor before making changes in your medication.)

In addition, the patients' total and LDL cholesterol levels dropped. Plus, the bad side effects of taking blood pressure medication—such as low blood potassium, muscle cramps, sexual dysfunction, and bad moods—vanished.

Researchers speculate that it all has to do with a complex array of interactions that affect insulin resistance, but the details aren't clear yet. Soluble fiber slows partially digested food in your intestines. That traps cholesterol and bile so that your body can't reabsorb them.

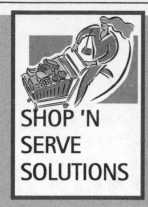

SHOP 'N SERVE SOLUTIONS

Keep a variety of cereals on hand, and day-trade. You'll be nutrionally rich!

WHEN SELECTING CEREAL:

■ Check the "best-used-before" date.

■ Look for packages that are well sealed and undamaged.

WHEN STORING:

■ Store unopened cereals in a cool, dry place.

■ Once you've opened them, store whole grain cereals in the refrigerator. (Even bugs are smart enough to go for the good stuff!)

WHOLE GRAIN GOODNESS

Here's how to enjoy whole grain cereal often:

◆ **Start the day bran-new.** Microwave a bowl of oat bran, then stir in chopped apples, walnuts, and a dash of ground nutmeg.

◆ **Eat nuttin', honey.** Microwave a bowl of whole wheat cereal, then stir in 1 tablespoon of peanut butter and 2 teaspoons of honey. Yummy!

◆ **Go bananas.** Whip up a bowl of farina, then stir in a mashed overripe banana and a sprinkle of brown sugar. This is tops when your tummy's funky.

◆ **Stash a pack.** Keep instant cereal packets in your desk drawer at work. Heat and eat when you need to warm up or chill out.

HOW SWEET IT ISN'T

Meanwhile, that slow-moving digestive mix is gradually releasing food energy for a gentle blood sugar rise, requiring only a minimal amount of insulin to help the blood sugar get into cells. (This is unlike what happens with a highly processed food that is quickly digested and dumped into your bloodstream, causing a sharp blood sugar rise and an insulin surge.)

NAME THAT CEREAL!

There are plenty of hot cereals out there, each with its own benefits. Check them out:

■ **Oat bran** is made from the finely ground outer layer of the oats. Just $\frac{1}{2}$ cup of dry oat bran packs 6 grams of fiber—3 soluble and 3 insoluble. Oat bran is also rich in vitamin B_1 (thiamin), iron, magnesium, phosphorus, and zinc. It's tops for keeping cholesterol at bay.

■ **Oatmeal** is made from thinly sliced whole oats, and it contains everything good in the oat—bran, germ, and endosperm. Cooking speed depends on the thickness of the slices. About $\frac{1}{2}$ cup of dry quick-cooking oats serves up 4 grams of fiber—2 soluble and 2 insoluble.

■ **Whole wheat cereal** (such as Wheateena) is made from whole wheat kernels that have been ground for cereal. It delivers all the goodness of other whole wheat products—bran, germ, and endosperm. (See "Wheat Germ: Harvest the Goodness!" on page 464 and "Whole Wheat Bread: The Real Staff of Life" on page 469.) Just $\frac{1}{2}$ cup of dry whole wheat cereal delivers 4 grams of fiber, 1 soluble and 3 insoluble. It's great for regularity.

■ **Harvest Mornings** cereals are instant multigrain cereals made from oatmeal, whole wheat, and barley flakes. One packet supplies 3 grams of fiber.

Insulin's basic job is to coordinate the way your body uses and stores the energy from the foods you eat. It's beneficial to have low levels of circulating insulin, because the insulin gets used up doing its good work.

Excess insulin, however, causes mischief, such as teasing your liver into producing more cholesterol. Insulin resistance and diabetes happen when cells balk at using insulin correctly. But over three to four weeks on a high-oat diet, insulin sensitivity improves, thus reducing the risk of developing diabetes. This diet also can decrease sodium retention, which may be the mechanism that lowers blood pressure.

Fresh-Start Breakfast

Change the fruits and nuts in this breakfast dish to reflect the season, but make the power-packed grains a staple. This stick-to-your-ribs breakfast provides goodness that lasts until lunch.

½ cup dry quick-cooking oats
1 tablespoon toasted wheat germ
½ cup calcium-fortified soy milk
½ cup skim milk
1 tablespoon honey
1 tablespoon toasted pecans
½ cup fresh blueberries
¼ teaspoon ground cinnamon

In a microwaveable cereal bowl, combine the oats, wheat germ, and milks. Stir to blend well. Microwave on high for 2 minutes, or until the cereal is hot and the oats are cooked. Stir in the honey, pecans, blueberries, and cinnamon.

Yield: One serving.

Nutritional data per serving: Calories, 415; protein, 16 g; carbohydrates, 71 g; fiber, 8 g; fat, 11 g; saturated fat, 1 g; cholesterol, 2 mg; sodium, 70 mg; folate, 15% of Daily Value; vitamin B_1 (thiamin), 35%; vitamin B_2 (riboflavin), 32%; calcium, 35%; magnesium, 40%; manganese, 108%; zinc, 23%.

Cheese:

Grate for Bones

BATTLES:
- colon cancer
- premenstrual syndrome
- tooth decay

BOLSTERS:
- bones

Here's a confession: Karen doesn't drink milk. She hasn't since she was about two years old. But throughout her life, she has always managed to get enough calcium—thanks largely to cheese.

It's a good thing, too. Why? "The single best thing women can do to ward off osteoporosis is to make sure they get plenty of calcium," says Felicia Kausman, M.D., clinical director of the National Osteoporosis Foundation. "Dairy products such as milk, cheese, and yogurt are some of the most significant sources of the mineral."

A COURSE IN CALCIUM

Here's a quick lesson about the way your body uses calcium: Most of your body's calcium is stored in your bones, where it gives

NUTRITION IN A NUTSHELL

Parmesan cheese
(2 tablespoons grated)

Calories: 57

Fat: 4 g

Saturated fat: 2 g

Cholesterol: 10 mg

Sodium: 233 mg

Total carbohydrates: 0 g

Dietary fiber: 0 g

Protein: 5 g

Calcium: 17% of Daily Value

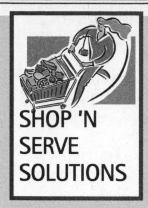

SHOP 'N SERVE SOLUTIONS

Ahhhh, don't you love the aroma in a cheese store? It's as if you can taste the Parmesan with your nose!

WHEN SELECTING CHEESE:

Check the expiration date on the package before buying.

WHEN STORING:

■ Preserve your purchase by refrigerating it as soon as possible.

■ Store cheese in its original wrapper or in an airtight container. Hard cheeses, such as cheddar, should keep for several months, while fresh or soft cheeses, such as ricotta, may last for only one to three weeks.

HOW TO HANDLE "GOLDEN MOLDIES":

■ If you notice mold on fresh or soft cheese, discard the cheese.

■ If you spot a single spot of mold on hard cheese, cut off $\frac{1}{2}$ inch beneath the mold and eat the rest of the cheese as soon as possible.

■ Throw out any hard cheese that has more than two spots of mold.

Serving tip: Most cheese aficionados prefer to leave hard cheeses at room temperature for about an hour before serving, which gives them a chance to warm up and "breathe," thus heightening their flavor. But don't do the same with fresh, unripened cheeses, such as ricotta or cottage cheese, because they might spoil.

CHEESY CREATIONS

Now that you know how to care for your cheese, see how to get creative with it:

◆ **Get your goat.** Instead of mayo, spread a thin layer of goat cheese on your deli sandwich.

◆ **Follow the French.** Don't dig into a piece of cake for dessert. Instead, have a few cubes of fromage and fruit.

them the strength to support your body, protect your internal organs, and work with your muscles so that you can move.

About 1 percent of your calcium resides in your bloodstream, where it regulates cell walls and sends messages between cells.

When it comes to calcium intake, here's what you should know:

▶ **Don't break the bank.** It's crucial that you meet your calcium requirements, because if you fall short, your bones sacrifice some of their stores of the mineral and give it to your bloodstream. If your bones are continually called upon to make up your dietary deficit, they become weak and prone to fractures. Unfortunately, research shows that one in two women suffer an osteoporosis-related fracture sometime in their lives.

▶ **Set more aside.** Before you hit the big Five-O, you require about 1,000 milligrams of calcium daily. After that, your needs increase to 1,200 milligrams a day. Most 1-ounce servings of cheese provide about 170 to 210 milligrams of calcium, a good chunk of what you require daily. And, lovers of Italian food, rejoice: Parmesan cheese offers a whopping 330 milligrams!

▶ **Focus on low-fat.** Unfortunately, many women have cut cheese out of their diets—or trimmed it back considerably—because they are counting fat grams. While some cheeses, especially soft varieties such as Havarti, pack 10 grams of fat in an ounce, others, such as part-skim mozzarella or part-skim ricotta, contain a more reasonable 5 grams.

Quick Fix:

Muscle Cramps

If you're plagued by muscle cramps every time you do something strenuous, research suggests that you may not be getting enough calcium. Make sure you get more of the mineral—and ditch those annoying cramps—by eating a few bites of cheese every day.

Calcium Bargains and Busts

Sure, cheese is loaded with calcium. Trouble is, some types contain a lot of calories, too. To determine which cheeses are calcium bargains—and which are busts—we divided the calcium content by the number of calories. The result: a calcium quotient. Of course, the higher the quotient, the better.

Cheese	Calcium Quotient
Cream cheese, fat-free	3.4
Parmesan	3
Ricotta, part-skim	2.9
Swiss	2.7
Mozzarella, part-skim	2.6
Romano	2.6
Edam	2.3
Gouda	2.1
Asiago	2
Monterey Jack	2
Feta	1.9
Muenster	1.9
Cheddar	1.8
Colby	1.7
American	1.5
Blue cheese	1.5
Goat cheese	0.52
Cream cheese, regular	0.22

For everyday meals, focus on cheeses that are naturally lower in fat and calories. Save the high-fat baked Brie for holidays and other special occasions.

THIS JUST IN

The latest research suggests that while you're striving to come up with enough calcium to protect your bones, you might be helping out your body in other ways. Consider this:

▶ A study of more than 400 women found that getting 1,200 milligrams of calcium daily reduced symptoms of premenstrual syndrome, such as irritability and bloating, by half.

▶ Another study suggests that calcium may lower the risk of colon polyps, which can lead to cancer.

▶ Finally, research has shown that eating a small piece of cheese after a meal stimulates the production of saliva, which washes away harmful acids that trigger tooth decay.

All that research is really something to smile about. So, say "Cheese!"

Guilt-Free Grilled Cheese

Love the taste of melted cheese oozing out of slices of crunchy bread? Everyone does! Try this guilt-free, grown-up version of the classic grilled cheese sandwich. It will become a lunch favorite!

Canola oil cooking spray
4 slices part-skim mozzarella cheese
2 halves roasted red pepper
4 slices whole wheat bread

Coat a large nonstick skillet with cooking spray and place over low to medium heat. Layer 1 slice of cheese, 1 pepper half, and another piece of cheese on a slice of the bread. Top with a second slice of the bread. Repeat with the remaining ingredients. Lightly coat the outside of the bread, top and bottom, with cooking spray. Place the sandwiches on the heated skillet. Cook until the bottom of each sandwich is light brown, 2 to 3 minutes, and flip. Continue to cook until the other side begins to brown, about 2 minutes. Remove from the skillet. Let cool for 1 minute and then slice each sandwich in half.

Variation: Substitute reduced-fat or 2% American cheese slices for the mozzarella.

Yield: Two servings.

Nutritional data per serving: Calories, 242; protein, 13 g; carbohydrates, 34 g; fiber, 4 g; fat, 7 g; saturated fat, 3 g; cholesterol, 11 mg; sodium, 540 mg; calcium, 20% of Daily Value; iron, 20%.

Blackberry Cheese Dip

If you're tired of serving ranch or onion dip at parties, try this tasty alternative. One caveat: Have copies of the recipe made in advance. Your guests will want it—guaranteed!

¾ cup part-skim ricotta cheese
¼ cup low-fat plain yogurt
3 tablespoons blackberry jam
¼ teaspoon vanilla extract
⅓ cup blackberries, lightly crushed with a fork

In a food processor, mix the cheese, yogurt, jam, and vanilla extract until very smooth. Add the blackberries and just combine. Chill until thickened.

Yield: Six servings.

Nutritional data per serving: Calories, 80; protein, 4 g; carbohydrates, 10 g; fiber, 0 g; fat, 3 g; saturated fat, 2 g; cholesterol, 10 mg; sodium, 47 mg; calcium, 11% of Daily Value; iron, 2%.

Cherries:
Health Is Just
a Bowlful Away

BATTLES:
- arthritis pain
- cancer
- heart disease

BOLSTERS:
- bones

We've always thought that life without cherries would be the pits. Now we know that, healthwise, it's true. While their nutritional profile never seemed outstanding in any vitamin or mineral, the good news about cherries is finally leaking out: They're packed with powerful disease-fighting nutrients!

NEWLY FOUND NUTRIENTS

Dark red cherries, both sweet and sour, are packed with flavonoids called anthocyanins. These natural plant chemicals create the blue, pink, red, mauve, and violet colors that help flowers attract insects for pollination. Later, anthocyanins defend fruits and vegetables against attacks from invading germs and hungry bugs.

NUTRITION IN A NUTSHELL

Fresh cherries (10)

Calories: 49

Fat: 1 g

Saturated fat: 0 g

Cholesterol: 0 mg

Sodium: 0 mg

Total carbohydrates: 11 g

Dietary fiber: 2 g

Protein: 1 g

Vitamin C: 5% of Daily Value

In your body, anthocyanins seem to act as antioxidants that protect against cancer and heart disease. But Americans consume only an estimated 200 milligrams of anthocyanins a day—probably nowhere near enough—considering that our record for eating fruits and veggies is the pits.

So chomp on cherries, and double your pleasure as well as your protection. Just six juicy, dark red cherries a day will deliver an additional 200 milligrams of anthocyanins.

CHERRIES EQUAL APPLES

Cherries are just quivering with quercetin, another flavonoid that fights cancer and heart disease. How high are they in quercetin? As high as apples, which are the top bananas when it comes to fruits that deliver the goods. And the best news is that processed cherries, the kind you get in cans and as prepared pie filling, deliver double the quercetin of fresh cherries. That means you can get cherry-good protection all year long.

BUT WAIT, THERE'S MORE

Cherries are also a good source of perillyl alcohol, which has been shown to prevent the development of breast and pancreatic cancer in rats, and of the mineral boron, which seems to be important for bone health.

What's more, cherries may help relieve the pain of arthritis. Recent laboratory research at Michigan State University in East Lansing has shown that, at least in the test tube, tart cherry juice is 10 times better than aspirin at reducing pain and swelling —and it won't irritate tender tummies as aspirin can.

Quick Fix:

Gout

Many people report that eating cherries helps relieve gout, although there's no science to explain why they would.

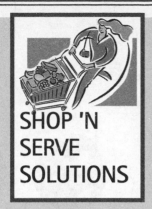

SHOP 'N SERVE SOLUTIONS

Fresh sweet cherries have a very short season, so grab them when you can. They won't last long!

WHEN SELECTING CHERRIES:

■ Look for fruits that are shiny, plump, and firm enough to pop when you bite them.

■ Choose those that still have their stems. Stemless cherries are ripe for spoilage—and besides, it's more fun to eat them from the stem!

■ Avoid cherries that are underripe, soft, cut, or moldy.

WHEN STORING:

Store your cherries in a covered container, and eat them within a few days. (As if we had to tell you that. At Colleen's house, they usually wash and eat them while they're unpacking the rest of the groceries!)

CHEW ON CHERRIES

We cannot tell a lie—here are some fun things to do with cherries:

◆ **Mix them into muffins.** Substitute freeze-dried cherries in any muffin or quick-bread recipe that calls for raisins.

◆ **Guzzle them down.** Buy all-natural sour cherry juice at your local health food store or over the Internet. Drink it plain, or mix it with other favorite fruit juices. For instance, mix your own orange-cherry, grape-cherry, or cranberry-cherry blend. Or use it instead of water in your next cup of hot chocolate.

◆ **Whirl them around.** Toss frozen or canned cherries and a ripe banana into your blender with a little skim milk and a few ice cubes for a frosty cherry cooler.

Cherry Pork Wrap

8 flour tortillas
3 cups pitted dark sweet cherries
2 tablespoons chopped fresh basil
2 teaspoons grated fresh ginger
½ teaspoon garlic powder
½ teaspoon ground cayenne pepper
¼ teaspoon salt
⅛ teaspoon freshly ground black pepper
1 tablespoon canola oil
12 ounces lean boneless pork tenderloin,
cut into 2-by-2-by-4-inch strips
2 cups cooked brown rice
2 cups finely shredded romaine lettuce

Preheat the oven to 350°F. Wrap the tortillas tightly in heavy foil and heat in the oven for 10 to 15 minutes. Meanwhile, in a food processor, coarsely chop 2 cups of the cherries. Stir in the basil, ginger, garlic power, cayenne pepper, salt, and black pepper. Set aside.

Heat the oil in a heavy skillet. Add the pork and the remaining 1 cup of cherries. Sauté just until the pork is cooked through, about 5 minutes. Stir in the cooked rice and heat through. Top each warm tortilla with ¼ cup of the pork-rice mixture, a spoonful of the cherry sauce, and ¼ cup of the lettuce. Fold in the sides of each tortilla and roll into a bundle.

Yield: Eight servings.

Nutritional data per serving: Calories, 404; protein, 18 g; carbohydrates, 61 g; fiber, 5 g; fat, 10 g; saturated fat, 2 g; cholesterol, 28 mg; sodium, 438 mg; folate, 29% of Daily Value; vitamin B$_3$ (niacin), 54%; manganese, 52%.

Chicken:

Helps You Be a Featherweight

BATTLES:
- colds
- heart disease
- high cholesterol

BOLSTERS:
- energy
- immune function
- weight control

Even though we make chicken at least four nights a week, our families hardly ever whine, "Chicken *again?*" Sure, they're being considerate. But even they admit that chicken—unlike many other foods—can taste incredibly different, depending on the recipe.

Think about it: Season steamed asparagus with Italian herbs or top it with hollandaise sauce, and it still tastes, well, like asparagus. But if you grill chicken and toss it into a warm flour tortilla with salsa, peppers, and onions, it takes on an entirely different flavor than if you roasted it with rosemary and garlic.

Versatility is the beauty of chicken—not only in cooking, but also in the nutrition it provides. A 3-ounce piece of chicken contains at least 5 percent of the Daily Value for eight different vitamins and minerals that are crucial to maintaining good health.

143

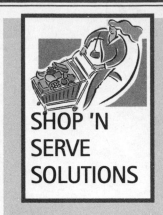

SHOP 'N SERVE SOLUTIONS

It's important to handle chicken with care to keep your family healthy. Here's how to give it the TLC it deserves.

WHEN SELECTING CHICKEN:

■ Pick out all your meat last—so that it won't be unrefrigerated as you check out the magazines, look for a new lipstick, compare nutrition labels on crackers, and do other time-consuming stuff.

■ Immediately put your package of chicken into a plastic bag. (Good supermarkets have these bags in the meat department. If yours does not, snag some from the produce section.) Just in case the outside of the package has become contaminated with salmonella or another type of bacteria, the plastic bag will keep the bugs from spreading to your other groceries.

■ Ask the checkout clerk to bag your meat separately from your other foods.

■ In warm weather, place your groceries in the car (not the trunk) to keep them as cool as possible.

WHEN STORING:

■ When you get home, unpack your meat first, immediately putting it in the refrigerator. Store it in the coldest part of your refrigerator.

■ Freeze it if you're not planning to use it within two days or more.

GIVE YOUR HEART A LEG UP

The most abundant nutrient in chicken is niacin, or vitamin B_3. Just a single chicken breast packs nearly 60 percent of what you need for the entire day. Studies suggest that niacin may lower cholesterol and drop your risk of heart disease.

WHEN YOU'RE READY TO USE:

■ Thaw frozen chicken in the fridge (never on the countertop!) or by immersing it in cold water.

■ Remove the skin either before or after you cook your chicken. Leaving the skin on while cooking doesn't increase the calorie or fat content of the meat.

■ Use a meat thermometer to check for doneness. Whole chickens should reach 180°F; bone-in chicken parts should reach 170°F; and boneless parts need to register 165°F. Immediately refrigerate any extra chicken. Whew—that's it!

VARIATIONS ON A THEME

You probably have plenty of recipes for chicken, so we won't bore you with the basics. But we'll pass along some ways that you can get creative with this basic food. C'mon, don't be chicken!

◆ **Throw a pizza party.** Karen tops her crust with tomato sauce, roasted peppers, grilled chicken pieces, and a sprinkling of Parmesan and smoked mozzarella cheeses. This version of pizza—minus the usual coating of high-fat cheese and pepperoni—becomes a healthy meal.

◆ **Tuck it into tacos.** Sure, your taco recipe calls for ground beef. But you can substitute shredded chicken breast—and have your taco taste every bit as good.

◆ **Dish out spaghetti and chicken.** When you stir grilled chicken pieces into your pasta dishes, no one will miss the meatballs. Even Karen's meatball-lovin' husband doesn't complain.

And if you're substituting chicken for beef, your heart will appreciate that, too. Three ounces of roasted chicken has just a single gram of saturated fat, while the same amount of ground beef is brimming with 6 grams or more! When you slice the saturated fat in your diet, you also drop your risk of ticker trouble.

NUTRITION IN A NUTSHELL

Skinless chicken breast (3 ounces, roasted)

Calories: 140

Fat: 3 g

Saturated fat: 1 g

Cholesterol: 72 mg

Sodium: 63 mg

Total carbohydrates: 0 g

Dietary fiber: 0 g

Protein: 26 g

Vitamin B_2 (riboflavin): 7% of Daily Value

Vitamin B_3 (niacin): 59%

Vitamin B_6: 20%

Vitamin B_{12}: 5%

Iron: 5%

Magnesium: 6%

Phosphorus: 19%

Zinc: 6%

Swapping chicken breast for beef also saves on calories. A serving of roasted chicken breast sans the skin contains about 100 fewer calories than a portion of ground beef and about 50 fewer than steak. Over time, the calorie cutting will add up and you'll lose weight—another bit of good news for your heart.

NO MORE SICK DAYS!

Chicken is also peppered with vitamin B_6, vitamin B_{12}, and zinc—a trio that keeps your immune system strong, so you're less likely to catch the virus of the week. Plus, poultry packs a little iron, the mineral that prevents you from becoming anemic.

Quick Fix:

Upper Respiratory Infection

If you're coming down with a cold, whip up a batch of chicken soup—or, better yet, get your loved one to do it. Chicken contains the amino acid cysteine, which is chemically similar to the bronchitis drug acetyl-cysteine. Plus, new research suggests that chicken soup helps block the production of neutrophils, white blood cells that contribute to upper respiratory cold symptoms, says study author Stephen Rennard, M.D.

Grandma's Old-World Chicken Soup

Stephen Rennard, M.D., a researcher at the University of Nebraska Medical Center, studied his wife's Lithuanian grandmother's chicken soup recipe. He found that it helped ease cold symptoms—just like his grandma said it would.

1 baking chicken (5–6 pounds), cleaned
1 package chicken wings (1–2 pounds), cleaned
3 large onions
1 large sweet potato
3 parsnips
2 turnips
12 carrots
6 stalks celery
1 bunch parsley
40 matzo balls
Salt and ground black pepper to taste

Put the baking chicken in a large pot and cover it with cold water. Bring the water to a boil. Add the chicken wings, onions, sweet potato, parsnips, turnips, and carrots. Boil for about 90 minutes, removing the fat from the surface as it accumulates. Add the celery and parsley and boil for about 45 minutes longer. Remove the chicken. Transfer the vegetables to a food processor and whirl until finely chopped. Return the vegetables to the pot, add the matzo balls, and season with salt and pepper. Simmer until the matzo balls are heated through.

Yield: Twenty-four 1-cup servings.

Nutritional data per serving: Calories, 163; protein, 5 g; carbohydrates, 18 g; fiber, 2 g; fat, 8 g; saturated fat, 1 g; cholesterol, 89 mg; sodium, 50 mg; folate, 13% of Daily Value; vitamin C, 10%; iron, 6%.

Chiles:
They're Hot for Colds

BATTLES:
- heart disease
- stuffy nose
- ulcers

BOLSTERS:
- mood
- pain management

Learning to eat chile peppers is a lot like learning to drink alcohol. When you first taste alcoholic beverages, you're taken aback by their fiery breathlessness. But with experience, you taste different flavors in red and white wines, beer, and bourbon. So it is with chiles.

Each type boasts a unique flavor. Some have a mild fruit flavor with tones of coffee, licorice, dried plum, and raisin. And each type is armed with its own amount of fire-power. The biggest chiles are fairly mild. It's those tiny chiles that will take your head off!

Now, don't be threatened. Once you eat chiles regularly, you develop a tolerance for their heat. Some people say you become "addicted" to them. Here's why.

NUTRITION IN A NUTSHELL

Red chile (1 pod)

Calories: 18

Fat: 0 g

Saturated fat: 0 g

Cholesterol: 0 mg

Sodium: 0 mg

Total carbohydrates: 4 g

Dietary fiber: 1 g

Protein: 1 g

Vitamin A: 97% of Daily Value

Vitamin C: 121%

Calcium: 1%

Iron: 3%

148

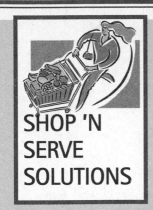

SHOP 'N SERVE SOLUTIONS

Chiles are available fresh, dried, frozen, canned, and ground.

WHEN SELECTING FRESH CHILES:

■ Choose pods that are firm and bright-looking.

■ Avoid those with any signs of bruising or decay.

Warning! Don't touch your eyes or nose after handling fresh chiles. No matter how tolerant your taste buds become, your mucous membranes never get used to capsaicin.

Looking for a mild chile? Banana peppers, cherry peppers, and jalapeños show up, sliced or whole, in jars in your supermarket. You almost can't go wrong with them. And there's always paprika, crushed red pepper, and ground cayenne pepper in the spice section. These should be a deep red color and a little lumpy (because they've hung on to their fresh, natural flavoring oils), rather than dusty and dry.

LIGHTING THE FIRE

Here are a few quick ways to spice up your life with chiles. (If the fire gets too hot, have milk, yogurt, or frozen yogurt available to douse the flames.)

◆ **Go Italian.** Sprinkle crushed red pepper and a small amount of anise seeds on your pizza to mimic the taste of Italian sausage—without the fat. Add pepperoncini to your salad.

◆ **Go Mexican.** Spice up a can of vegetarian chili with a dash of ground cayenne pepper, chopped onions, and a little cilantro.

◆ **Go Thai.** Mix chilled, thinly sliced filet mignon with garlic, ginger, soy sauce, and fish sauce. Toss with sliced red onions and jalapeños and some lime juice. Serve on Butterhead lettuce.

◆ **Go Hungarian.** Add Hungarian cherry peppers (they're sweet and mild—usually!) to your next pickle and olive tray.

FEEL BETTER FAST

The ribs and seeds of chiles are packed with capsaicin, a heat-producing chemical with bountiful benefits. While your body is feeling the heat, your brain is chilling out with a flood of endorphins—high-flying, mood-lifting natural painkillers that create a sense of well-being (a sort of "eater's high"!). One Thai dish called Drunken Noodles contains not a drop of alcohol, but packs enough heat from chiles to make diners downright woozy!

WARM YOUR HEART

Capsaicin also turns out to be an antioxidant that helps lower bad low-density lipoprotein (LDL) cholesterol and reduce the stickiness of blood platelets so that they don't clot and cause a heart attack or stroke. And each chile also comes packed with plenty of additional heart-smart ingredients. One fresh chile provides 126 percent of the vitamin C and 95 percent of the vitamin A you need daily, creating a powerful antioxidant team that fights the kind of cell damage that sets you up for heart disease, cancer, and (worse!) premature aging.

Quick Fix: Stuffy Nose

Cold got you all stuffed up? Cook up a pot of chicken soup (canned will do), then add fresh garlic and plenty of ground cayenne pepper. Inhale the fumes while you eat the soup. You'll be breathing freely in no time. But keep the tissues handy. Your nose will run freely, too!

What's more, capsaicin is heat-stable, so if you don't want to be bothered with fresh chiles, dried or ground peppers will do.

And here's some funny news: For years, part of ulcer treatment was to avoid hot, spicy foods. Now chiles are being explored as a treatment for ulcers because of their bacteria-fighting ability.

Chile Shrimp and Melon Salad

¼ **cup olive oil**
1 **tablespoon cayenne chili powder**
½ **teaspoon salt**
2 **cloves garlic, pressed or minced**
¼ **cup chopped fresh cilantro**
12 **very large shrimp, deveined, with shells and tails on**
Peel of 1 lime, grated
Juice of 1 lime
1 **cup fat-free vanilla yogurt**
2 **cups diced watermelon**
2 **cups shredded red leaf lettuce, washed and patted dry**

In a medium bowl, combine the oil, cayenne powder, salt, garlic, and cilantro. Add the shrimp, cover, and marinate overnight in the refrigerator. When you're ready to eat, preheat the grill. Remove the shrimp from the bowl, reserving the marinade. Grill the shrimp over high heat for 3 to 5 minutes, depending on the size of the shrimp. Do not overcook. Allow to cool at room temperature, then peel. Boil the reserved marinade for 5 minutes to kill any bacteria from the raw shrimp, so that the marinade can be used as salad dressing. Allow to cool. In a medium bowl, stir the lime peel and lime juice into the yogurt, mixing well. Add the watermelon and chill for 30 minutes.

To assemble the salad, toss the lettuce with 2 tablespoons of the cooled marinade and arrange on two salad plates. Top each with half of the watermelon mixture and then half of the shrimp.

Yield: Two servings.

Nutritional data per serving: Calories, 303; protein, 13 g; carbohydrates, 30 g; fiber, 4 g; fat, 15 g; saturated fat, 2 g; cholesterol, 67 mg; sodium, 747 mg; vitamin A, 48% of Daily Value; vitamin B_6, 16%; vitamin C, 33%; vitamin E, 14%; calcium, 24%; iron, 10%.

Chives:
The Single-Calorie Seasoning

BATTLES:
- cancer
- heart disease
- high cholesterol

BOLSTERS:
- immune function
- weight control

Until recently, Karen rarely ate chives—except for an occasional sprinkle on her baked potato. But now, they're often in her kitchen. The reason for the about-face: She discovered that this often-overlooked herb gives dishes an incredible flavor. And chives pack a lot of health benefits, too.

Chives have pretty darn good genes. Depending on the type you choose, they're related to either onions or garlic. Whatever your choice, chives contain compounds that curb cancer, head off heart disease, and more.

The most-studied compound in chives is called allium. Research suggests that allium has antibacterial and antifungal properties that may help stave off infections. What's more, allium guards against cancers of the stomach and colon, and also lowers cholesterol.

NUTRITION IN A NUTSHELL

Chives (1 tablespoon)

Calories: 1

Fat: 0 g

Saturated fat: 0 g

Cholesterol: 0 mg

Sodium: 0 mg

Total carbohydrates: 0 g

Dietary fiber: 0 g

Protein: 0 g

Vitamin C: 3% of Daily Value

152

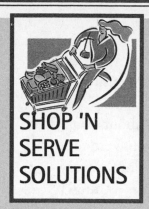

SHOP 'N SERVE SOLUTIONS

Fresh chives are available year-round in the produce section of your supermarket. When buying them, you first need to decide whether you want onion or garlic chives. Onion chives, the most common type, taste like a mild onion. Garlic chives have the air of the "stinking rose," but they're not quite as strong. Choosing a good bunch of either kind isn't a challenge.

WHEN SELECTING FRESH CHIVES:

■ Choose those that have uniformly green leaves.

■ Avoid those that show any signs of wilting.

WHEN STORING:

Store fresh chives in your fridge, where they'll keep for up to a week.

Frozen chives. If you can't find fresh chives in the produce section, head to the freezer case, where you might be able to snag a bag of frozen ones.

BRING YOUR FOODS ALIVE WITH CHIVES

Ready to add some spice to your life? Try these uses for chives:

◆ **Spark your salad.** Karen likes to line a plate with romaine lettuce leaves and then top them with red grapes, chopped pecans, a little blue cheese, a splash of olive oil vinaigrette, and fresh garlic chives.

◆ **Add zip to your dip.** Mix 1 tablespoon of onion chives with 1 cup of low-fat sour cream or low-fat plain yogurt. Serve with baked chips at your next party.

◆ **Sensationalize your shrimp.** For an extra kick, top your cooked shrimp with a sprinkling of garlic or onion chives.

◆ **Give your breakfast a boost.** Throw some onion chives into your egg-white omelette. Or mix them into some low-fat cream cheese for a great bagel topping.

SKINNY-DIPPING

If you try to cut back on fat in your diet, as we have, your taste buds will probably cry foul. Ours sure did—but only until it dawned on us to add fresh herbs to our dishes.

Think about it: One tablespoon of butter has about 100 calories; 1 tablespoon of chives has just 1 calorie. If you were to replace a tablespoon of butter with a tablespoon of chives every day, you'd lose about a pound a month and not miss a thing!

Chive Baked Potatoes

If you have never cooked with chives before, this recipe, courtesy of the Idaho Potato Commission, is a great place to start.

¼ **cup low-fat plain yogurt**
½ **cup low-fat cottage cheese**
1½ **teaspoons chopped fresh parsley**
1½ **teaspoons chopped onion chives**
¼ **teaspoon salt**
¼ **teaspoon ground black pepper**
4 **potatoes, baked**

In a blender, process the yogurt, cottage cheese, parsley, chives, salt, and pepper until smooth. Split the potatoes open and spoon one-fourth of the mixture on top of each.

Yield: Four servings.

Nutritional data per serving: Calories, 251; protein, 9 g; carbohydrates, 53 g; fiber, 5 g; fat, 1 g; saturated fat, 0 g; cholesterol, 2 mg; sodium, 275 mg; calcium, 7% of Daily Value; iron, 16%.

Chocolate:

A Gift-Wrapped Assortment of Health Benefits

BATTLES:
- heart disease

BOLSTERS:
- longevity
- mood

When a roomful of registered dietitians, nutrition researchers, and health writers sit down for dinner, the scene is pretty much as you'd expect. Everybody wants salad dressing on the side. Nobody touches the saltshaker. They all fill their plates with more broccoli than most people eat in a week.

But when the main course has been eaten, something surprising happens: They start whispering about dessert—and how they hope it's chocolate. Chocolate! Not fruit, not angel food cake, not sugar-free Jell-O. Chocolate!

Men and women (but mostly women) who know by heart the calories, fat, and nutrients in virtually every food still want chocolate.

The point: If nutritionists aren't phobic about chocolate, maybe you don't have to feel guilty about reaching for a Russell Stover, digging into a Dove, or going for a Godiva. In fact, new research suggests that chocolate may even be healthy. It's not wishful thinking. Really!

HEALTH BY CHOCOLATE

No doubt you've heard about fruits such as strawberries being superior sources of antioxidants, compounds that battle cancer and heart disease. Five strawberries offer about 2,400 antioxidant units.

Well, chocolate offers more! Dark chocolate packs 5,700 antioxidant units in 1½ ounces (about the size of a standard candy bar), and milk chocolate weighs in at nearly 3,000.

"Ounce for ounce, dark chocolate has 10 times the antioxidants in strawberries," says Penny Kris-Etherton, Ph.D., R.D., distinguished professor of nutrition at Pennsylvania State University in State College. "But when you look at serving sizes, it's more like twice as many."

What do these antioxidants have to offer? For one thing, they may help us live longer. At Harvard University, a study of nearly 8,000 men found that those who ate chocolate and other candy—regardless of how much they indulged—lived a year longer than those who passed up these treats.

Dr. Kris-Etherton's research suggests that the type of saturated fat in cocoa butter—called stearic acid—doesn't raise bad low-density lipoprotein (LDL) cholesterol. In one study, she gave men 1⅓ ounces of cocoa powder (added to milk or pudding) and 2 tablespoons of chocolate chips. As expected, their levels of bad cholesterol remained steady. But surprisingly, their levels of good high-density lipoprotein (HDL) cholesterol increased.

"We used to think all saturated fat was bad for your heart," she says. "But now we know that there are some types of saturated fat, like the kind found in chocolate, that have neutral or beneficial effects."

Quick Fix:

Lactose Intolerance

If you have trouble digesting milk, stirring in a few teaspoons of cocoa may help, according to a study at the University of Rhode Island in Kingston. How? The cocoa may stimulate an enzyme that breaks down lactose, the compound in milk that may be responsible for your bloating and gas.

Test-tube research has shown that chocolate may prevent bad cholesterol from undergoing a process that makes it more damaging to your heart. Animal studies suggest that an antioxidant in cocoa powder may halt the growth of skin tumors. And scientists have long known—although they didn't need a study to tell you this—that chocolate contains a chemical that improves mood!

A KISS CAN MAKE IT BETTER

Given all the good news about chocolate, how often should you pass the candy dish? No one knows for sure, but the Harvard study indicated that moderate candy eaters—those who reached for one to three candy bars a month—fared the best, reducing their risk of dying by 36 percent over those who didn't eat chocolate.

"It also has a lot to do with the portions," points out Judith Stern, Ph.D., R.D., nutrition researcher at the University of California-Davis. "You can have a full-size chocolate bar a couple of times a month or a mini one every day." Her choice? You guessed it—the mini.

Researchers figure that you're also better off reaching for either solid chocolate candies or those with nuts rather than those with creamy fillings, which contribute calories but very few antioxidants. Also be careful of chocolate in desserts such as cake, cookies, and ice cream. Although you get the health benefits of the chocolate, they come with a lot of calories and other ingredients that could spell trouble for your heart.

The bottom line: Settle for a kiss.

NUTRITION IN A NUTSHELL

Dove Promises Dark Chocolate (1 miniature)

Calories: 31

Fat: 2 g

Saturated fat: 1 g

Cholesterol: 0 mg

Sodium: 5 mg

Total carbohydrates: 4 g

Dietary fiber: 0 g

Protein: 0 g

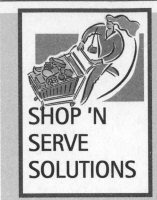

SHOP 'N SERVE SOLUTIONS

Shopping for chocolate is almost always fun! In general, look for chocolate that's made with cocoa butter rather than palm kernel oil. Cocoa butter won't raise your cholesterol, says Margo Denke, M.D., professor of internal medicine at the University of Texas Southwestern Medical Center in Dallas and one of the first researchers to break the news that chocolate has redeeming health qualities. Let your taste buds decide the rest.

Dr. Denke would rather opt for a single piece of wonderful chocolate than an entire bar of something that tastes just so-so. You can apply her suggestion to chocolate chips, too. The more flavorful they are, the fewer you'll need to feel satisfied.

CHOCOLATE MORNING, NOON, AND NIGHT!

Since you're already a pro at using chocolate in desserts, we thought you'd appreciate these healthier options:

◆ **Go skinny-dipping.** For an easy dessert, melt chocolate chips in the microwave on medium heat, stirring once or twice. Dunk the tips of strawberries, orange slices, pineapple rings, or prunes into the melted chocolate.

◆ **Accent your apples.** Core and slice an apple. Give the slices a thin coat of peanut butter, then sprinkle with a few mini chocolate chips. It makes a great snack.

◆ **Sweeten your cereal.** Love those sugar-laden kiddie cereals? We won't tell, but you have to try this instead. Deal? Pour yourself a bowl of low-sugar, high-fiber cereal, and add a tablespoon of mini chocolate chips and a tablespoon of mini marshmallows along with low-fat milk.

◆ **Make your sorbet snazzy.** Trade ice cream for sorbet or low-fat frozen yogurt, and drizzle it with a little chocolate syrup. Karen's favorite: raspberry sorbet with a teaspoon of chocolate sauce and a few fresh berries.

Cheery Chocolate Slush

A summertime alternative to hot chocolate, this fast-to-fix drink packs lots of calcium.

2 cups low-fat chocolate milk
2 tablespoons instant espresso powder
3 tablespoons unsweetened cocoa
¼ cup sugar
¾ teaspoon almond extract
2 cups ice cubes
¼ cup low-fat whipped cream

In a blender, combine the milk, espresso powder, cocoa, sugar, and almond extract until the sugar dissolves. Add the ice cubes and blend until smooth. Pour into four glasses. Top each serving with 1 tablespoon of the whipped cream.

Yield: Four servings.

Nutritional data per serving: Calories, 153; protein, 5 g; carbohydrates, 29 g; fiber, 3 g; fat, 3 g; saturated fat, 2 g; cholesterol, 4 mg; sodium, 78 mg; calcium, 15% of Daily Value; iron, 6%.

Cinnamon:

Old Spice
with a New Twist

BATTLES:
- food poisoning
- heart disease
- ulcers

BOLSTERS:
- healthy eating

Remember the aroma of fresh-from-the-bakery cinnamon buns on Sunday mornings long, long ago? Back then, of course, they accompanied bacon and eggs—not exactly what we're touting in this book! Nowadays, we use the scent of cinnamon to lure hungry eaters to healthier foods, such as fruits, vegetables, and rice.

Actually, the saga of cinnamon began with the birth of civilization. The Egyptian spice trade was booming in 2500 B.C. and included cinnamon, which came from Ceylon and eventually made its way to Greece and Rome. Citizens of the Eternal Empire developed a real "spice tooth," which they spread to all the territories they conquered. Not only did cinnamon and other spices taste good, but rumor has it, they also helped cover up the smell of rotting meat. But, hey, you shouldn't listen to rumors.

Researchers now think that cinnamon, along with cardamom, cloves, and other spices typically used in Asian cuisine, may actually prevent food spoilage. In one study, high doses of cinnamon

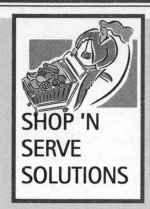

SHOP 'N
SERVE
SOLUTIONS

Cinnamon is the dried inner bark of two trees in the laurel family that grow in Asia. One is true cinnamon and is pale tan. But most of the cinnamon in our grocery stores comes from the other, and that's okay. This cinnamon is darker in color and has a stronger fragrance.

You can buy it ground or in sticks. When selecting cinnamon, look for a sealed container, and check the freshness date. Store your cinnamon in a cool, dark place.

WAKE UP YOUR TASTE BUDS

Keep your cinnamon handy, because there are so many ways to use it. Try these:

◆ **Go with the grain.** Cinnamon delivers a wake-up call at breakfast. Stir ground cinnamon into hot whole grain cereal, or sprinkle it on a whole grain waffle topped with fresh strawberries.

◆ **Update cinnamon toast.** Start with 100 percent whole wheat bread, spread with reduced-fat ricotta cheese, and sprinkle with ground cinnamon. Intense!

◆ **Squash fat.** Season winter squash, such as acorn or butternut, with ground cinnamon and toasted nuts, and you won't have to worry about whether butter or margarine is better. (See "Cinnamon Acorn Squash" on page 163.)

◆ **Get your just desserts.** Dust deli custard, pudding, or rice pudding with ground cinnamon for a homemade touch.

◆ **Cause a stir.** Use a cinnamon stick to stir your hot chocolate or hot apple cider for a little fun and a lot of taste.

◆ **Savor the daily grind.** Toss in a piece of cinnamon stick when you grind your coffee beans. Exotic!

NUTRITION IN A NUTSHELL

Ground cinnamon (1 teaspoon)

Calories: 6

Fat: 0 g

Saturated fat: 0 g

Cholesterol: 0 mg

Sodium: 0 mg

Total carbohydrates: 2 g

Dietary fiber: 1 g

Protein: 0 g

Calcium: 3% of Daily Value

Iron: 5%

Manganese: 19%

bark oil stopped mold from growing in lab dishes. (Hmmmm. Think this might work in our refrigerators?)

JUNK THAT GUNK

The other surprising news is that cinnamon seems to have some antioxidant activity. In one laboratory study, cinnamon and cloves turned out to be the nicest spices for preventing fatty acid oxidation. This chemical change turns cholesterol into the gunk that clogs your arteries, increasing heart disease risk. Other research suggests that cinnamon and cardamom may act by waking up antioxidant enzymes and sending them off to work.

BAN THE BLOAT

Cinnamon is also being tested for its ability to knock out *H. pylori*, the bacteria that cause most stomach ulcers. Stay tuned for more on that front. But in the meantime, if you have an upset stomach, bloating, or gas, try a cup of cinnamon tea. The German Commission E, which studies herbal medicines in Europe, says it really works.

Cinnamon Acorn Squash

When the cold winds blow, cook up this simple vegetable side dish. It'll warm your tummy and make your kitchen smell terrific!

1 medium acorn squash, halved and seeded
½ teaspoon ground cinnamon
2 tablespoons chopped toasted walnuts

Place the squash halves on a paper plate and microwave on high for 5 minutes. Turn the squash, then microwave for another 5 minutes, or until it is easily pierced with a fork. Place each half on a dinner plate and sprinkle with the cinnamon and walnuts.

Yield: Two servings.

Nutritional data per serving: Calories, 136; protein, 3 g; carbohydrates, 24 g; fiber, 4 g; fat, 5 g; saturated fat, 0 g; cholesterol, 0 mg; sodium, 7 mg; vitamin B_1 (thiamin), 22% of Daily Value; vitamin B_6, 19%; vitamin C, 27%; magnesium, 20%; manganese, 34%.

Corn:

A Bite for Sore Eyes

BATTLES:
- cancer

BOLSTERS:
- vision

Let's face it: A lot of men don't like many vegetables—corn and potatoes are pretty much it. So most cooks end up making a lot of corn, despite the fact that it doesn't offer much in the way of traditional vitamins and minerals. Fortunately, however, new research shows that corn packs a wad of antioxidants that are essential for your health. And that's good news for everyone!

NOW EAR THIS

Fresh yellow corn contains lutein and zeaxanthin, antioxidants that eye doctors are raving about. And it contains more than just a kernel of them, mind you. Corn is one of the best nongreen sources of these plant compounds. Even canned corn contains lutein and zeaxanthin, although it offers only about half the amount found in fresh yellow kernels.

So what's the fuss about? Here's what these nutrients can do for your eyes:

NUTRITION IN A NUTSHELL

Corn on the cob
(1 medium ear)

Calories: 75

Fat: 1 g

Saturated fat: 0 g

Cholesterol: 0 mg

Sodium: 15 mg

Total carbohydrates: 17 g

Dietary fiber: 1 g

Protein: 3 g

Folate: 9% of Daily Value

Vitamin A: 5%

Vitamin C: 10%

Iron: 3%

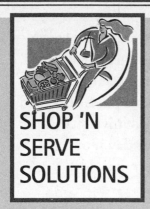

SHOP 'N SERVE SOLUTIONS

Want the freshest, sweetest corn? Be a cob snob: Skip the supermarket, and buy it directly from a farmer. Because corn begins to lose its sweetness after it's picked, much of what you find at the supermarket is already past its prime. Instead, head to the country or to the local farmers' market. And take a cooler with you.

WHEN SELECTING CORN:

■ Look for tight, bright green husks.

■ Strip back part of the husks to check the kernels. Be sure the kernels at the tip are smaller than those in the middle. If not, that's a sign that the corn might not be as sweet as you'd like.

■ Once you purchase the perfect ears, stash them in a cooler if you have a long trip home. Heat saps corn's sweetness, too.

WHEN STORING:

Ideally, you should cook corn the same day you buy it. But you can put the unhusked ears in a plastic bag and then store them in the fridge for up to three days.

GET CORNY

Now here are a couple of cooking ideas:

◆ **Brush with vinaigrette.** Instead of blasting your corn with butter—it's not exactly heart-friendly—season it with herb vinaigrette.

◆ **Make a gourmet salsa.** Sure, you could pay $5 a jar for one, but that's not necessary. Instead, buy one of the buck-a-bottle brands, and mix in corn that's fresh from the cob or straight from the can. We won't tell.

▶ **Derail macular degeneration.** Researchers have found that people with low levels of lutein and zeaxanthin in their diets are more likely to suffer from age-related macular degeneration (ARMD)—the leading cause of blindness in older Americans—than those with higher levels. A study at Harvard University showed that consuming 6 milligrams of lutein per day reduced the risk of ARMD by 43 percent! (One ear of corn provides about 1 milligram of lutein.)

▶ **Cancel cataracts.** Corn also may help protect your peepers by warding off cataracts. Another Harvard study concluded that men and women who ate a lot of lutein-rich foods cut their risk of cataracts by about one-fifth.

THE LATEST RESEARCH

Scientists in other areas of medicine also are exploring the health benefits of these antioxidants. And their results are pretty amazing, as well. Consider this:

▶ Preliminary research suggests that lutein and zeaxanthin may help protect against the sun damage that leads to skin cancer.

▶ Another recent study found that men and women with the highest levels of lutein in their diets had a 17 percent lower risk of colon cancer than those with the lowest levels.

The bottom line: The ears have it!

Super Summer Quesadillas

Put your corn to good use in this healthy version of a Mexican favorite. How does it taste? In a word: fantástico!

Canola oil cooking spray
1 tablespoon canola oil
½ cup chopped red onion
2 cloves garlic, minced
½ cup chopped sweet red pepper
1½ cups yellow sweet corn, freshly cut
from the cob (about 2 ears)
¼ cup chopped fresh basil
⅓ cup grated smoked cheddar cheese
4 flour tortillas (8-inch diameter)
½ cup salsa (garnish)

Coat a large nonstick skillet with cooking spray and the oil. In the skillet over medium heat, sauté the onion and garlic for 5 minutes, or until the onion begins to soften. Add the pepper and cook for 3 to 4 minutes. Add the corn and basil. Sauté, stirring often, for 4 to 5 minutes, or until the vegetables are cooked to the desired tenderness. Remove from the heat. Stir in the cheese and cover until melted.

Meanwhile, coat another nonstick skillet with cooking spray. In the skillet over medium heat, grill the tortillas for 20 to 30 seconds on each side, or until crisp. Spread the filling on 2 of the tortillas. Top with the remaining tortillas. Cut each quesadilla into quarters. Garnish with the salsa.

Yield: Four 2-piece servings.

Nutritional data per serving: Calories, 244; protein, 7 g; carbohydrates, 33 g; fiber, 4 g; fat, 10 g; saturated fat, 3 g; cholesterol, 10 mg; sodium, 554 mg; calcium, 13% of Daily Value; iron, 14%.

Cranberries:

Concentrated Power
That Protects

BATTLES:
- allergies
- colon cancer
- heart disease
- urinary tract infections

Hey, girlfriend, are you tired of UTIs—you know, what your doctor calls urinary tract infections? They're fairly common, accounting for seven million doctor visits each year. Most women get them at one time or another, but for some of us, they're a constant companion.

If you're ready for relief, it's time to start juicing up with cranberries.

THEY'RE FLUSH WITH TANNINS

Maybe you think that the stories about the protective power of cranberries are just old wives' tales. But they are true! Research done at Harvard Medical School showed

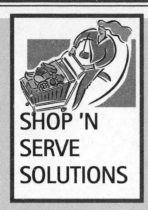

SHOP 'N SERVE SOLUTIONS

Fresh cranberries are available from September through December, just in time to make your own cranberry sauce for Thanksgiving.

WHEN SELECTING CRANBERRIES:

Look for berries that are plump, firm, and dark red. As with most fruits and vegetables, the darker the color, the greater the amount of antioxidants they contain.

WHEN STORING:

■ Store cranberries in their original bag in the refrigerator. They'll keep for up to two weeks.

■ Alternatively, freeze them in their original bag wrapped in extra plastic (to protect against freezer burn and dehydration). Then use them all year long.

WHEN YOU'RE READY TO USE:

Just before eating your refrigerated or frozen berries, rinse and sort them under running water.

CRAVE THOSE CRANBERRIES!

Use cranberries in these tasty ways:

◆ **Gobble up cranberry sauce.** Spread cranberry sauce on your turkey sandwich. It's a deliciously fat-free way to enjoy Thanksgiving leftovers and also a pretty good way to dress up deli sandwiches year-round. Try it on pork chops, too. They're leaner and drier now, and zesty cranberry sauce keeps them juicy and flavorful.

◆ **Go wild.** Cook up a batch of wild rice, and toss in some chopped celery, chopped dried apricots, and fresh or frozen cranberries. If company is already knocking at your door and you want to make a splash, use a white rice–wild rice quick mix.

that elderly women who drank 1¼ cups of cranberry juice every day for a month were only 42 percent as likely to have a UTI as those who did not. And if they continued drinking the tangy thirst quencher, their chances dropped even more.

Now researchers at Rutgers University's blueberry and cranberry research center in Chatsworth, New Jersey, think they've found the reason why. *E. coli* bacteria (the usual cause of UTIs) grow little hooks, like Velcro, that latch onto urinary tract walls. Instead of being washed away by the water you drink, they hang around and multiply, causing a massive infection. Fortunately, cranberry juice packs a powerful antidote, called condensed tannins, that appears to detach the hooks, so the bacteria can be washed away.

A SLENDER ALTERNATIVE

To get enough condensed tannins, you'll need a drink that's 27 percent cranberry juice. The cranberry juice you find in the supermarket measures up, but it has added sugar. Usually, a sweetened juice would not be considered a healthy food, but cranberry juice is an exception. In its natural state, this juice is so sour that you can't drink it straight.

Unfortunately, the sweetened variety packs 175 calories in the 10 ounces you'll need each day to flush the bugs. If you're calorie-conscious, switch to Ocean Spray Lightstyle Cranberry Juice Cocktail. This juice is sweetened with Splenda (sucralose) and weighs in at just 50 calories per 10-ounce serving.

THE DAILY DILEMMA

By now you're probably thinking, "Yes, I love that tart, refreshing taste, but *every day?*" Cheer up— you have other options:

Quick Fix:

Allergy Sneezes

Cranberries are naturally rich in quercetin, a natural antihistamine that can help cut down on the sneezing that comes with airborne allergens.

BORN IN THE U.S.A.

Cranberries are an all-American fruit that Native Americans used for food and medicine long before the *Mayflower* landed. The Pilgrims, however, did invent the name we use today.

As ships sailed between the Old World and the New, American sailors packed a couple of buckets of vitamin C-rich cranberries to prevent scurvy. British sailors relied on limes, hence the nickname "limey."

While there are more than 100 different varieties of cranberries, only 4 are commonly harvested: Early Blacks, Howes, McFarlins, and Searles.

▶ **One-fourth cup of Craisins** (dried cranberries infused with cranberry concentrate and sugar) also packs enough tannins to get the job done.

▶ **One cup of fresh or frozen blueberries** also does the job.

▶ **Ten ounces of cranberry/blueberry cocktail** provides the same bacteria-squelching power as straight cranberry juice.

But don't go too far astray. Mixing peach, kiwifruit, or other nonberry fruits with cranberries tastes delicious, too, but waters down the tannins' power, leaving you unprotected.

MORE BERRY MAGIC

Cranberries also contain ellagic acid, now being explored as a colon cancer fighter. And in lab dishes, cranberry extract prevents cholesterol from becoming sticky enough to clog arteries. Since cranberries are low in the ingredients now known to fight arterial gunk, researchers are still playing "Name That Antioxidant." But a rose (or antioxidant) by any other name still gets the job done. Just call it all cranberry magic—and enjoy!

Cranberry Muffins

When Thanksgiving rolls around, bake up a batch of these muffins. Of course, nobody eats them with dinner, because there's just too much turkey and trimmings. Instead, suggest that your guests take the muffins home for breakfast the next morning.

2 cups whole wheat flour
¾ cup sugar
1½ teaspoons baking powder
½ teaspoon salt
½ teaspoon baking soda
¼ cup canola oil
1 medium egg, beaten
1 teaspoon grated orange peel
¾ cup calcium-fortified orange juice
3 cups fresh cranberries, chopped
½ cup pecans, coarsely broken

Preheat the oven to 400°F. Line a large muffin pan with cupcake papers. Sift the flour, sugar, baking powder, salt, and baking soda into a large bowl. In a small bowl, combine the oil, egg, orange peel, and orange juice. Quickly stir into the flour mixture, just until the mixture is evenly moist. Fold in the cranberries and pecans. Fill the muffin cups two-thirds full with the batter. Bake for 15 minutes, or until a toothpick inserted in the center of a muffin comes out clean. Remove the muffins from the pan and cool on a wire rack.

Yield: 12 muffins.

Nutritional data per serving: Calories, 220; protein, 4 g; carbohydrates, 34 g; fiber, 4 g; fat, 9 g; saturated fat, 1 g; cholesterol, 16 mg; sodium, 104 mg; vitamin A, 1% of Daily Value; vitamin C, 11%; calcium, 7%; iron, 7%; manganese, 13%.

Cucumbers:
They're Way Cool

BATTLES:
- cancer
- heart disease
- puffy eyes

BOLSTERS:
- hydration
- weight control

For a long time, we thought cucumbers were, well, blah. They were just one more green ingredient in a salad. Nothing special, really. But we've learned that when you give cucumbers a starring role in your dish, they come alive.

Nutritionists have made an about-face with cucumbers, too. While they once regarded them as a nothing vegetable—few calories, but also few nutrients—dietitians now realize that there's more to cucumbers than meets the eye.

DREAMS COME TRUE
Let's start with the basics. One-third of an average-size cucumber contributes about 10 percent of the vitamin C and roughly 5 percent of the potassium you need for the day. We know that sounds paltry, but it's practically for free—costing you only 13 calories. Both vitamin C and potassium chip away at your risk of heart disease.

HIDDEN BENEFITS
Several years ago, Colleen pointed out that although cucumbers don't have much in the way of traditional vitamins and

minerals, she wouldn't be surprised if scientists uncovered beneficial phytochemicals—plant compounds—in them. She was right on the money.

Researchers now know that cucumbers contain phytosterols and terpenes, both believed to diminish the risk of cancer.

LOW-CALORIE CRUNCH

Not a convert yet? See how this one grabs you: Cucumbers may help you lose weight. Research at Pennsylvania State University in State College has shown that foods with a low energy density—that is, they take up a lot of room in your stomach for few calories—can help you shed some pounds. The theory suggests that when you eat these foods, you feel full on fewer calories, and so you stop eating.

Cucumbers and romaine lettuce are tied for the position of vegetable with the lowest energy density. So toss them in to your sandwiches and salads for extra bulk. Oh, and pack them in your picnic basket, especially on hot days. Cucumbers are mainly water and may provide you with the extra fluid you need to ward off dehydration.

NUTRITION IN A NUTSHELL
Cucumber (⅓ medium)
Calories: 13
Fat: 0 g
Saturated fat: 0 g
Cholesterol: 0 mg
Sodium: 2 mg
Total carbohydrates: 3 g
Dietary fiber: 1 g
Protein: 1 g
Vitamin C: 9% of Daily Value

Quick Fix:

Puffy Eyes

If you have puffy allergy eyes (as Karen sometimes does), place a cucumber slice on each eye for a couple of minutes. The cucumber slices cause blood vessels to constrict, which may reduce the puffiness.

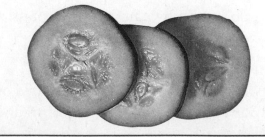

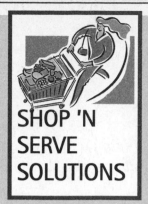

SHOP 'N SERVE SOLUTIONS

Good news: You can usually find a wide variety of cucumbers at your supermarket all year long.

WHEN SELECTING CUCUMBERS:

■ Choose cukes that are very firm and rounded right to the ends.

■ Opt for those that are a rich green.

■ If you're not a big fan of the seeds (who is, really?), pick up one of the slender European varieties, because they are usually seedless—or close to it.

WHEN STORING:

Keep all cucumbers in the fridge's crisper. If they're waxed and uncut, they'll last for about a week. Otherwise, check your cucumbers every day or two.

WHEN YOU'RE READY TO USE:

Before you dig in, wash your cucumber—even if you're planning on peeling it. That way, you won't transfer bacteria from the outside to the delicious inside. Waxed cukes should be peeled. With unwaxed ones, it's your choice.

GETTING CUTE WITH CUKES

Now here's what to do with your cucumbers besides adding them to plain old green salad:

◆ **Go British.** Spread thin slices of pumpernickel bread with light cream cheese and top it with cucumber slices. Add a little grated carrot for extra crunch. Makes a great "tea sandwich" to serve at high tea.

◆ **Make a cucumber sauce.** Stir chopped peeled cucumber into low-fat plain yogurt seasoned with your favorite herbs. (We like to use chives.) Serve with grilled chicken or fish.

◆ **Invigorate pasta.** Add diced cucumbers and diced tomatoes to your favorite pasta salad.

Five-Ingredient Cucumber Toss

It never fails: Whenever Karen plans a picnic, the mercury soars. So she often makes this refreshing cucumber salad to beat the heat.

2 medium cucumbers, peeled and chopped
2 large tomatoes, chopped
2 tablespoons chopped fresh basil
¼ cup reduced-fat Italian dressing
¼ cup feta cheese

In a large mixing bowl, toss the cucumbers, tomatoes, basil, dressing, and cheese. Chill for an hour or two before serving, to blend the flavors.

Yield: Four servings.

Nutritional data per serving: Calories, 76; protein, 3 g; carbohydrates, 11 g; fiber, 2 g; fat, 3 g; saturated fat, 1 g; cholesterol, 6 mg; sodium, 171 mg; calcium, 7% of Daily Value; iron, 6%.

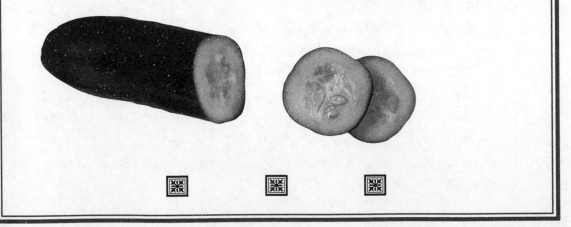

Curry Powder:

The Spice for Life

BATTLES:
- cancer
- diabetes
- heartburn
- stuffy nose

BOLSTERS:
- digestion
- immune funcion

We love to eat at a local Indian restaurant. Why, besides not having to wash dishes? Curry powder, of course! This Indian seasoning, made from as many as 20 different spices, including cinnamon, coriander, nutmeg, and turmeric, plays a starring role on the menu at all Indian restaurants.

KICK CANCER

Turmeric, the spice that lends curry powder its distinctive yellow color, is probably a potent cancer crusader. Preliminary studies from India suggest that two compounds in the spice—curcumin I and II—may possess cancer-fighting properties and also boost the immune system.

Researchers around the world are trying to pin down the details. Here's what they've learned so far:

▶ A British study found that turmeric may inhibit production of an enzyme found in high levels in certain types of cancer, including bowel and colon.

▶ Research at Columbia University College of Physicians and Surgeons in New York City suggests that turmeric may help in the fight against prostate cancer, too.

Stay tuned. You'll probably hear about more studies on the news soon.

DEFY DIABETES

Not to scare you, but people are getting type 2 diabetes earlier and earlier. We know people in their 20s with the condition. This type of diabetes can be the result of your bad habits catching up with you—too much high-calorie, high-fat food and not enough exercise. But with a better diet, regular exercise, and maybe a few spices, you may be able to ward off this condition, or at least diminish the severity of it.

When you have diabetes, your body doesn't make enough insulin, the hormone that delivers blood sugar to your cells. Turmeric, along with bay leaves, cinnamon, and cloves, can help regulate your body's level of insulin. In lab studies, this foursome spice creation tripled the ability of insulin to metabolize glucose, the blood sugar that supplies us with energy. More research is underway, but in the meantime, it can't hurt to be, well, a spice girl.

Quick Fix:

Heartburn

If heartburn has its evil spell on you, sprinkle a little curry powder on your food. Turmeric, a key ingredient in curry powder, stimulates the flow of digestive juices, which helps stave off the buildup of heartburn-provoking acid.

NUTRITION IN A NUTSHELL

Curry powder (1 teaspoon)

Calories: 7

Fat: 0 g

Saturated fat: 0 g

Cholesterol: 0 mg

Sodium: 1 mg

Total carbohydrates: 1 g

Dietary fiber: 1 g

Protein: 0 g

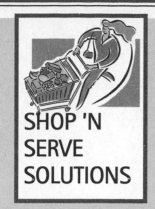

SHOP 'N SERVE SOLUTIONS

There are up to 20 different spices in traditional curry powder, so unless you have a big budget and a lot of time (neither one of which we are blessed with), we suggest that you buy the prepackaged spice rather than make your own.

Curry powder is readily available in your supermarket. Almost every spice manufacturer makes it—although some with more success than others. The Seattle Times *recently taste-tested several brands of curry powder and thought these two were tops:*

■ **Spice Islands Curry Powder.** Described as having a "smooth quality and soft golden color."

■ **Trikona Mild Curry Powder.** Described as having a "rich golden color and deep, spicy flavor."

Whatever your choice, store your curry powder in a cool, dry, dark place. If you reseal it after each use, it'll last for a few months before losing its kick.

ENJOY A TASTE OF THE TAJ MAHAL

Now here are some all-American approaches to using this exotic Indian flavor:

◆ **Dips ahoy!** Stir a teaspoon or two of curry powder into a cup of low-fat plain yogurt. Serve with baked tortilla chips or warm pita bread.

◆ **Charge chickpeas.** Mix a can of rinsed and drained chickpeas with a couple of teaspoons of curry powder. Bake in the oven at 375°F for 12 to 15 minutes.

◆ **Pump up popcorn.** Sprinkle curry powder on air-popped corn or even on low-fat chips. It'll give these foods a shot of flavor!

Curry Rice Pilaf

We snagged this recipe, a feast for the eyes and the taste buds, from the U.S.A. Rice Federation.

1 cup uncooked long-grain white rice
⅓ cup seedless raisins
⅓ cup chopped dried apple
2 tablespoons chicken bouillon granules
2 teaspoons curry powder
1 tablespoon butter
1¾ cups water

In a large bowl, combine the rice, raisins, apple, bouillon granules, and curry powder. Mix well. In a 2- to 3-quart saucepan, combine the rice mixture with the butter and water. Bring to a boil, stirring once or twice. Reduce the heat, cover, and simmer for about 15 minutes, or until the water is absorbed. Fluff with a fork and serve.

Yield: Six servings.

Nutritional data per serving: Calories, 167; protein, 3 g; carbohydrates, 34 g; fiber, 1 g; fat, 2 g; saturated fat, 1 g; cholesterol, 5 mg; sodium, 22 mg; calcium, 2% of Daily Value; iron, 10%.

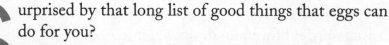

Eggs:

Incredible! Edible! And Good for You!

BATTLES:
- age-related macular degeneration
- heart disease
- hypoglycemia
- stroke

BOLSTERS:
- bones
- brain development in infants
- brain function
- immune function
- memory
- vision

Surprised by that long list of good things that eggs can do for you?

Years ago, Woody Allen made one of his funniest movies, called *Sleeper,* in which he awoke from a coma to find that everything that was "bad for you" when he fell asleep was now "good for you."

Well, things aren't quite that bad in the nutrition world, but sometimes it seems like it, especially when we start to talk about eggs. Eggs, especially the yolks, are loaded with nutrients that everybody needs, but many of us don't get enough of.

WHICH CAME FIRST?

Want a baby with a great memory that lasts forever? Be a good mom while you're pregnant and nursing, and eat some eggs.

NEWS FROM THE NEST

If you've been avoiding eggs, you may have missed these new arrivals:

■ **Davidson's Pasteurized Eggs.** These eggs are gently heat-treated to eliminate 99.999 percent of salmonella bacteria, making them safe for anyone to eat any way he or she wants (including folks at high risk). Prepare them soft-cooked or sunny-side up. Make Caesar salad or eggnog with them. You can even safely eat cookie dough! Use them as you would any regular in-shell egg.

■ **Eggland's Best.** These patented eggs come from chickens fed a vegetarian diet, canola oil, and extra vitamin E. As a result, two eggs deliver 50 percent of the Daily Value for vitamin E (important for heart health and immune function), about six times more than standard eggs provide.

■ **EggsPlus.** The chickens producing these eggs are fed vitamin E and flaxseeds, pushing vitamin E content for two eggs to 50 percent of the Daily Value and providing 200 milligrams of omega-3 fatty acids (the kind you usually only get from fatty fish). Omega-3s have been shown to reduce the risk of heart disease and stroke.

Their yolks are the top source of choline, a recently recognized essential nutrient for brain development.

Here's what we know: Rats whose moms chow down on choline during pregnancy and lactation learn mazes faster and with fewer mistakes. Getting choline early, while its brain is developing, permanently changes and enlarges a rat's hippocampus, where memory resides. Even in old age, choline-fed rats have better memories.

LET'S GET CRACKING

So, do human brains work the same way? We don't know yet. But changes in blood levels of choline in human and rat moms during pregnancy and breast-feeding are similar, suggesting that it's possible. So research is underway. Meanwhile, get cracking. A two-egg meal doubles blood choline levels. Milk is another good source.

DON'T RUN OUT OF EGGS

Athletes in heavy training should shake a leg and hard-boil some eggs. Recent research has shown that blood choline can drop by 40 percent after heavy exercise. And choline supplements boosted performance in marathon runners and helped maintain blood choline levels in triathletes.

Why not just take a supplement? "It takes several grams of choline supplements to cross the blood brain barrier, and that much makes you smell like fish!" says Jim Joseph, Ph.D., chief of the neuroscience laboratory at Tufts University in Boston. So break an egg, and you'll get other benefits, too, such as high-quality protein.

GRANDMA'S PERFECT FOOD

Older adults need more protein, B vitamins, vitamin D, calcium, and zinc than younger people do. Yet many don't even meet the Daily Values, much less get bonus amounts. And they probably need more choline for memory, says the Institute of Medicine in Washington, D.C.

Why are they falling short? Older

Quick Fix:

Low Blood Sugar

Have hypoglycemia? Eat three small meals a day, with high-protein snacks in between. A hard-boiled egg fills the bill for lifting you out of a midafternoon slump.

NUTRITION IN A NUTSHELL

Egg (1 medium)

Calories: 68

Fat: 5 g

Saturated fat: 1 g

Cholesterol: 186 mg

Sodium: 55 mg

Total carbohydrates: 0 g

Dietary fiber: 0 g

Protein: 6 g

Vitamin A: 9% of Daily Value

Vitamin B$_{12}$: 13%

Vitamin D: 11%

Calcium: 2%

Iron: 3%

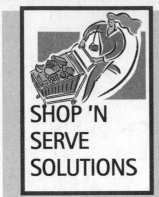

SHOP 'N SERVE SOLUTIONS

Eggs are available in sizes from small to jumbo. Medium eggs, however, are the size called for in most recipes. And they are the most economical to buy.

WHEN SELECTING EGGS:

■ To prevent salmonella poisoning, buy only eggs that have been kept cold in the dairy case.

■ Check each egg in the carton and don't buy any that are cracked or dirty.

WHEN STORING:

■ Stash eggs deep in the fridge (not in the door!), where they'll stay plenty cold.

■ If you hard-boil a batch of eggs, cool them under running water and then put them right back in the fridge for safekeeping.

ADDING EGGS-TRA OOMPH TO MEALS

You probably know just what to do with an egg, but here are a few more ideas:

◆ **Top a tossed salad.** Peel and slice a hard-boiled egg to add protein to your veggies.

◆ **Highlight cooked spinach.** Chop your hard-boiled egg, then scatter the pieces on cooked spinach for eye appeal and lutein-rich eye protection.

◆ **Brighten a waffle.** Toast a whole grain waffle and top it with a poached egg.

people require fewer calories, which means every bite has to be jam-packed with nutrients. So it's eggs to the rescue! They come in single-serving packages (no leftovers!) stuffed with easy-to-digest protein for maintaining muscle and building immunity against pneumonia and flu.

The yolks (the part that you've been throwing away!) are loaded with these important nutrients:

▶ **B vitamins.** These vitamins boost germ-fighting immunity, maintain memory, and prevent heart attack and stroke.

▶ **Vitamin D.** It builds bone and boosts memory and clear thinking.

▶ **Lutein and zeaxanthin.** These two carotenoids are critical for preventing age-related macular degeneration, the major cause of blindness in adults. These sight-saving nutrients are absorbed more easily from eggs than from green vegetables.

So scramble to the kitchen and cook yourself—and your mom—an egg.

EGG ON OUR FACE?

In defense of nutritionists, we'd like to say that no one ever advised the nation to stop eating eggs entirely. Cut down? Yes. And change their surroundings? Definitely! Forget fried eggs with bacon and sausage and white toast slathered with butter. All that saturated fat could send your cholesterol soaring.

But if you boil or poach your egg, for example, and then serve it with whole wheat toast smeared with peanut butter and wash it down with a glass of orange juice, your heart will jump for joy!

MORE EGGS-ACT SCIENCE

Thirty years ago, when the drive to defeat heart disease went into high gear, we were told to limit cholesterol intake to 300 milligrams per day. Since an egg yolk packs 186 milligrams, it might have seemed reasonable to just ditch eggs. But even the American Heart Association said that folks on a cholesterol-lowering diet may eat two or three eggs (with yolks) a week.

After years of scientific research, we've learned that it's not the cholesterol in foods, but the saturated fat oozing from bacon, burgers, and ice cream that raises our blood cholesterol. In fact, most people (except for those with very high cholesterol) can eat an egg a day without a problem.

Egg studies abound, but you may find two of particular interest. One followed 38,000 men for 8 years, and the other tracked 80,000 women for 14 years. Both studies found that—except for people with diabetes—those who ate an egg a day were no more likely to have a heart attack or stroke than those who ate less than one a week. So don't be hard-boiled—enjoy an egg now and then!

WHAT ABOUT RAW EGGS?

In recent years, the risk of salmonella poisoning from eating raw eggs has risen dramatically. Although most healthy people can withstand the onslaught, some risk death by dehydration from prolonged diarrhea. Fortunately, thorough cooking makes eggs perfectly safe.

Avoid eggs with runny yolks, raw cookie dough, real Caesar salad (which is made with raw egg), and traditional eggnog if you're in one of these high-risk groups:

▶ pregnant women

▶ young children

▶ the elderly

▶ those who are immune-compromised (undergoing chemotherapy or HIV-positive)

Egg Salad Sandwich

Remember that good old-fashioned egg salad? It was mostly eggs and mayo. Now you can have a big, fat sandwich that's a phytochemical feast by bulking up your egg with veggies.

1 hard-boiled egg, chopped
1 tablespoon light mayonnaise
¼ cup chopped celery
¼ cup chopped red radishes
½ cup diced, peeled cucumber
⅛ teaspoon celery seeds
¹⁄₁₆ teaspoon salt
Dash of freshly ground black pepper
2 slices whole wheat bread
2 slices tomato
Lettuce

In a small bowl, combine the egg, mayonnaise, celery, radishes, cucumber, celery seeds, salt, and pepper. Stir until well blended. Pile the mixture on 1 slice of the bread, and top with the tomato, lettuce, and the remaining slice of bread. Cut in half diagonally.

Yield: One serving.

Nutritional data per serving: Calories, 282; protein, 12 g; carbohydrates, 33 g; fiber, 6 g; fat, 12 g; saturated fat, 3 g; cholesterol, 192 mg; sodium, 350 mg; folate, 19% of Daily Value; vitamin B$_2$ (riboflavin), 23%; vitamin C, 21%; vitamin D, 14%; vitamin E, 12%; zinc, 12%.

Fennel:

Seeds of Cancer Destruction

BATTLES:
- cancer
- inflammation

BOLSTERS:
- weight control

Several years ago, while vacationing in the Sonoma Valley in northern California, Colleen stumbled upon some fennel growing wild. She collected the seeds and planted them in her own backyard in Maryland. They grew into tall, top-heavy plants that reseed every year, so she always has fresh fennel to add to pork dishes. Eventually, she gave some of the seeds to her daughter Bobbi, and now she has grandchild fennel!

Each fall, after Colleen harvests her seeds, she cuts the plants off at the ground, gathers them into a bunch, and then stands them in a large pot that Bobbi made in ceramics class. At nearly 6 feet tall, the arrangement is quite impressive. And it makes the house smell so good! To enhance the natural room-freshening effect, Colleen adds last year's bundle to the woodpile and burns it bit by bit in the fireplace over the winter.

ANCIENT SEEDS, MODERN MEDICINE

Fennel seeds have been around practically forever. Ancient Egyptians called the fennel plant "fragrant hay," but it's actually

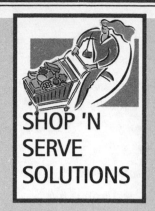

SHOP 'N SERVE SOLUTIONS

Fennel bulb is available in large grocery stores, mostly in winter. The finest fennel bulb looks nice and clean, is firm with straight stalks, and sports fresh-looking green, feathery leaves. Take it home, trim the stalks off at the bulb, wrap each in a plastic bag, and then store the fennel in the fridge, where it'll keep for four to five days.

You'll find fennel seeds in the spice section of your grocery store. They should be fresh-looking and deeply colored, rather than dried-out and pale.

FUN WITH FENNEL

Here are a few neat ways to add a different taste to everyday dishes:

◆ **Dice it.** Instead of celery, dice a fennel bulb into your chicken or tuna salad.

◆ **Sliver it.** Thinly slice a fennel bulb, mix with chopped onion and garlic, and then simmer in chicken broth for about 15 minutes. Drain and serve with a squeeze of fresh lemon juice. It's great with chicken or lean pork!

◆ **Shave it.** Toss fennel bulb shavings with red onion shavings and green leaf lettuce. Dress with oil and balsamic vinegar, and garnish with freshly grated Parmesan cheese.

◆ **Clip it.** Snip fennel leaves into salad.

◆ **Toss it.** Throw some fennel seeds into bread dough just before shaping and baking.

part of the carrot clan. Close relatives include anise (you'll find it in Italian sausage), caraway (in rye bread), coriander (the seed from which you grow cilantro), cumin (essential for Mexican and Indian dishes), parsley (the worldwide garnish), and dill (the best in red-skin potato salad). When they all get together, what a flavorful family!

But although fennel seeds are ancient, scientists with their test tubes and lab mice have just started discovering natural ingredients in the seeds that may help keep you alive and well long enough to enjoy all that delicious flavor.

One recent discovery is anethole, which has been shown to block inflammation and to prevent cancer formation. Fennel seeds also provide modest amounts of flavonols, including quercetin, a more powerful antioxidant than vitamin E, suggesting that these seeds may add to the protective army of fruits and vegetables such as apples, onions, and tea that ward off heart disease. And, of course, flavoring with fennel instead of saturated fat such as butter or cream is heart-smart and waist-conscious, too!

NUTRITION IN A NUTSHELL

Fennel seeds
(1 tablespoon)

Calories: 20

Fat: 1 g

Saturated fat: 0 g

Cholesterol: 0 mg

Sodium: 5 mg

Total carbohydrates: 3 g

Dietary fiber: 2 g

Protein: 1 g

Calcium: 7% of Daily Value

Iron: 6%

Magnesium: 6%

Manganese: 19%

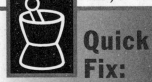

Quick Fix:

Icky Breath

Need a breath mint? Chew on a few fennel seeds. They'll make you kissing-sweet! Hint: They're often served for free at the end of a meal in Indian restaurants.

ENJOY THE LIGHT BULB

Fennel bulb is the edible base of one type of fennel plant. It looks like fat celery with green feathers. Like celery, it's very low in calories (about 27 per cup), but it packs more fiber (about 3 grams) and a little vitamin A (about 2 percent of Daily Value), which is important for protecting all your mucous membranes against invading bacteria and viruses. Fennel bulb makes a top-notch diet food because it tastes a lot like licorice, is bulky and filling, and, best of all, is nearly calorie-free!

One-Dish Fennel Pork

Pork tenderloin is about as lean a meat as you can get. But it's way too large a cut for two people to eat in one meal, so there are always delicious leftovers. Here's a quickie supper that uses up those leftovers. It sings with the flavor of fennel, so it resonates with Colleen's Eastern European ancestors, but it drains the fat from the good old days.

2 cups low-sodium sauerkraut, rinsed and drained
½ cup water
1 tablespoon fennel seeds
2 cups baby carrots, split
4 whole small canned potatoes
6 ounces cooked, leftover pork tenderloin, thinly sliced

Place the sauerkraut in a large nonstick skillet with the water. Sprinkle the fennel seeds evenly over the sauerkraut. Top with the carrots, potatoes, and pork. Cover, bring to a boil, and then simmer for about 5 minutes, or until the carrots are tender and all the ingredients are hot.

Yield: Two servings.

Nutritional data per serving: Calories, 304; protein, 28 g; carbohydrates, 36 g; fiber, 11 g; fat, 5 g; saturated fat, 1.5 g; cholesterol, 67 mg; sodium, 902 mg; vitamin A, 792% of Daily Value; vitamin B_1 (thiamin), 65%; vitamin C, 46%; iron, 28%; potassium, 38%.

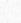

Figs:
An Ancient Health Food

BATTLES:
- cancer
- heart disease
- high blood pressure
- high cholesterol
- stroke

BOLSTERS:
- regularity
- weight control

When Karen worked on her college newspaper, the staff had an official cookie: Fig Newtons. You could find an open bag in the office every Monday, when the team of kids was frantically assembling the weekly issue. At the time, Karen turned her nose up at figs, often baking cupcakes for the marathon sessions. Now, a decade later, Karen still likes (and bakes) cupcakes. But she's wild about figs, too. She's fig-ured out that this ancient fruit tastes fabulous—and not just in cookies!

GO FIG-URE!
Never tried a fig? You don't know what you're missing. Figs supply a boatload of nutrients, benefiting your body in different ways:

▶ **Fiber.** Each serving of dried figs (three Calimyrna or four or five Mission figs) contributes about 5 grams of fiber. About one-quarter of that fiber is the soluble type that works to reduce cholesterol levels. A recent study also found that soluble fiber may

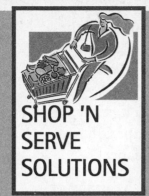

SHOP 'N SERVE SOLUTIONS

During summer and early fall, you'll be able to buy fresh figs, as well as dried. And you should buy them, because the taste of fresh figs is unbelievable.

WHEN SELECTING FRESH FIGS:

■ Look for figs that are plump and unblemished.

■ Buy ones that are soft to the touch, but not mushy.

■ Sniff figs, too, because a sour smell tips you off to spoilage.

WHEN STORING:

The one drawback to fresh figs is that they have the shortest shelf life on the planet. Once they're harvested, they last no longer than a week. By the time you pick them up at the store, they may have only two good days left. So handle them with care: To prevent bruising, place fresh figs in a container lined with paper towels, then refrigerate them immediately.

FIGGY FUN

Now you're ready to add figs to your menu. Try these techniques:

◆ **Sweeten your oatmeal.** Stir chopped fresh or dried figs into your morning oatmeal for a natural hint of sweetness. If you haven't refrigerated your figs, do so for an hour to make them easier to cut.

◆ **Perk up your greens.** Top a bed of greens with chopped walnuts and sliced figs. Season with a vinaigrette dressing, such as "Basil Balsamic Vinaigrette" on page 106.

◆ **Bulk up your bread.** Toss chopped figs in a little flour and add them to bread or muffin batter just as you would dried apricots or berries. What's the flour for? It prevents the figs from settling to the bottom of the baked goods.

◆ **Stick 'em up.** Skewer figs along with bananas and your other favorite fruits. Serve the kebabs as a side dish along with grilled chicken or pork.

NUTRITION IN A NUTSHELL

Dried figs (about 4)

Calories: 120

Fat: 0 g

Saturated fat: 0 g

Cholesterol: 0 mg

Sodium: 5 mg

Total carbohydrates: 28 g

Dietary fiber: 5 g

Protein: 1 g

Calcium: 6% of Daily Value

Iron: 8%

help you lose weight. When overweight women were given a soluble fiber supplement, they began eating fewer calories and reported feeling fuller.

The other kind of fiber in figs, the insoluble form, staves off constipation and may drop your risk of colon cancer.

▶ **Potassium.** What's more, a serving of figs provides more potassium than a banana does. This mineral manages to lower your blood pressure, reducing your risk of heart disease and stroke.

▶ **Phenols.** But perhaps the most exciting nutrients found in figs are polyphenols. These compounds may be able to curb cancer, head off heart trouble, and more. Just one serving of dried figs packs 444 milligrams of this disease-fighting army. That's twice as much as the average American gets from vegetables in an entire day!

Add to that the fact that figs contain coumarin and benzaldehyde, two other potent cancer fighters, and you'd be silly not to dig into figs at least a couple of times a week.

Brie-Stuffed Figs

Since figs are the ultimate finger food, why not serve them as an appetizer? This recipe, passed on to us by the folks at Valley Fig Growers, was a hit at our last family party. And we have picky relatives, too!

16 dried Calimyrna or Mission figs
6 ounces Brie cheese, cut into small pieces
⅓ cup chopped fresh rosemary

Preheat the oven to 350°F. Trim the stems from the figs. If using Calimyrna figs, peel the figs, as well. With the tip pointing up, slice each fig vertically, but don't cut all the way through. Stuff each fig with a piece of the cheese. Sprinkle with the rosemary. Place the figs cheese side up in a large pan. Bake for 7 minutes, or until hot.

Yield: Eight servings.

Nutritional data per serving: Calories, 193; protein, 6 g; carbohydrates, 30 g; fiber, 6 g; fat, 7 g; saturated fat, 4 g; cholesterol, 21 mg; sodium, 139 mg; calcium, 15% of Daily Value; iron, 13%.

Fish:

Get Hooked on It

BATTLES:

- depression
- heart disease
- high blood pressure
- irregular heartbeat
- menstrual pain
- rheumatoid arthritis
- stroke

BOLSTERS:

- brain and vision development in infants
- menstrual regularity

We're always surprised when we talk to folks who admit that they'd like to eat more fish, but they just don't know how to cook it. Nothing could be easier. Fish is so thin and tender that it requires minimal fuss. And nothing could be healthier. Fish arrives packed with omega-3 fatty acids—essential fats that our bodies can't make, so we have to get them from foods.

JOIN THE OMEGA-3 FRATERNITY

Strangely, omega-3s actually come from green plants, such as plankton and tree leaves. We get our omega-3s by eating the fish that ate the plankton. Our forebears got their omega-3s from the meat of animals that fed on tree leaves, such as deer and antelope. But those days are long gone. Nowadays, our meat comes from the feedlot, where the cattle grow fat eating silage and hay,

Angling for the Fattiest Fish

When you're fishing for omega-3 fatty acids, net these beautiful swimmers for a bountiful catch. The fat grams for each are based on a 3-ounce raw edible portion.

Fish	Omega-3 Fatty Acids (g)
Sardines in sardine oil	3.3
Atlantic mackerel	2.5
Lake trout	1.6
European anchovy	1.4
Bluefish	1.2
Pink salmon	1.0
Striped bass	0.8
Pacific oysters	0.6
Tuna	0.5
Shrimp	0.4
Alaska king crab	0.3
Northern lobster	0.2
Scallops	0.2
Swordfish	0.2

which contain only very small amounts of omega-3s.

A few other foods, such as canola oil, flaxseeds, walnuts, and some green leafy vegetables, deliver alpha-linolenic acid), which our bodies can use to create omega-3s.

DON'T CELL YOURSELF SHORT

Why focus on fish? Numerous studies have shown that people who eat just two 3-ounce fish portions weekly have lower rates of heart disease, stroke, irregular heartbeat, and high blood pressure. Researchers speculate that omega-3s are the source of fish's

(Continued on page 200)

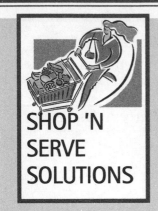

SHOP 'N SERVE SOLUTIONS

Buying delicious fresh fish is easier than you might think.

WHEN SELECTING FRESH FISH:

■ Look for plump, moist fish that smells fresh and breezy, not fishy.

■ Look for whole fish with bright, clear eyes and clean, tight scales.

■ Choose moist-looking steaks and filets.

WHEN STORING:

■ Store fresh fish in its original wrapper in the coldest part of your refrigerator. Use it within two days.

■ Keep raw fish and cooked fish separate to avoid contamination from the uncooked juices.

Frozen fish. If you buy your fish frozen, follow these guidelines:

■ Be sure the packaging is intact and there's no freezer burn.

■ Put it in your freezer immediately.

■ Thaw it safely by transferring it to the fridge the day before you want to use it.

FROM HOOKED TO QUICK-COOKED

Baked, broiled, poached, fried, or stewed fish will take about 10 minutes cooking time per inch of thickness. You can tell fish is done when it changes from translucent to opaque and also flakes easily when tested with a fork.

Fish is very tender—so don't marinate it for more than 10 minutes, or it will become mushy. Also, don't overcook fish, because that makes it tough. However, do make sure the fish is completely cooked. Eating "medium-rare" fish can be risky because fish can harbor parasites and bacteria that cause food poisoning. But relax: Thorough cooking makes fish perfectly safe.

SAFE SUSHI

The USDA says raw fish dishes, such as sushi and sashimi, can be safe for most people (except for those with diabetes) if the dishes are made with very fresh fish, commercially frozen (at temperatures lower than those of home freezers) and then thawed before eaten. Commercial freezing kills any parasites that may be present. Once killed, they are no longer a danger to you.

HAVE A FISH DISH

If you're ready to boost the health quotient of every cell in your body, reel in some fish. Two little servings each week will do it. For the best nutritional catch, mix and match different varieties. Here are some simple and tempting ways to begin. Take the bait!

◆ **Hook up with vegetable soup.** Add fresh fish bits to commercial vegetable soup to make a chunky chowder. Simmer at least 5 minutes to be sure the fish is cooked through. You can also use leftover cooked fish pieces.

◆ **Munch a tuna lunch.** White albacore tuna packs more omega-3s than light tuna or the yellow fin sold in most restaurants. To make tuna salad, use light mayo and plenty of fresh veggies, such as chopped celery, grated carrots, chopped cucumber, and sliced radishes. Stuff into a whole wheat pita pocket.

◆ **Just say yes to anchovies.** Along with peppers, onions, and olives, order anchovies on your pizza. Have them on your Caesar salad, too.

◆ **Make "planned-overs."** When you're grilling salmon, cook a double batch. Chill the leftovers to mix into pasta salad to take to work the next day.

◆ **Get cracking with sardines.** Have a couple of sardines with some whole grain crackers for lunch or a snack.

(Continued from page 197)
power because these fats are incorporated into cell walls throughout your body and change the way cells work.

When omega-3s become part of blood platelets, for instance, the platelets are less sticky, less likely to clump, and so, less likely to block an artery and cause a heart attack.

REAP THE O-3 BENEFITS
Here are some other findings:

▶ A Danish study found that women with severe menstrual pain tended to have low fish intake.

▶ In a study at Albany Medical College, 33 patients with rheumatoid arthritis who took fish oil had much less joint pain. Some were able to stop taking their non-steroidal anti-inflammatory drugs (NSAIDs), such as ibuprofen and naproxen sodium.

▶ Finnish research suggests that people with low levels of omega-3s in their neural membranes are more likely to suffer from depression.

BRAIN FOOD FOR BABY
On the child development front, researchers have learned that when a pregnant woman eats fish, the omega-3s are passed on to her baby, who uses them for brain and vision development. Later, during breast-feeding, omega-3s are again passed on to the infant. Currently, there is great debate over adding omega-3s to infant formula in the United States, as is being done in Europe.

Quick Fix:

Irregular Periods

Constantly worried about ruining your clothes because you can never tell when your period is due? Fish to the rescue! Researchers have found that supplementing women's diets with omega-3 fatty acids makes their menstrual cycles more regular—which means you'll know when you can wear white pants!

NUTRITION IN A NUTSHELL

Broiled wild Atlantic salmon (3 ounces)

Calories: 155

Fat: 7 g

Saturated fat: 1 g

Cholesterol: 60 mg

Sodium: 48 mg

Total carbohydrates: 0 g

Dietary fiber: 0 g

Protein: 22 g

Vitamin E: 13% of Daily Value

Iron: 5%

Zinc: 13%

Grilled Salmon Primavera

Olive oil cooking spray
2 tablespoons olive oil
1 pound wild Atlantic salmon filet
Salt to taste
½ pound rotini or other pasta
1 clove garlic, minced
½ pound fresh snow peas
1 cup each 2-inch strips red and yellow bell peppers
¼ cup thinly sliced scallions
1 cup evaporated skim milk
½ cup freshly grated Parmesan cheese
4 tablespoons thinly sliced fresh basil (garnish)

Spray the grill with cooking spray, then, preheat it. Adjust the heat so that you can hold your hand 14 inches from the flame for 20 seconds. Place the salmon skin-side down on the grill and close the lid. Slowly grill for 10 to 20 minutes, depending on the thickness, or until the salmon flakes easily. Remove to a clean plate and divide into four equal pieces.

While the salmon is grilling, fill a large pot with water, add salt to taste, and bring the water to a boil. Add the pasta and boil until al dente. Drain and return to the pot to keep warm.

Heat the olive oil in a large, heavy skillet over high heat. Add the garlic, snow peas, peppers, and scallions, and cook for 1 minute, stirring constantly. Add the milk and heat just until bubbly. Add the cooked pasta and the cheese. Stir gently to combine. Divide the pasta and vegetables among four plates. Top each with a piece of salmon. Garnish with the basil.

Yield: Four servings.

Nutritional data per serving: Calories, 367; protein, 34 g; carbohydrates, 17 g; fiber, 3 g; fat, 18 g; saturated fat, 4 g; cholesterol, 72 mg; sodium, 359 mg; calcium, 41% of Daily Value.

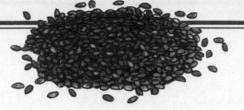

Flaxseeds:

Nutty Nuggets

BATTLES:
- cancer
- heart disease

BOLSTERS:
- brain and vision development in infants
- regularity

When Colleen and Ted got married just a few years ago, they ended up with lots of kitchen doubles—silverware, dishes, pots, pans, corn poppers, even coffee grinders. A major yard sale restored order. They got rid of all their doubles—except for those coffee grinders. Colleen refused to sell either one. Why? She uses one to grind fresh coffee beans for that one perfect cup each morning. The other is for grinding the flaxseeds she adds to the turkey burgers that keep her heart happy.

Flaxseeds? Yep, the seeds of the flax plant. Admittedly, they're an oddball food. But the reason we recommend flaxseeds is that they contain a special oil that most Americans don't get enough of in their diets.

Public health officials have harangued us for a good 30 years to cut down on saturated fat from burgers, cheese, butter, and ice cream so that we'll cut our risk of heart disease, the number one killer of men and women. And a lot of us did. So that should be the end of the problem, right? Wrong! Now another fat problem is rearing its ugly head: polyunsaturated fat imbalance.

FATS OUT OF KILTER

It turns out that there are two kinds of fat that we must eat (yes, we have to eat some fat!) because our bodies can't make them. They're called essential fatty acids. The one called omega-6 comes from the vegetable oils in our fried foods, cookies and cakes, and highly processed foods. As you can probably guess, we get way too much of it. The other, omega-3, comes mostly from fish—and, of course, we get too little of that.

This imbalance—too much of one, too little of the other—creates problems with blood clotting, constricted arteries, and irregular heart rhythms. Some studies also suggest that it sets us up for arthritis, autoimmune disorders, and cancer. That's why the American Heart Association and the *Dietary Guidelines for Americans* recently suggested that we eat two servings of fish each week.

THE FACTS ABOUT FLAX

So what does this have to do with flaxseeds? They're loaded with alpha-linolenic acid, which your body can turn into the same kind of fat it needs so desperately from fish.

Are we sure flaxseeds are as good as fish? Flaxseed studies are in their beginning stages, so a lot more needs to be done before we have an absolute Yes. But in a University of Toronto study of nine healthy women, their total cholesterol

QUICK EGG SUBSTITUTE

Need an egg for your pancake, muffin, or cookie recipe? Mix 1 tablespoon of milled flaxseeds with 3 tablespoons of water and let stand for a minute or two. Add to the recipe in place of an egg.

NUTRITION IN A NUTSHELL

Flaxseeds (1 tablespoon)

Calories: 42

Fat: 4 g

Saturated fat: 1 g

Cholesterol: 0 mg

Sodium: 4 mg

Total carbohydrates: 2 g

Dietary fiber: 2 g

Protein: 2 g

Calcium: 2% of Daily Value

Iron: 5%

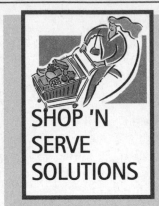

SHOP 'N SERVE SOLUTIONS

The flaxseed is a shiny, red-brown, flat oval with a pointed tip. It's a little bigger than a sesame seed. It's hard and chewy, but it adds an enjoyable light, nutty taste to foods.

Unfortunately, you probably won't find flaxseeds in your supermarket. So you'll have to make a trip to your favorite health food or natural food store. That's okay. They're worth going out of your way for. If all else fails, call toll-free (877) BUY-FLAX. They'll ship you a pound of flaxseeds for about $6, just to get you started.

You can buy whole flaxseeds, milled flaxseed flour to use in baked goods, or flaxseed oil.

WHEN STORING FLAXSEEDS:

■ Store whole flaxseeds in the pantry, at room temperature. They'll keep for up to a year.

■ Keep milled flaxseeds in an airtight container in the fridge, where it'll keep for up to 30 days.

■ Place flaxseed oil, which is cold-pressed from the seeds and filtered, in a lightproof bottle in the refrigerator. Then use it up fast, because it doesn't keep long.

USING FLAX TO THE MAX

Now here's how to make flaxseeds a delicious part of your life:

◆ **Bolster your bread.** Toss flaxseeds into quick-bread or muffin dough before baking. Or brush yeast bread with egg white and top with flaxseeds instead of sesame or poppy seeds before baking.

◆ **Give your cookies crunch.** Stir flaxseeds into oatmeal cookie batter for a nutty crunch.

◆ **Change your oil.** Replace oil or shortening with milled flaxseeds in your baked goods. Add 3 tablespoons of milled flaxseeds for each tablespoon of fat that you're replacing.

dropped by 9 percent and their bad low-density lipoprotein (LDL) cholesterol dove by 18 percent when they ate 2 ounces of flaxseeds daily for just four weeks. That's a great way to protect your heart.

Omega-3 fatty acids are also critical to brain and vision development, both before and just after babies are born. Mothers who eat plenty of fish, flaxseeds, and walnuts deliver these brain builders through the placenta and through breast milk.

BENEFITS ABOUND

Beyond their fishlike oil, flaxseeds contain up to 800 times more lignans than any other plant food. Lignans? They're plant compounds that act like weak estrogens. They've been shown to tie up the body's estrogen receptors, the way telemarketers tie up your phone line. Lignans prevent human estrogen from being absorbed, which may prevent breast, prostate, and endometrial cancers from getting started.

Flaxseeds also are rich in insoluble fiber, the roughage that keeps you going and prevents constipation.

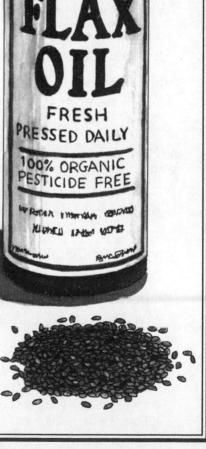

Flax Prairie Bread

If you're tired of white "balloon" bread, this bread's for you, compliments of the Flax Council of Canada.

3 cups enriched all-purpose flour
2½–3 cups whole wheat flour
⅓ cup whole flaxseeds
2 tablespoons sunflower seeds
1 tablespoon poppy seeds
2 tablespoons fast-rising instant yeast
2 teaspoons salt
1½ cups water
½ cup 2% milk
3 tablespoons honey
2 tablespoons shortening

In a large bowl, mix 2 cups of the all-purpose flour, the whole wheat flour, flaxseeds, sunflower seeds, poppy seeds, yeast, and salt. Heat the water, milk, honey, and shortening until hot to the touch (125° to 130°F). Stir the hot liquids into the dry mixture. Mix in enough of the remaining all-purpose flour to make a soft dough that does not stick to the bowl. Turn out onto a floured board, and knead until smooth and elastic, about 8 minutes. Cover the dough and let rest for 10 minutes. Cut the dough in half and shape each half into a loaf. Place each in a greased 8½-by-4½-inch loaf pan. Cover and let rise in a warm place until double in volume, 40 to 50 minutes. Preheat the oven to 400°F. When the dough has risen, bake for 30 to 35 minutes. Remove from the pans and let cool on wire racks.

Yield: Two loaves (32 slices).

Nutritional data per slice: Calories, 113; protein, 4 g; carbohydrates, 20 g; fiber, 2 g; fat, 3 g; saturated fat, less than 1 g; cholesterol, 0 mg; sodium, 150 mg; folate, 10% of Daily Value; vitamin B$_1$ (thiamin), 12%; iron, 4%; magnesium, 6%; zinc, 4%.

Garlic:
The Clove
That Loathes Cancer

BATTLES:
- athlete's foot
- cancer
- heart disease
- high cholesterol

BOLSTERS:
- immune function
- mood
- weight control

While vacationing in San Francisco a few years ago, Karen and her husband, John, visited Garlic World, a market that carries every product made from garlic, including garlic ice cream and garlic jelly. That sounded just as wild to us as it does to you. What's not wild, however, is garlic's amazing ability to keep us well.

CUTS CANCER RISK

In a recent analysis of medical studies, for instance, researchers from the University of North Carolina found that people who consumed six or more garlic cloves per week had a 30 percent lower risk of colon cancer

NUTRITION IN A NUTSHELL

Garlic (5 cloves)

Calories: 22

Fat: 0 g

Saturated fat: 0 g

Cholesterol: 0 mg

Sodium: 3 mg

Total carbohydrates: 5 g

Dietary fiber: 0 g

Protein: 1 g

Vitamin C: 8% of Daily Value

Quick Fix:

Athlete's Foot

It's the ultimate irony: You may be able to end athlete's foot with none other than the "stinking rose." Just soak your tootsies in a basin of warm water with a few crushed garlic cloves and a splash of rubbing alcohol, suggests James Duke, Ph.D., retired USDA researcher and author of THE GREEN PHARMACY. "Because of its anti-fungal properties, garlic is my first choice of treatment," says Dr. Duke.

and a 50 percent lower risk of stomach cancer than those who ate a clove or less weekly. Other studies have hinted that garlic staves off breast and prostate cancers, too, but the evidence is still preliminary.

How does garlic ground cancer? It contains allicin, a cancer-fighting sulfur compound.

Garlic supplements, by the way, don't seem to have an effect on cancer, because they have only trace amounts of allicin, according to the North Carolina researchers.

MORE BULB BENEFITS

People have used garlic since ancient times to help ward off dozens of health problems. The ancient Greeks actually ate garlic before a race to get a competitive advantage. (Maybe no one wanted to be near them!)

Scientists haven't checked out the validity of every use, but besides fighting cancer, garlic seems to help in these four areas:

▶ **Heart disease.** A review of studies found that consuming one-half to one clove of garlic daily lowers total cholesterol level by about 9 percent, reducing the risk of heart disease by about 20 percent.

▶ **Immune function.** Garlic is loaded with compounds that may be able to kill some bacteria and viruses. A study at Brigham Young University in Provo, Utah, reported that crushed garlic in oil killed rhinovirus type 2 (a common cause of the common cold), two forms of herpes, and several other common viruses.

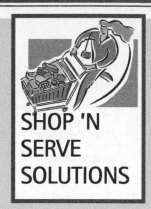

SHOP 'N SERVE SOLUTIONS

There's nothing complicated about buying any variety of garlic.

WHEN SELECTING GARLIC:

- Choose plump, firm bulbs.
- Look for tightly closed cloves.

WHEN STORING:

Keep your garlic in a cool, dark place until you're ready to use it.

THE ABCs OF PEELING

- Peeling garlic cloves is a cinch with this method:
- Place the cloves on a cutting board.
- Lay the flat side of a knife on top of them.
- Tap the knife gently with your closed fist to split the peels. And, like magic, the cloves will pop out.

To get rid of the odor on your hands, rub them with salt or lemon juice and wash with warm, soapy water. (To ditch garlic breath, chew on a parsley sprig.)

QUICK GARLICKY GOODIES

Now cast your cloves on these dishes:

◆ **Dress up your mayo.** Think low-fat mayo tastes blah? Mix 2 tablespoons with 1 teaspoon of minced garlic, and watch it come alive. Spread it on a veggie sandwich.

◆ **Slip it into your chicken.** When you're roasting a chicken, tuck a few peeled garlic cloves into the cavity for extra flavor.

◆ **Baste your bread.** Most prepackaged garlic bread piles on the fat and calories. Make your own by slicing a loaf of Italian bread in half horizontally and brushing on a tad of olive oil, a few crushed garlic cloves, and some parsley flakes. Bake in the oven until it begins to brown slightly.

▶ **Mood.** We're not kidding here. A recent study found that when garlic is served at a meal, families are more likely to be nice to each other. A possible explanation: Garlic evokes positive childhood memories, making people chill out.

▶ **Weight control.** Plain old steamed broccoli or cooked carrots come alive when you add some minced garlic. And the more you like your veggies, the more likely you will be to eat them—and that's good news for your hips and your heart.

Mom's Garlic Pasta

Karen's mom, Linda, can't seem to get enough garlic. Even when dining at restaurants that the rest of her family thinks have a generous hand, Mom says, "I can barely taste it." So now she makes her own garlic-laden pasta dishes, such as this one. Warning: It's not for the faint of heart!

1 pound medium-size pasta, such as rigatoni, rotini, or shells
1 bulb garlic, peeled and minced
¼ cup chopped fresh basil
2 tablespoons dried oregano
5 large ripe tomatoes, chopped
¼ cup extra virgin olive oil
¼ cup grated Parmesan cheese

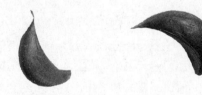

Cook the pasta according to package directions. Meanwhile, in a large skillet over medium-low heat, sauté the garlic, basil, oregano, and tomatoes in the oil for 8 to 10 minutes. Drain the pasta, toss with the sauce, and sprinkle with the cheese.

Yield: Six servings.

Nutritional data per serving: Calories, 257; protein, 7 g; carbohydrates, 33 g; fiber, 3 g; fat, 12 g; saturated fat, 2 g; cholesterol, 3 mg; sodium, 94 mg; calcium, 12% of Daily Value; iron, 15%.

Ginger:

It Makes Good Health a Snap!

BATTLES:
- cancer
- heart disease
- infections
- inflammation
- nausea
- stroke

BOLSTERS:
- digestion
- weight control

When Colleen's kids were little, her family spent a lot of time camping. And there was one treat they always brought along from home: Colleen's famous ginger-bread, a simple one-bowl cake that she could whip up just before they left for camp and allow to cool in the car. Little did the kids know that their mom stuffed the sweet treat with some whole wheat flour and heart-healthy canola oil! They thought they were in cake heaven.

The secret, of course, was the pungent ginger that gave the cake its unforgettable flavor. That cake got all three kids addicted

NUTRITION IN A NUTSHELL

Ground ginger
(1 teaspoon)

Calories: 7

Fat: 0 g

Saturated fat: 0 g

Cholesterol: 0 mg

Sodium: 0 mg

Total carbohydrates: 1 g

Dietary fiber: 0 g

Protein: 0 g

Iron: 2% of Daily Value

to the zingy taste of ginger. Now they can't get enough Thai or Chinese food, where the ancient flavor is essential to so many dishes.

GINGER IS PEACHY

The good news is that ginger is more than just a potent flavor enhancer. Asians have long used it to tame troubled tummies. And now researchers are discovering that, while ginger doesn't look very promising when you're weighing its vitamins and minerals, it's packed with a cool array of phytochemicals that protect just about every cell in your body:

▶ **Zingerone.** This phytochemical, for instance, protects polyunsaturated fat from being oxidized, so the fat can work its heart-protective magic.

▶ **Gingerol.** It fights cancer by preventing cancer cells from multiplying—and even by encouraging them to just drop dead. Gingerol also prevents platelets in your blood from clotting, which reduces your chance of a heart attack or stroke.

▶ **Glucosides.** These appear to have antioxidant activity that protects against cancer and heart disease.

▶ **Phenolic substances.** The pungent phenolic substances in ginger fight inflammation.

In addition, ginger appears to have mild antibacterial properties that may help prevent infection. What a spoonful—tasty *and* powerful!

WEIGHTY MATTERS

With obesity becoming an increasingly bigger problem in the United States, many of us are looking for ways to keep our weight under control. One way to do it is to eat smaller portions of better-tasting food that's more satisfying. Another way is to eat big piles

Quick Fix:

The Queasies

Troubled by a queasy tummy when you travel? Simply begin your travels with a cup of ginger tea. Not strong enough? Ginger capsules will deliver a more-standardized dose. Need help along the way? Carry some candied ginger.

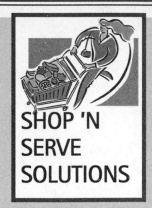

SHOP 'N SERVE SOLUTIONS

Gingerroot is a misnomer. Ginger is actually a rhizome, an underground stem that looks like a thick, lumpy root. But both new roots and new stems can grow out of it.

You'll find fresh ginger in the specialty section of the produce department of most grocery stores. You'll find ground ginger in the baking section of your store. You may find crystallized ginger there, too. It makes a tasty snack.

You'll almost always buy more fresh ginger than you can use at one time, but that's okay. The leftovers will keep for months in your freezer, double-wrapped in plastic. Grating and slicing are actually easier when the ginger is frozen.

SNAP YOUR FOODS TO ATTENTION

Use ginger to make your foods a little more exotic—and healthier! Here are some ideas:

◆ **Add sizzle to stir-fries.** Finely chop fresh ginger and add it with the onions and garlic when you stir-fry.

◆ **Make a mean meat marinade.** Add chopped fresh ginger or ground ginger to any marinade to perk up the flavor of lean beef, pork, or chicken.

◆ **Stir up soup with a spark.** Add ground ginger to carrot or squash soup. It'll bring the soup to life.

◆ **Clear your head.** Add thin slices of fresh ginger to chicken soup when you're congested. It'll help clear your nose.

of highly seasoned vegetables. Ginger can be a star player here, spicing up stir-fries and even small portions of lean meat. And ginger can help reduce your weight control woes when you use it to spice up your meals instead of burying them in tons of fat.

Colleen's Famous Gingerbread

Colleen is famous for making this incomparable gingerbread. It's amazingly easy for a "from-scratch" cake—and healthy, too, for a sweet treat. And it's great served with applesauce!

1 cup enriched white flour
1 cup white whole wheat flour
1 cup molasses
¾ cup buttermilk
½ cup canola oil
1 large egg
1 teaspoon baking soda
1 teaspoon ground ginger
1 teaspoon ground cinnamon
½ teaspoon salt

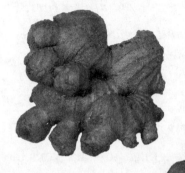

Preheat the oven to 325°F. Grease and flour a 9-inch-square baking pan. In a large mixing bowl, combine the flours, molasses, buttermilk, oil, egg, baking soda, ginger, cinnamon, and salt. With an electric mixer on low speed, gently beat until well blended. Increase the speed to medium and beat for 3 minutes. Pour the batter into the prepared pan. Bake about 1 hour, or until the top springs back when gently pressed with your finger. Cool completely.

Yield: 12 servings.

Nutritional data per serving: Calories, 241; protein, 3 g; carbohydrates, 36 g; fiber, 2 g; fat, 10 g; saturated fat, less than 1 g; cholesterol, 18 mg; sodium, 233 mg; vitamin E, 13% of Daily Value; calcium, 8%; iron, 13%; magnesium, 18%; potassium, 13%.

Grapefruit:

Sour on Cancer

BATTLES:
- asthma
- cancer
- heart disease
- high cholesterol
- stroke

BOLSTERS:
- cellular repair

Quick Fix:

Asthma

Asthma driving you nuts? Preliminary studies suggest that adding grapefruit to your daily diet can help reduce asthma symptoms.

The grapefruit may play second fiddle to the orange in some houses—but not in ours! That's because grape-fruit—especially the red and pink varieties—is tccming with antioxidants that fend off cancer, heart disease, and other significant health problems.

ANTIOXIDANTS AT YOUR SERVICE

The antioxidants in grapefruit work both solo and in tandem to fight disease. So eat your grapefruit, and enjoy these advantages:

▶ **The value of vitamin C.** The bigwig of these antioxidants, as you undoubtedly know, is vitamin C. Just half a grapefruit guarantees you all the vitamin C you need for the entire day! In addition to clobbering free radicals, substances that cause cell

NUTRITION IN A NUTSHELL

Pink grapefruit
(½ medium)

Calories: 60

Fat: 0 g

Saturated fat: 0 g

Cholesterol: 0 mg

Sodium: 5 mg

Total carbohydrates: 16 g

Dietary fiber: 6 g

Protein: 1 g

Vitamin A: 15% of Daily Value

Vitamin C: 110%

damage, vitamin C helps maintain collagen, which repairs your body's tissues.

▶ **The benefits of beta-carotene.** Pink and red grapefruits also are packed with beta-carotene. Studies have shown that this antioxidant may play a valuable role in fending off cancer and heart disease when it's consumed in foods (but not in vitamin supplements).

▶ **The promise of lycopene.** Both of these colorful grapefruit varieties, but especially red, also are loaded with lycopene, an antioxidant that seems promising in the prevention of prostate cancer. (See "Tomatoes: A Man's Best Friend" on page 448.)

▶ **The package deal.** What's more, the antioxidants in grapefruit may team up to stave off strokes. A Harvard University study found that drinking a glass of grapefruit juice or orange juice daily lowered the risk of a common type of stroke by 25 percent.

FOREVER FIBER

Finally, there's fiber. All grapefruit varieties supply a lot of fiber, mostly the soluble type. This kind of fiber helps lower your level of low-density lipoprotein (LDL) cholesterol—the bad kind—

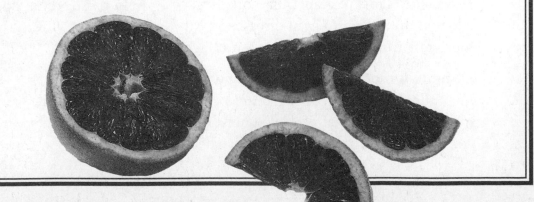

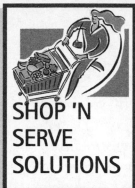

SHOP 'N SERVE SOLUTIONS

For the most cancer-fighting beta-carotene and lycopene, choose pink or, better yet, red grapefruit.

WHEN SELECTING GRAPEFRUIT:

■ Lift the grapefruit. The heavier it feels for its size, the more yummy juice it contains.

■ Avoid rough-looking fruit that has puffy skin and protruding ends, because it'll probably be fairly dry.

WHEN STORING:

Store your beautiful bounty on the kitchen counter if you're planning to eat it within a few days. If not, put your grapefruit in the fridge, where it'll keep for as long as six weeks.

GRAPEFRUIT GOODIES

Once you check out these ideas, you'll never have grapefruit hanging around for very long:

◆ **Brighten your salad.** Toss Ruby Red grapefruit pieces into your green salad for an extra boost of color and fiber. Drizzle with citrus vinaigrette.

◆ **Make a rainbow.** Combine segments from white, pink, and red grapefruits in a fruit salad. It'll light up your eyes.

◆ **Accent your fish.** Sprinkle your shrimp with grapefruit juice instead of lemon juice. Or top broiled or grilled fish filets, such as salmon or flounder, with grapefruit pieces. Or stir-fry shrimp and grapefruit pieces.

◆ **Sweeten the deal.** Fresh grapefruit not sweet enough for you? Drizzle it with a little maple syrup or honey.

thus protecting your heart. And to get the most fiber, don't skip the walls that separate the grapefruit segments—they contribute at least half of the total amount.

Cookout Citrus Splash

This refreshing thirst quencher will be a huge hit—you might even say, a splash—at your summer picnics. In just one serving, it packs all the vitamin C you need for the entire day. Give the drink a calcium boost by using calcium-fortified orange juice and a mineral water such as Gerolsteiner, which contains more calcium than most other brands.

1½ cups frozen grapefruit juice concentrate, thawed
1½ cups frozen orange juice concentrate, thawed
2 liters sparkling mineral water, chilled
Crushed ice
2 lemons, thinly sliced
¼ cup fresh raspberries (optional)

Pour the juices into a large punch bowl. Stir in the water and crushed ice. Top with the lemon slices and, if using, the raspberries.

Yield: 14 servings.

Nutritional data per serving: Calories, 136; protein, 1 g; carbohydrates, 33 g; fiber, 0 g; fat, 0 g; saturated fat, 0 g; cholesterol, 49 mg; sodium, 7 mg; vitamin C, 101% of Daily Value; calcium, 2%; iron, 2%.

Grapes:
A Bunch
of Health Benefits

BATTLES:
- cancer
- heart disease
- morning sickness

BOLSTERS:
- cardiovascular function

There's something so indulgent about eating a bunch of grapes. Picture yourself leaning back at your desk and popping one after another into your mouth. It calls up images of reclining Romans feasting at a bacchanal, doesn't it? Yet, while we might not enjoy grapes in such opulent luxury, we do have one thing in common with those feasting residents of ancient Rome: We reap the health benefits provided by grape skins.

Grape skins are *the* richest known source of resveratrol, a naturally occurring compound that puts the brakes on an enzyme that cancer cells need in order to grow. Not only that, resveratrol appears to interfere with the kinds of gene mutations that create cancer cells in the first place!

INDULGE IN A PURPLE PASSION

Purple grape juice, like red wine, is bursting with flavonoids. These are naturally occurring plant compounds that help prevent

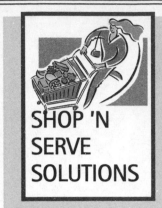

SHOP 'N SERVE SOLUTIONS

Grapes ripen on the vine, but the ripening process comes to a screeching halt when grapes are picked. So shop carefully, because the moment of purchase is as good as it gets.

WHEN SELECTING GRAPES:

■ For the sweetest grapes, look for green ones that are yellow-green, red ones that are deep crimson, and purple ones that are nearly black.

■ Choose plump grapes that seem to be bursting with goodness.

■ Look for stems that are green and supple.

WHEN STORING:

Store grapes in the refrigerator, where they'll last about a week. Wash them just before serving.

GRAPE IT UP

Now you can enjoy your grapes in all these delicious ways:

◆ **Eat like a kid.** Want a quickie lunch? Have a good old-fashioned peanut butter and purple grape jelly sandwich. The peanut butter packs the kind of fat that's heart-healthy, and the jelly is loaded with flavonoids that protect against heart disease and cancer.

◆ **Add crunch to salads.** Seedless grapes add a sweet, crispy crunch to chicken, tuna, or shrimp salad. Sprinkle a little curry powder on, too, for a spicy contrast.

◆ **Create a gala garnish.** Skip the parsley and go for the grapes when you garnish the plates and platters at your next dinner party.

◆ **Bob for grapes.** Serve fruit kebabs for dessert. Skewer grapes, banana circles, whole strawberries, and pineapple chunks. Drizzle with honey, lime juice, and allspice, and broil just until warm.

◆ **Focus attention on grapes.** Replace that candy dish with a grape centerpiece. Combine small bunches of white, red, and purple grapes for a color extravaganza.

unnecessary platelet aggregation. (When platelets in your blood "aggregate," they form tiny blood clots that can get stuck in a clogged coronary artery, cutting off the blood supply to that part of your heart. That's a heart attack.)

A small clinical study of five men and five women showed that drinking 5 ounces of 100 percent purple grape juice every day for a week reduced platelet aggregation by 60 percent, a reduction even better than that brought about by taking aspirin.

LATE-BREAKING NEWS

Here are some of the latest scientific findings that reveal other health benefits of eating grapes:

▶ Clinical studies have shown that drinking grape juice makes arteries more flexible, which can improve blood flow.

▶ In addition, both purple and red grape juices have been shown to make bad low-density lipoprotein (LDL) cholesterol less likely to oxidize, a chemical process that makes cholesterol stick to artery walls.

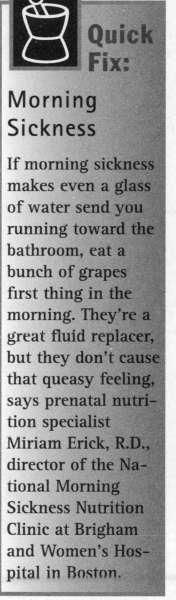

Quick Fix:

Morning Sickness

If morning sickness makes even a glass of water send you running toward the bathroom, eat a bunch of grapes first thing in the morning. They're a great fluid replacer, but they don't cause that queasy feeling, says prenatal nutrition specialist Miriam Erick, R.D., director of the National Morning Sickness Nutrition Clinic at Brigham and Women's Hospital in Boston.

NUTRITION IN A NUTSHELL

Tokay, Empress, or Red Flame grapes (1 cup)

Calories: 114

Fat: 1 g

Saturated fat: 0 g

Cholesterol: 0 mg

Sodium: 3 mg

Total carbohydrates: 28 g

Dietary fiber: 2 g

Protein: 1 g

Vitamin B$_1$ (thiamin): 10% of Daily Value

Vitamin C: 19%

Copper: 7%

Hearty Purple Cow

Whip up this simple frosty treat that's packed with calcium for your bones and flavonoids for your heart. It tastes so yummy that you'll forget it's good for you.

1 cup fat-free frozen cherry yogurt
½ cup purple grape juice
3 purple grapes in a cluster, still on the stem (garnish)

In a blender, whirl the yogurt and grape juice until creamy smooth. Pour into a tall glass. Garnish with the grape cluster. Serve with a wide straw.

Yield: One serving.

Nutritional data per serving: Calories, 257; protein, 7 g; carbohydrates, 57 g; fat, 0 g; saturated fat, 0 g; cholesterol, 0 mg; sodium, 94 mg; calcium, 61% of Daily Value; manganese, 23%.

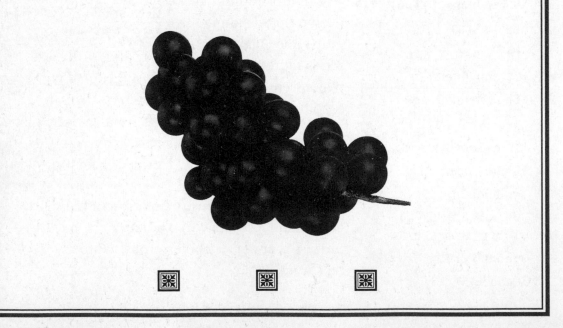

Green Beans:

Health with
No Strings Attached

BATTLES:
- cancer
- heart disease

BOLSTERS:
- weight control

Green beans have always been a part of Karen's life. She remembers, as a little girl, snapping off the ends of green beans at her grandparents' house. (Her grandmother makes a mean green bean and ham soup.) In high school, Karen often cooked green beans Lyonnaise-style, following a recipe from her French teacher. Now, she steams and seasons green beans for a quick side dish or orders chicken and green beans from her local Chinese restaurant.

While green beans don't have one standout nutrient, they pack a sprinkling of lots of goodies. Take a look at what they have to offer.

NUTRITION IN A NUTSHELL

Cooked Green beans (½ cup)

Calories: 22

Fat: 0 g

Saturated fat: 0 g

Cholesterol: 0 mg

Sodium: 2 mg

Total carbohydrates: 5 g

Dietary fiber: 2 g

Protein: 1 g

Folate: 5% of Daily Value

Vitamin A: 7%

Vitamin C: 10%

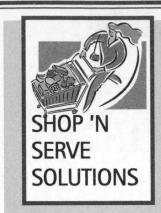

SHOP 'N SERVE SOLUTIONS

Fresh green beans are available in the produce department of your supermarket all year long. Choosing great fresh beans is, well, a snap.

WHEN SELECTING FRESH GREEN BEANS:

■ To buy the best, make sure the pods are bright green, firm, and smooth.

■ If the pods feel bumpy, it's probably because the beans were picked past their prime and the seeds have grown very large. Leave these at the store.

WHEN STORING:

Once you get your beans home, refrigerate them. They'll keep for about three days.

WHEN YOU'RE READY TO USE:

Rinse the beans, scrub off any dirt with a veggie brush, and remove the stem ends before cooking.

Frozen and canned green beans. If you can't find the fresh variety, there are always plenty of frozen and canned green beans to meet your needs. They aren't bad choices, either. Despite common myths, studies show that they have about the same amount of nutrients as fresh. (In case you're curious: This is true for all the veggies that we've tested.) Just be careful of the sodium content of canned veggies if you're following a low-salt diet.

SNAPPY SERVING SUGGESTIONS

Now here are some delicious ways to eat your green beans:

◆ **Follow the French.** Cook green beans, toss them with olive oil, and top with a little bit of goat cheese.

◆ **Chill out.** Make a cold green bean salad for a summer picnic. Just marinate cooked beans in vinaigrette (we like Ken's Basil and Balsamic Vinaigrette), then add a little minced garlic and chopped fresh garden tomatoes.

THE BOUNTY IN BEANS

Green beans contribute fiber, potassium, folate, and vitamins A and C. Many of these nutrients work toward the same purpose: protecting your heart. Here's how they do it:

▶ Fiber helps reduce your cholesterol level.

▶ Potassium lowers blood pressure.

▶ Folate decreases your level of an amino acid that researchers suspect contributes to ticker trouble.

▶ Vitamins A and C also contribute, gobbling up free radicals, bad guys that may trigger both heart disease and cancer.

The bottom line: With green beans, your ticker is in good hands.

Scientists have also identified two additional cancer-fighting compounds in green beans—coumarin and quercetin. Researchers aren't sure yet *exactly* how much green beans contain, and *specifically* how the compounds work. But they know that coumarin and quercetin do work!

Quick Fix: That Big Appetite!

Do you always order Sweet-and-Sour Chicken at a Chinese restaurant—or some other dish that has no vegetables? Too bad. Loading up on veggies, including green beans, helps you feel full, so you won't polish off that entire carryout pint of Kung Pao Chicken.

Holiday Green Beans

We love to make this festive green-and-red side dish for holiday parties. But it's so simple, you can whip it up for dinner any night of the week.

¾ pound fresh green beans, cleaned and stems removed
2 tablespoons extra virgin olive oil
2 cloves garlic, minced
½ cup roasted red peppers
2 tablespoons lemon juice

In a large pot, boil the green beans for 4 to 7 minutes, or until tender, but not mushy. Meanwhile, heat the oil in a large skillet over medium heat. Add the garlic and sauté for 1 to 2 minutes. Add the beans and peppers, and heat for 2 minutes, tossing frequently. Transfer to a bowl and stir in the lemon juice. Serve immediately.

Yield: Four servings.

Nutritional data per serving: Calories, 98; protein, 2 g; carbohydrates, 8 g; fiber, 3 g; fat, 7 g; saturated fat, 1 g; cholesterol, 0 mg; sodium, 51 mg; calcium, 3% of Daily Value; iron, 8%.

Greens:

They're Glorious!

BATTLES:
- cancer
- heart disease

BOLSTERS:
- bones
- vision

Some greens are wallflowers: They just don't seem to attract a lot of attention. But if you look a little closer, you find that they're worth your time and attention. Now, kale, spinach, and even bok choy are greens that most of you know. But here we're talking about another set of greens: collard, mustard, and turnip. Please read on. You'll be pleasantly surprised.

NOW SEE THIS

Like kale and spinach, collard, mustard, and turnip greens are loaded with lutein and zeaxanthin, two important compounds for eye health. Two Harvard University studies—one of 36,000 men, the other of 50,000 women—found that those who ate foods richest in these compounds had about a 20 percent lower chance of needing cataract surgery.

These foods also help protect your vision in another way: They may help ward off age-related macular degeneration (ARMD), the leading cause of blindness in people over age 65. In this disease, the macula of the eye—a small spot on the retina—starts to fizzle. As a result, people have a tough time

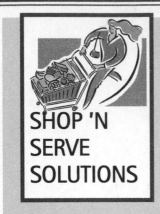

SHOP 'N SERVE SOLUTIONS

Fresh greens are available most of the year in all parts of the country, although you're sure to find them everywhere from Thanksgiving to Christmas.

WHEN SELECTING GREENS:

■ Look for plants—no matter which type of green you're buying—that have small leaves. These will be more tender and have a milder flavor than larger leaves.

■ Make sure the greens have been chilled while on display.

■ Check that the leaves are fresh and green, not wilting or yellow.

■ Avoid leaves that have little holes—a sign of insect damage.

WHEN STORING:

Store your greens, unwashed, in a plastic bag in your fridge, where they'll keep for up to five days.

WHEN YOU'RE READY TO USE:

■ Cut off and discard stems, roots, and any discolored leaves.

■ Swish the leaves in a large bowl of cold water, rinse them, and then drain. If your greens are very gritty, rinse them a few times.

■ Dry the greens in a salad spinner or roll them up in several sheets of paper towels and put them in the fridge for a few minutes.

■ Now boil, steam, microwave, or stir-fry your greens. Whichever method you choose, cook them for the least amount of time possible, so that they retain more of their nutrients.

COOKING THE GREEN WAY

Try these ideas to make your family keen on greens:

◆ **Cool 'em.** Cook collards. Chill and serve with lemon juice, olive oil, pine nuts, and garlic.

◆ **Bury 'em.** Place greens in between the layers in your favorite lasagna.

NUTRITION IN A NUTSHELL

Cooked mustard greens
(½ cup)

Calories: 11

Fat: 0 g

Saturated fat: 0 g

Cholesterol: 0 mg

Sodium: 11 mg

Total carbohydrates: 2 g

Dietary fiber: 1 g

Protein: 1 g

Folate: 13% of Daily Value

Vitamin A: 43%

Vitamin C: 30%

Vitamin E: 10%

seeing straight ahead. Turns out, the macula is loaded with the same two compounds abundant in these leafy green vegetables.

One small study found that 13 of 14 people with ARMD who ate ½ cup of cooked spinach four to seven times a week showed improvements in their vision. Collard greens, turnip greens, and kale actually have more of these compounds than spinach does.

DON'T BREAK A LEG (OR A HIP!)

You've heard it a zillion times: Make sure you get enough calcium to prevent osteoporosis, a disease that makes your bones weak and more likely to fracture at the slightest slip. While calcium certainly is crucial, researchers also are investigating the role of another nutrient: vitamin K.

Research at Tufts University in Boston shows that vitamin K activates at least three proteins involved in bone health. And which foods are rich in vitamin K? You guessed it—greens.

BRAVO TO BETA-CAROTENE

As if that weren't enough reason to eat your greens, you also should know that they fight heart disease and cancer. All greens are loaded with beta-carotene and vitamin C, antioxidants that gobble up free radicals, those compounds that spell trouble for your heart and increase your risk of cancer.

Indian-Style Greens

Karen snagged this recipe from a friend where she used to work. She's modified it to make it healthier.

1 tablespoon olive oil
1 red onion, sliced
4 cloves garlic, sliced
1 tablespoon sliced peeled fresh ginger
1 teaspoon coriander seeds
1 teaspoon cumin seeds
1½ teaspoons curry powder
1½ pounds mustard greens, cleaned and cut into 2-inch strips
½ cup water
1½ pounds spinach, cleaned and cut into 2-inch strips

Heat the oil in a large wok over medium-high heat. Add the onion and garlic, and sauté, stirring frequently, for 4 to 5 minutes. Stir in the ginger, coriander, cumin, and curry powder, and cook for 1 minute. Add the mustard greens and water, cover, and cook for 3 to 4 minutes, or until the greens are tender. Uncover and cook for 2 minutes to evaporate the water. Add the spinach, and cook, stirring constantly with tongs, for about 3 minutes, or until the spinach is wilted.

Yield: Four servings.

Nutritional data per serving: Calories, 142; protein, 11 g; carbohydrates, 21 g; fiber, 9 g; fat, 5 g; saturated fat, 1 g; cholesterol, 0 mg; sodium, 180 mg; calcium, 37% of Daily Value; iron, 47%.

Horseradish:
The Cancer-Fighting Condiment

BATTLES:
- cancer
- food poisoning
- heart disease
- stuffy nose

BOLSTERS:
- wound healing

Horseradish is pretty easy to dismiss. It's just that mushy gray stuff that you dump into a Bloody Mary or spread on a roast beef sandwich.

But this condiment is one that you should respect more—and use more. Just a dab of this powerful root vegetable provides a surprising amount of good nutrition.

A HEART HELPER AND A HEALER
Fresh or prepared, just 2 tablespoons of horseradish provide 12 percent of the vitamin C you need daily. Who would have guessed it?

NUTRITION IN A NUTSHELL
Prepared horseradish (2 tablespoons)

Calories: 14

Fat: 0 g

Saturated fat: 0 g

Cholesterol: 0 mg

Sodium: 94 mg

Total carbohydrates: 3 g

Dietary fiber: 6 g

Protein: 1 g

Folate: 4% of Daily Value

Vitamin C: 12%

Over the long haul, vitamin C seems to fend off heart disease and cancer. In the short run, it speeds up wound healing, so that you recover from your razor cuts or even your root canal a little faster.

But vitamin C isn't why researchers are excited about horseradish. After all, citrus fruits and red bell peppers pack much more vitamin C than horseradish does.

A TOXIN NEUTRALIZER

What has nutrition researchers doing cartwheels is a group of compounds whose name doesn't exactly roll off your tongue: isothiocyanates. Research has found that, at least in test tubes, isothiocyanates seem to deactivate chemicals before they trigger cancer. Scientists think that isothiocyanates may be especially helpful in staving off cancers of the mouth, pharynx, lung, stomach, colon, and rectum.

A BACTERIA BUSTER

And that's not the only promising news about these compounds. Research suggests that they help fight *Listeria, E. coli,* and other harmful bacteria that cause food poisoning. There's no telling when these bacteria may end up in your food, especially sandwiches. So why not top your sandwich with some horseradish? It'll taste great, and you can rest a little easier.

Quick Fix:

Stuffy Nose

Head cold got you down? Can't breathe, either? Slather a teaspoon of prepared horseradish on a cracker, then eat it slowly. The horseradish vapors will reach into the back of your nose and liquefy the stuffy stuff. Even the stuffiest nose will respond to three crackers' worth!

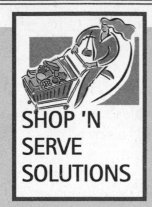

SHOP 'N SERVE SOLUTIONS

When you're in the market for horseradish, you have three choices: the prepared version, the fresh root, or horseradish sauce.

Most people choose prepared horseradish. It comes in a jar and is usually mixed with vinegar. (If the horseradish is red, it has been mixed with vinegar and beet juice.)

WHEN SELECTING FRESH HORSERADISH:

Rather take the fresh route? Be warned: Fresh horseradish is much more pungent than the prepared version. If you opt for fresh, follow these guidelines:

■ Select firm roots.

■ Store them in a plastic bag in the refrigerator, where they'll keep for up to a week.

■ Just before you're ready to grate the fleshy, white roots, clean them, removing their outer skin.

START HORSING AROUND

Here's how horseradish can take root in your kitchen:

◆ **Mix it with mustard.** Sure, you could buy prepared horseradish mustard, but it costs more and may have too much or too little horseradish for your taste. So stir some horseradish into your favorite brand of mustard. It'll breathe new life into your roast beef, turkey, or ham sandwich!

◆ **Concoct a cream sauce.** Stir 3 tablespoons of horseradish into 1 cup of low-fat sour cream, plain yogurt, or French dressing. It makes a tangy dip for red bell pepper strips, broccoli florets, and baby carrots.

Tuna Tucks

*Sorry, Charlie, but we get bored with the same old tuna.
Horseradish gives a standard can of tuna a well-deserved
flavor boost.*

1 can (6 ounces) tuna packed in water, drained
⅓ cup fat-free or low-fat mayonnaise
⅓ cup low-fat plain yogurt
¼ cup prepared horseradish
1 red onion, diced
½ cup shredded carrots
2 tablespoons pickle relish
2 leaves romaine lettuce
4 slices tomato
2 whole wheat pita pockets, warmed

In a medium bowl, mix the tuna, mayonnaise, yogurt,
horseradish, onion, carrots, and relish. Cover and refrigerate
for at least 1 hour to blend the flavors. Tuck half of the
tuna salad, 1 lettuce leaf, and 2 tomato slices into each of
the pita pockets.

Yield: Two servings.

*Nutritional data per serving: Calories, 337; protein, 28 g; carbohydrates, 51 g;
fiber, 6 g; fat, 3 g; saturated fat, 1 g; cholesterol, 26 mg; sodium, 961 mg; calcium, 13% of Daily Value; iron, 23%.*

Kale:
Your Eyes Will See the Glory

BATTLES:
- allergies
- cancer
- heart disease
- age-related macular degeneration

BOLSTERS:
- bones
- vision

Kale is Colleen's favorite vegetable, an idiosyncrasy passed down from her mom and on to Colleen's daughter Bobbi. So Colleen is always surprised when the grocery store clerk asks, "Now what is this?"

Well, unless you're from the Deep South, you probably don't know. But you should, because kale is king when it comes to providing carotenoids, substances that protect your eyes against cataracts and age-related macular degeneration (ARMD). ARMD is the leading cause of blindness among older Americans.

A SIGHT SAVER
Your eyes may be the windows of your soul, but they're also important for seeing the light.

Quick Fix:
Sneezin' and Wheezin'

When your allergies to airborne pollens act up, eat some kale. It's rich in quercetin, a natural antihistamine—and it doesn't cost as much as those drugstore antihistamines!

Unfortunately, seeing the light has its downside. The very act of "looking" produces dangerous, unpaired free-radical oxygen. While seeking an oxygen mate, these free radicals can damage the macula of your eye.

The macula, a tiny spot in the center of your retina, is critical for straight-ahead vision. It is packed with the antioxidant pigments lutein and zeaxanthin, which scavenge free radicals before they can harm vision.

Early studies suggest that eating foods such as kale and spinach, which are rich in these carotenoids, makes the macular pigments denser, protecting against ARMD, which—fortunately—takes decades to develop. So start now to get to know and love kale.

But hold your nose when you're cooking kale, and turn on the exhaust fan before the pot begins to boil. Otherwise, the cabbagelike smell may dampen your enthusiasm for this sweet, tender powerhouse vegetable.

A CANCER FIGHTER

Cruciferous (cabbage family) vegetables, such as kale, have long been known to reduce the risk of cancer, and now scientists are beginning to understand a little of the "why." Kale is packed with phytochemicals, naturally occurring elements in plants that help your body fight disease and infection.

A HEART HELPER

Despite all the progress being made in reducing deaths from heart disease, it remains the number one killer of both women

NUTRITION IN A NUTSHELL

Cooked kale (½ cup)

Calories: 17

Fat: 0 g

Saturated fat: 0 g

Cholesterol: 0 mg

Sodium: 15 mg

Total carbohydrates: 4 g

Dietary fiber: 1 g

Protein: 1 g

Vitamin A: 120% of Daily Value

Vitamin C: 44%

Vitamin K: 400%

Calcium: 5%

Iron: 4%

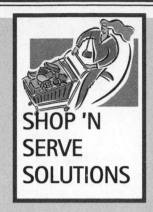

SHOP 'N SERVE SOLUTIONS

You can buy kale frozen in blocks or loose in bags, but it's definitely best when it's cooked fresh.

WHEN SELECTING FRESH KALE:

■ Look for very curly, smaller leaves that are medium to dark green. They'll be far more tender and delicately flavored than those big, tough, leathery leaves.

■ Avoid any leaves that look moldy or have yellow spots.

WHEN STORING:

At home, rinse the kale, shake off the excess water, wrap the kale in paper towels, and then store it in a plastic bag in a cold, dark area of your refrigerator to protect its fragile vitamins. Cook your kale within three to four days, because it can turn bitter if it's stored any longer.

NEW WAYS TO COOK KALE

Substitute kale for spinach anytime. Or try these uses:

◆ **Make a bed.** Use kale, for example, as a bed for grilled chicken with mango salsa.

◆ **Make supersoup.** Toss leftover cold, cooked kale into bean, lentil, or vegetable soup.

◆ **Make it Italian.** Shred kale and add it to baked lasagna.

and men in the United States. The big problem stems from excess cholesterol in your blood. It clings to the walls of your arteries, blocking the flow of blood.

But cholesterol can't latch on unless it's combined with

dangerous free-radical oxygen—formed in a process called oxidation—and that's where kale comes to the rescue. In laboratory tests, kale outranked all other vegetables in its ability to prevent this process from getting started.

GOT KALE?

Certainly you know that you need milk for strong bones, but what about kale? Of course! Recent research at Tufts University in Boston suggests that you may need 110 micrograms of vitamin K daily to activate a bone protein called osteocalcin, which is needed to make bones strong. A ½-cup serving of raw kale more than doubles that dose, providing 274 micrograms of vitamin K.

One caveat: If you're taking Coumadin (warfarin sodium) or any other blood-thinning medication, talk to your doctor before you start eating more kale and other green leafy vegetables. Your medication and these foods could work against each other, because the vitamin K in these veggies helps blood to clot.

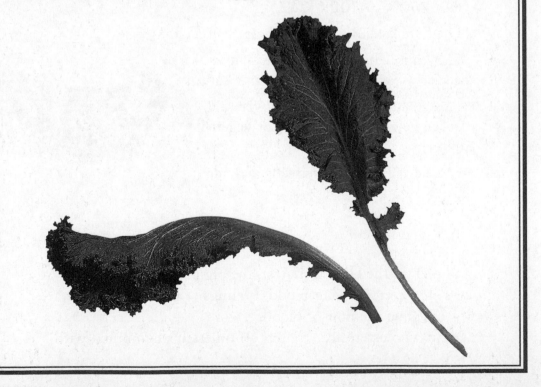

No-Fail Kale

The typical southern approach to cooking kale is to boil it with a ham hock. Common sense suggests that you should eliminate the ham hock, since the hock is mostly fat. But if you like that smoky, meaty taste that ham adds, you can add some chopped lean ham, chopped Canadian bacon, or even just a dash of liquid smoke instead.

1 pound fresh kale
1 cup water
¼ teaspoon salt
Freshly ground black pepper to taste
2 ounces lean ham or Canadian bacon, chopped (optional)

Remove and discard the heavy central stem from each kale leaf. Tear the leaves into bite-size pieces. (You'll have about 16 cups.) To remove any dirt or sand, wash the torn leaves several times in lukewarm water until the water is clear. Place the leaves in a large pot or pasta cooker. Add the cup of water. Sprinkle with the salt and pepper. Top with the ham or Canadian bacon, if using. Cover and cook over high heat just until the water boils. Reduce the heat to medium-high, and cook for 5 to 8 minutes, or until the kale is tender and bright green.

Serve with a splash of your favorite vinegar, or add a little crushed pepper that has been sautéed in a tablespoon of olive oil.

Yield: 12 servings.

Nutritional data per serving (if using Canadian bacon): Calories, 26; protein, 2 g; carbohydrates, 4 g; fiber, 1 g; fat, 1 g; saturated fat, 0 g; cholesterol, 0 mg; sodium, 131 mg; vitamin A, 67% of Daily Value; vitamin C, 75%; calcium, 5%; iron, 3%.

  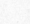

Kiwifruit:
The Down Under Disease Fighter

BATTLES:
- birth defects
- cancer
- cataracts
- diabetes
- heart disease
- stroke

BOLSTERS:
- immune function
- vision

Know which food we reach for when we need a little extra vitamin C? Hint: It's not an orange. Sure, Valencias, navels, and other orange varieties pack close to 70 milligrams of vitamin C, making them an excellent source of the nutrient. But another kind of fruit offers even *more* C. Stumped? We'll give you another clue: It's green. One medium kiwifruit, barely 2½ ounces, delivers 75 milligrams of vitamin C—5 milligrams more than an orange twice its weight. An added bonus: A kiwifruit offers three times the amount of vitamin E that an orange does.

E-C DOES IT

By now, you know that vitamins C and E act as powerful antioxidants in your body, gobbling up substances that can cause the cell damage responsible for cancer, heart attack, stroke, diabetes, and even cataracts. But USDA data show that many Americans don't meet the minimum intake requirements for these nutrients—especially vitamin E. The numbers are startling: A whopping 71 percent of women over age 20 and more than 60 percent of men over age 50 fall short of the recommended daily amount of vitamin E.

The unfortunate consequence is that you tremendously raise your risk of getting some of your most-feared diseases. For instance, research reported in the *Journal of the National Cancer Institute* showed that women who didn't eat a lot of foods rich in vitamin E and beta-carotene had a 21 percent increased risk of developing breast cancer. Likewise, a study of more than 1,600 men, published in the *British Medical Journal*, found that those with the lowest intake of vitamin C were at the highest risk for a heart attack.

NUTRITION IN A NUTSHELL

Kiwifruits (2 medium)

Calories: 90

Fat: 0.5 g

Saturated fat: 0 g

Cholesterol: 0 mg

Sodium: 10 mg

Total carbohydrates: 23 g

Dietary fiber: 5 g

Protein: 2 g

Folate: 14% of Daily Value

Vitamin C: 250%

Copper: 12%

Magnesium: 12%

Potassium: 14%

A FAR SIGHT BETTER

In addition to its powerful antioxidant vitamins, kiwifruit holds another disease-fighting weapon: lutein, a powerful carotenoid that's also found in your eyes. In a recent study, kiwifruit ranked higher than spinach and all other produce except yellow corn for its lutein content.

Recent research suggests that lutein may protect your eye tissues from damage that leads to age-related macular degeneration, the leading cause of blindness in older Americans. Unfortunately, a study published

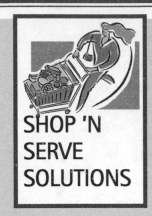

SHOP 'N SERVE SOLUTIONS

Used to be that finding good kiwifruit year-round was as hard as finding a pair of jeans that really fit. But, with imports from Chile and New Zealand, plus California's crop, you can now buy kiwifruit 365 days a year.

WHEN SELECTING KIWIFRUIT:

- Look for firm, unblemished kiwi.
- Buy kiwi that yields slightly to your touch.

WHEN STORING:

- Place ripe kiwi in the fridge, where it'll keep for up to a month—far longer than most other fruits.

- Place hard, unripe kiwi in a vented plastic bag with an apple or a banana, and leave the bag on your kitchen counter for a day or two.

QUICK KIWI CREATIONS

But if you try any of these mouthwatering creations, your kiwifruit will never be in cold storage for very long:

◆ **Play matchmaker.** Strawberries and kiwifruit make a great team. To enjoy this winning combination, mix 1 cup of sliced strawberries, 1 cup of sliced kiwi, 1 cup of low-fat milk, and 1 cup of low-fat yogurt in a blender until smooth.

◆ **Perk up your pancakes.** Instead of drowning them in maple syrup (1 tablespoon alone packs 52 calories, and who stops there?), top your pancakes with chopped kiwifruit and your other favorite fruits.

◆ **Look like a gourmet.** Karen likes to slice kiwifruit lengthwise in $\frac{1}{4}$- to $\frac{1}{3}$-inch pieces and then use a small cookie cutter to make star shapes. It's an excellent—and easy—appetizer for a Fourth of July picnic.

◆ **Sweeten your swimmers.** Puree kiwifruit with a tad of lemon juice. Serve it with salmon, shrimp, or any fish for a great taste.

in the *Journal of the American Dietetic Association* found that lutein intake is decreasing among Americans—and particularly among Caucasian women.

GOOD THINGS, SMALL PACKAGES

With lutein and oodles of vitamins C and E, you'd think there wouldn't be room for anything more in one little kiwifruit. But there is! The fuzzy fruit also offers these nutrients:

▶ **Folate.** This B vitamin is important for preventing birth defects.

▶ **Copper.** It's essential for a strong immune system.

▶ **Magnesium.** This mineral is needed for bone formation and the regulation of heart rhythm.

▶ **Potassium.** It's critical for blood pressure control.

And, oh yeah, two kiwifruits supply 5 grams of fiber, about 20 percent of what you need daily. So what are you waiting for? Go ahead and dig in!

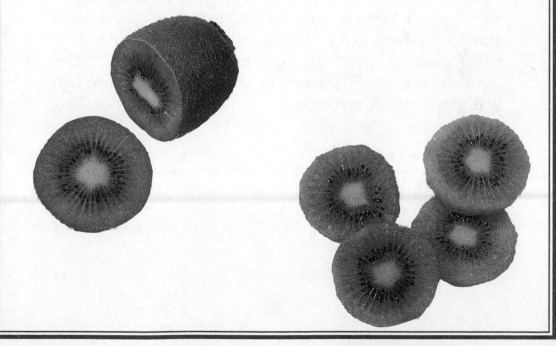

Chicken Kiwi

Forget about Chicken Kiev. This easy and enticing entrée, which delivers half of the vitamin C you need daily, will become a family favorite in no time at all!

2 tablespoons olive or canola oil
4 boneless, skinless thin-sliced chicken breast halves
¼ teaspoon freshly ground black pepper
¼ teaspoon dried rosemary
¼ cup white wine
2 kiwifruits, sliced

Preheat the oven to 300°F. Heat the oil in a large nonstick skillet over medium-high heat. Sprinkle both sides of the chicken breasts with the pepper and rosemary. Place the chicken in the skillet, and cook for 2 to 3 minutes on each side, or until done. Remove the chicken from the skillet and keep warm in the oven. Add the wine to the skillet, and heat, stirring constantly, for 2 to 3 minutes. Gently stir in the kiwifruits and cook for 1 minute. Remove the chicken from the oven and place the four pieces of chicken on four plates. Top with the kiwifruits and serve.

Yield: Four servings.

Nutritional data per serving: Calories, 223; protein, 28 g; carbohydrates, 6 g; fiber, 1 g; fat, 8 g; saturated fat, 1 g; cholesterol, 68 mg; sodium, 79 mg; calcium, 3% of Daily Value; iron, 8%.

Lentils:

Small Packages, Big Benefits

BATTLES:
- birth defects
- cancer
- heart disease
- high cholesterol

BOLSTERS:
- regularity

We like to cook dried beans. But the truth is that we don't always have the time or the foresight to plan ahead and presoak them. And that's why lentils are our savior. You don't have to remember to do anything in advance. You just take them out of the package, and in 5 to 30 minutes, depending on the variety, you have dinner on the table. The best part: You don't have to sacrifice a bit of nutrition for these speedy suppers.

FOLATE FINDS

When it comes to folate, lentils are a powerhouse, supplying 45 percent of your daily requirement in just a $\frac{1}{2}$-cup cooked serving.

NUTRITION IN A NUTSHELL

Cooked Lentils ($\frac{1}{2}$ cup)

Calories: 115

Fat: 0 g

Saturated fat: 0 g

Cholesterol: 0 mg

Sodium: 2 mg

Total carbohydrates: 20 g

Dietary fiber: 5 g

Protein: 9 g

Folate: 45% of Daily Value

Vitamin B$_3$ (niacin): 5%

Copper: 12%

Iron: 18%

Magnesium: 9%

Zinc: 8%

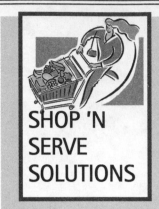

SHOP 'N SERVE SOLUTIONS

Dried lentils are always stocked in your supermarket. And, if you have a good market nearby, you may find more than one variety. Available options include the following:

■ **Regular lentils.** Also known as brewers' lentils, these are a good all-purpose choice.

■ **Red Chief lentils.** They're best in purees, dips, and other dishes where soft lentils work well.

■ **Pardina, or Spanish Brown, lentils.** These lentils tend to have a lighter flavor.

■ **Large green lentils.** They're excellent for salads.

WHEN SELECTING LENTILS:

■ Look for boxes containing lentils of uniform size.

■ If you buy lentils in bulk, examine them for pinhole marks—a sign of insect damage.

WHEN STORING:

■ Place lentils in well-sealed containers.

■ Store them in a cool, dry place (but not the fridge), where they'll keep for up to a year.

That's more than many fortified cereals provide! Folate and its synthetic form, folic acid, are crucial for warding off neural tube birth defects, such as spina bifida.

For the childbearing years: Moms-to-be need this nutrient before they even know they're pregnant. So we, along with nearly every government health organization, strongly urge all women who are capable of becoming pregnant to make sure they get 400 micrograms of folate from foods and another 400 micrograms of folic acid from fortified foods or supplements daily. Lentils will provide 179 micrograms in a ½ cup.

WHEN YOU'RE READY TO USE:

Unlike beans, you shouldn't presoak lentils. Simply sort, rinse, and then boil most varieties in unsalted water for 15 to 30 minutes; Red Chiefs require only 5 to 10 minutes. Follow the directions on your package for exact cooking times.

LEARNING TO LOVE THE GENTLE LENTIL

Here are a few ideas to get you started on adding these little packets of goodness to your life:

◆ **Jazz up a salad.** Add cooked lentils to a salad made with spinach or watercress.

◆ **Refill your potato.** Bake 2 medium potatoes, scoop out the insides, and mash with $1/4$ cup of low-fat milk, 2 tablespoons of low-fat plain yogurt, and $1/2$ cup of cooked lentils.

◆ **Top your pizza.** We kid you not—it's good! Mix a little bit of meat topping (such as sausage) with cooked lentils, and top your pie. Don't forget to pile on veggies, too.

◆ **Open a can.** For those days when you really have no time, buy a few cans of lentil soup.

For the later years: Even if babies are no longer a concern, you still need folate for your heart. Although researchers are still working to solidify the link, it appears that folate lowers your level of homocysteine, an amino acid that could trigger a heart attack when it rises too high. How much is enough? Researchers suspect that it's 400 to 800 micrograms daily.

Quick Fix:

Constipation

If you're often suffering from constipation, add $1/2$ cup of cooked lentils to your diet. They kick in 5 grams of fiber—roughly one-fifth of what you need for the day.

FIBER FACTORY

Lentils also are chock-full of fiber. Studies suggest that fiber lowers cholesterol and reduces your risk of developing cancer. In fact, a new study suggests that people who eat the most fiber-rich foods have about half the risk of developing mouth and throat cancers as those who consume the least.

Lentil-Stuffed Mushrooms

At your next shindig, try this recipe, courtesy of the U.S.A. Dried Pea and Lentil Council.

¼ cup dried lentils
16 medium mushrooms
¼ cup butter or margarine
¼ cup finely chopped onion
¼ teaspoon salt
⅛ teaspoon freshly ground black pepper
½ cup grated Parmesan cheese
½ cup dried plain bread crumbs

Cook the lentils according to package directions. Meanwhile, preheat the oven to 350°F. Remove the stems from the mushrooms. Chop the stems and set aside. Arrange the caps in an oiled baking dish. In a skillet, stir together the butter or margarine, chopped stems, onion, salt, and pepper. Cook until the onion is clear and soft. Stir in the lentils, cheese, and bread crumbs. Remove from the heat. Stuff the caps with the lentil mixture. Bake for 10 to 15 minutes (or broil for about 5 minutes). Serve hot.

Yield: Eight servings.

Nutritional data per serving: Calories, 135; protein, 6 g; carbohydrates, 10 g; fiber, 2 g; fat, 8 g; saturated fat, 5 g; cholesterol, 20 mg; sodium, 440 mg; calcium, 10% of Daily Value; iron, 8%.

Lettuce:
Go for the Green!

BATTLES:
- birth defects
- breast cancer
- heart disease

BOLSTERS:
- immune function
- regularity
- wound healing

Colleen grew up loving lettuce—you know, that sweet, crispy iceberg kind. So it wasn't easy for her to switch to the deeper, darker, more flavorful types such as red leaf lettuce and romaine. But iceberg lettuce itself helped her make the switch, because instead of going cold turkey, she mixed little bits of the dark stuff with the iceberg until her taste buds adapted. Now, she's gone totally dark. And that's good, because the darker the color, the deeper the nutrition.

PLAY YOUR CARDS RIGHT

Dark green lettuce deals out a luscious array of the antioxidant vitamins A, C, and E—your ACEs in the hole for better health, so to speak. Three decades of ongoing studies show that people who eat the most fruits and vegetables have the lowest rates of heart disease, hypertension, stroke, and cancer. As

Quick Fix:

A Hot Head

Suffering from the heat? Try this baseball players' trick: Put a chilled lettuce leaf under your cap. It'll cool you off!

researchers tease out the beneficial ingredients, these vitamin ACEs are usually part of the winning hand, because they rev up your immune system to fight invading bacteria, viruses, and pollutants.

Are we sure lettuce can do this? In one Mexican study, 198 women ages 21 to 79 were evaluated to see how their usual diet matched up with their risk of getting breast cancer. Among the premenopausal women, those who ate the most onions, lettuce, and spinach were the least likely to get breast cancer.

A Mix of Additional Greens

Certainly lettuce will make up the bulk of your salad. But markets are bursting with other "greens" (some red!) that add color, texture, and flavor interest to tossed salads. Here are those that you're most likely to see.

Green	Appearance	Flavor	Keeps Well For	Top Nutrients
Arugula	Tiny, flat leaves	Peppery	2–3 days	Magnesium
Chicory	Curly, feathery leaves	Bitter	7 days	Vitamin A
Endive	Pale green	Bitter	3–4 days	Vitamin A
Escarole	Broad, curved leaves	Mild	7 days	Folate, fiber
Radicchio	Little red cabbage	Slightly bitter	7 days	Vitamin A, vitamin E
Watercress	Tiny leaf bouquet	Delicate	3 days	Vitamin A, vitamin C, vitamin E, magnesium

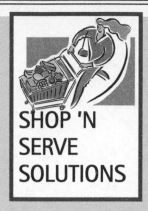

SHOP 'N SERVE SOLUTIONS

You'll find lots of lettuce year-round.

WHEN SELECTING LETTUCE:

■ Lettuce is 95 percent water, and it's the water that gives it crunch. If lettuce loses its water, it goes limp. Always skimp on limp lettuce.

■ To get the most vitamin C, go for the green. If lettuce looks pale for its type, don't buy it.

WHEN YOU'RE READY TO USE:

■ Except for the iceberg variety, lettuce tends to be pretty dirty, so you'll need to wash it well. And since salad dressing sticks best to dry leaves, do your washing well in advance of eating your lettuce.

■ After washing the leaves, whirl them around in a salad spinner to get them damp-dry. Wrap the lettuce in several layers of paper towels, then stuff the whole thing in a plastic bag. The paper towels will absorb the moisture, and the plastic will keep the leaves from drying out. Your lettuce will be so crisp and fresh, you won't believe it!

LET-TUCE MAKE A RHYME

Here's a poem about crispy things you can do with your lettuce:

◆ **Have a Thai treat.** Pile bits of seafood, vegetables, onions, and peanut sauce in a lettuce leaf. Roll up the leaf like a tortilla, and enjoy.

◆ **Skip the leftover beat.** Shred failing lettuce into soup or stir-fries.

◆ **Make it real neat.** Fold a large lettuce leaf and stuff it into your pita pocket sandwich.

◆ **Cool the heat.** Add shredded lettuce and chopped tomatoes to tacos and tortillas.

◆ **Watch fruit and greens meet.** Top a plate of salad greens with citrus sections, or add pear or apple chunks to your next bowlful.

◆ **Never retreat.** When you're too tired to chop, tear open a bag of mixed greens. But do wash it. Processed lettuce has been known to carry the vicious *E. coli* bacteria.

GREEN LIGHT

Green means "Go," and you'll keep going longer if you let a little lettuce into your life. Dark green lettuce serves up a serious dose of folate, the B vitamin that fends off heart disease and prevents neural tube birth defects.

LET-TUCE MAKE SALAD

As you shop your way through the produce section, you'll find four unique kinds of lettuce: iceberg, Butterhead, romaine (also called cos), and looseleaf. Regardless of which type you choose, color is key. The darker the color, the richer the vitamins and minerals. Here's a rundown on the four types:

■ **Iceberg** is nearly synonymous with lettuce in the United States. Its pale green, cabbagelike head is crisp and sweet, and almost anyone will eat it. It's sturdy, too, and will easily keep for a week in your vegetable crisper. Unfortunately, it pales in comparison with other lettuce types in nutrition.

■ **Butterhead** is a soft, tender, almost velvety head lettuce with a gentle green color. The Boston variety is shaped like an old-fashioned rose, while the Bibb variety is more cup-shaped. Both are quite fragile and will survive only two to three days at home. Butterhead lettuce packs twice as much magnesium as any other lettuce.

■ **Romaine**, or cos, is dark green lettuce that forms an elongated, rather than a round, head. Each leaf boasts a sturdy rib that is tender and sweet and always included in the salad. Romaine is the lettuce all-star, packing the most folate, vitamins A, B, and C, potassium, and zinc. And it's really sturdy—it'll last for 1½ weeks in your fridge.

■ **Looseleaf** is the wildest-looking lettuce, with its curly, ruffled leaves that barely agree to be joined at the stem. It can be dark green or tinged with red. While very pretty in a salad, it's delicate—so use it quickly. Looseleaf is the most fibrous lettuce and is second only to romaine in vitamin A and potassium.

Vitamin C is part of the package, too. It's part of the plant machinery that makes chlorophyll, the green color in plants. And vitamin C boosts collagen, the "glue" that holds your bones and cells together and helps heal all your little nicks and cuts, as well as your surgical incisions. And lettuce adds fiber to your diet to help keep you going you-know-where!

NUTRITION IN A NUTSHELL

Romaine lettuce (2 cups)

Calories: 16

Fat: 0 g

Saturated fat: 0 g

Cholesterol: 0 mg

Sodium: 8 mg

Total carbohydrates: 3 g

Dietary fiber: 2 g

Protein: 2 g

Folate: 38% of Daily Value

Vitamin A: 58%

Vitamin C: 30%

Calcium: 4%

Iron: 7%

Perfect Red Salad

What makes salad really great is fresh, crispy, crunchy leaves that are lightly, but evenly, coated with a small amount of dressing.

1 cup romaine lettuce
1 cup red leaf lettuce
½ cup chicory greens
½ cup radicchio
1 tablespoon olive oil
2 tablespoons red wine vinegar
⅛ teaspoon salt
⅛ teaspoon freshly ground black pepper

At least 2 hours before dining, or even the night before, thoroughly wash all the salad greens, changing the water several times if necessary, to remove every trace of grit or sand. Dry the leaves in a salad spinner until damp-dry. Wrap the leaves in several layers of paper towels, then store the wrapped leaves in a plastic bag in the refrigerator. (The paper towels will absorb all the remaining water, and the plastic will keep the leaves from drying out and make them unbelievably crunchy.) Just before you're ready to eat, tear or cut the leaves into bite-size pieces and put them in a very large salad bowl. Drizzle with the oil and toss thoroughly until every leaf is coated. Sprinkle with the vinegar and toss thoroughly again. Add the salt and pepper and toss once more. Perfect!

Yield: Two servings.

Nutritional data per serving: Calories, 87; protein, 2 g; carbohydrates, 6 g; fiber, 3 g; fat, 7 g; saturated fat, 1 g; cholesterol, 0 mg; sodium, 172 mg; folate, 27% of Daily Value; vitamin A, 61%; vitamin C, 26%; vitamin E, 16%.

Mangoes:
A Tropical Folk Remedy

BATTLES:
- cancer
- heart disease

BOLSTERS:
- digestion
- vision

Karen's taste buds first fell in love with mangoes at least 10 years ago (but who's counting?). She tried a variety of Snapple called Mango Madness—and was wild about it from the first sip. Because the drink had a lot of calories (and probably not very much mango), she saved it for special occasions. But she decided to try the fruit behind this incredible beverage. And she's been hooked on mangoes ever since.

MUCH ADO ABOUT MANGOES

One of the most commonly eaten fruits in the world, mangoes originated in southeast Asia more than 4,000 years ago, and have been used in folk remedies ever since.

Mangoes are loaded with vitamins A and C, nutrients that help fend off cancer and heart disease. In fact, just half a mango offers 40 percent of the vitamin A

(Continued on page 258)

NUTRITION IN A NUTSHELL

Mango (½)

Calories: 70

Fat: 0.5 g

Saturated fat: 0 g

Cholesterol: 0 mg

Sodium: 0 mg

Total carbohydrates: 17 g

Dietary fiber: 3 g

Protein: 1–3 g

Vitamin A: 40% of Daily Value

Vitamin C: 15%

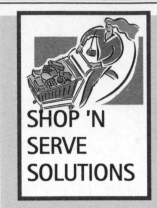

SHOP 'N SERVE SOLUTIONS

Chances are, you've never bought a mango. If you have, please pardon us as we give a lesson to the beginners. Mangoes are most plentiful from February through September (although Karen found some good ones last Christmas), and they come in several varieties that don't resemble each other very much. (See "The Many Faces of Mango" on page 258.) For that reason, you can never really judge a mango by its color. Fortunately, there are other ways to know you're getting the best fruit.

WHEN SELECTING MANGOES:

■ Use your nose. A good mango will have a lush fragrance. (The better the aroma, the better the flavor.)

■ Press the flesh. A ripe mango will yield slightly to gentle pressure (like a peach).

■ Avoid mangoes with lots of black spots. Some black specks on the skin are normal, but too many of them may indicate damage to the flesh underneath.

■ Put back any mangoes that have loose or shriveled skin.

WHEN STORING:

■ Place ripe mangoes in the refrigerator, where they'll keep for two to five days.

■ Put unripe mangoes in a paper bag on your kitchen counter for a couple of days. Then transfer them to the fridge.

FLESH IT OUT

Ready to dig in? Here's how: Most mango flesh clings to a large, flat pit. Your best bet is to get out a good, sharp, thin-bladed knife.

Begin by slicing off both ends of the fruit. Place the mango on one of the flat ends, and cut the peel from top to bottom along the curvature of the fruit. Never eat the peel. Slice away the fruit by carving lengthwise along the pit.

Some grocery stores even sell presliced mango, although it costs a little more. You also might find dried or frozen mango.

MANGO MANIA

Now that you have your supply of this tropical treasure, treat yourself to some healthy fun:

◆ **Wake up your morning.** You can incorporate mango into almost any breakfast. Stir small pieces into plain yogurt; top pancakes or waffles with mango slices instead of syrup; or stir chopped dried mango into your muffin or quick-bread mixes.

◆ **Tenderize your chicken or pork.** Simply marinate it (in the fridge, of course) in mango juice for about an hour. Then grill or broil it—and serve with mango slices. You'll think you've died and gone to a tropical paradise.

◆ **Swap 'em for peaches.** Mangoes have so much in common with peaches that you can substitute an equal amount of them in most of your recipes.

◆ **Have your just desserts.** Karen is a huge fan of dessert—no dinner is really complete without it. To have your dessert and still fit into your skirt, keep it simple. Drizzle mango slices with a teaspoon of melted chocolate or chocolate syrup. Top low-fat vanilla frozen yogurt with mango slices and a dollop of whipped cream. Or pick up a pint of Häagen-Dazs mango sorbet—it tastes incredible and delivers a big scoop of vitamin A.

The Many Faces of Mango

There are four common varieties of mangoes. Each differs in size, appearance, flavor, and fiber content from the other three. They are so different, in fact, they don't even look like they're related.

Mango	Color When Ripe	Flavor	Fiber Content	Availability
Harden	Yellow, with a red-orange blush	Mild	Medium	February–June
Keitt	Green; may have a slight yellow blush	Rich	Low	July–September
Kent	Green-yellow; may have a red blush	Very sweet	Low	June–August
Tommy Atkins	Red	Mild	High	April–July

(Continued from page 255)
that you need for the entire day.

To test the mango's anticancer potential, researchers from the University of Florida in Gainesville dropped either mango extracts or water on mice cells. The mango was 10 times more effective at inhibiting the development of cancerous cells than the water.

In humans, study after study has shown that vitamins A and C gobble up free radicals, substances that may contribute to cancer and heart disease.

What's more, mangoes contain the antioxidants lutein and zeaxanthin, which help protect vision by warding off age-related macular degeneration, a common cause of blindness in older Americans.

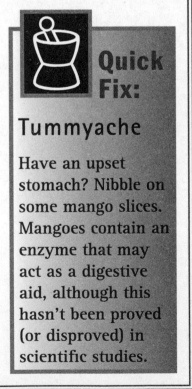

Quick Fix:

Tummyache

Have an upset stomach? Nibble on some mango slices. Mangoes contain an enzyme that may act as a digestive aid, although this hasn't been proved (or disproved) in scientific studies.

Mango Pops

*In the dog days of summer, we'll eat or drink just about any-
thing to cool off. Instead of buying vitamin-vacant, artificially
colored ice pops (c'mon, nature never intended food to be
neon blue!), make your own treats using this recipe, courtesy
of London Fruit. It takes just a couple of minutes—and once
you taste these mango pops, you'll never go back to ordinary
ice pops again.*

2 cups chopped mangoes
½ cup evaporated skim milk
¾ cup water
¼ cup frozen pineapple juice concentrate, thawed

In a blender, puree the mangoes until smooth. Add the milk,
water, and pineapple juice concentrate. Blend until well
mixed. Pour into freezer molds or paper cups and insert
wooden sticks. Seal and freeze until firm. Unmold and serve
immediately.

Yield: 4 servings.

*Nutritional data per serving: Calories, 111; protein, 3 g; carbohydrates, 26 g;
fiber, 2 g; fat, 0 g; saturated fat, 0 g; cholesterol, 1 mg; sodium, 39 mg; vitamin
C, 40% of Daily Value; calcium, 11%.*

Margarine:
Take Control of Cholesterol

BATTLES:
- heart disease
- high cholesterol

When Karen was growing up, her parents always kept margarine in the house—even though she preferred the taste of butter. Her mom would remind her that margarine was healthier for her than butter and that, if she preferred, she could always leave her bread dry.

But years later, Harvard University researchers shocked the country by saying that margarine could actually *increase* your risk of heart disease. Why? Unfortunately, when margarine manufacturers made liquid vegetable oils creamy, they created trans fat, a type that the brainiacs at Harvard believe is worse for you than the saturated fat in butter!

Now some manufacturers are offering margarines that don't contain any trans

NUTRITION IN A NUTSHELL

Benecol Light Spread
(1 tablespoon)

Calories: 45

Fat: 5 g

Saturated fat: 0.5 g

Cholesterol: 0 mg

Sodium: 110 mg

Total carbohydrates: 0 g

Dietary fiber: 0 g

Protein: 0 g

Vitamin A: 10% of Daily Value

Vitamin E: 20%

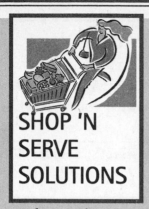

SHOP 'N SERVE SOLUTIONS

If you're in a hurry, the margarine aisle in your supermarket can be a nightmare. But if you bear with us for a minute, we'll get you through it in a flash.

WHEN SELECTING MARGARINE:

■ Choose a margarine such as Promise Ultra or Smart Beat, both of which are free of trans fat or close to it.

■ Consider a liquid margarine, which usually has far less trans fat than the stick variety.

■ Or, if you have high cholesterol, talk to your doctor about using Benecol or Take Control. These are specifically designed to lower your level of bad cholesterol.

COOKING WITH THE NEW MARGARINES

You can cook the same way with trans fat–free margarine (except Take Control) as you can with the regular stuff. Baking results, however, may vary depending on the brand and the recipe you're using. So you'll have to experiment. Take Control's manufacturer recommends that you don't use that particular product for baking.

fat—and a couple of these products are actually made with a compound to lower your cholesterol. Cool, huh?

MEET THE MARGARINES THAT LOWER CHOLESTEROL

Let's start with the trans fat–free margarines that lower cholesterol—Benecol and Take Control. They boast a cholesterol-like plant fat that blocks the absorption of cholesterol in the small intestine. As a result, the level of bad low-density lipoprotein (LDL) cholesterol in the blood drops. How much? The American Heart Association (AHA) says 2 tablespoons of Benecol or 3 tablespoons of Take Control daily lower LDL cholesterol

Sizing Up the Spreads

The following spreads are all trans fat–free (and that's fabulous), but their calories and fat content per tablespoon vary tremendously. We suggest sticking with the lower-calorie and lower-fat versions, especially if you're watching your weight. Take a look.

Spread	Type	Calories	Fat (g)	Saturated Fat (g)	Cholesterol	Sodium (mg)	Vitamin E (% of Daily Value)
Benecol	Tub	90	9	1	0	110	20
Benecol Light	Tub	45	5	0.5	0	110	20
Brummel & Brown	Tub	45	5	1	0	90	0
Fleisch-mann's Light	Tub	40	4.5	0	0	90	0
Promise	Stick	90	10	2.5	0	90	15
Promise	Tub	80	8	2	0	70	15
Promise Buttery Light	Tub	45	51	0	0	10	15
Promise Fat-Free	Tub	5	0	0	0	90	0
Promise Light	Stick	50	6	2	0	55	15
Promise Ultra	Tub	35	3.5	1	0	90	10
Smart Balance	Tub	80	9	2.5	0	90	10
Smart Beat	Tub	20	2	0	0	105	10
Take Control	Tub	50	6	1	Less than 5	110	6
Take Control Light	Tub	40	4.5	0.5	Less than 5	110	0

levels by 7 to 10 percent—more if used in conjunction with a heart-healthy diet.

Amazingly, these margarines don't seem to lower your level of good high-density lipoprotein (HDL) cholesterol. But the AHA warns that you should discuss trying these margarines with your doctor so that the two of you can monitor the impact and make adjustments to your medication if necessary.

What's more, Benecol and Take Control are really just for people with high cholesterol. The AHA recently emphasized: "Children and adults who have not been diagnosed as having elevated levels of LDL cholesterol should not consume the product as a 'preventive' measure. While cholesterol-lowering margarines may be used as part of a treatment plan, they do not prevent the underlying cause of elevated LDL."

Somewhere between the new cholesterol-reducing margarines and the old trans fat margarines, you'll find a few products that are trans fat–free, but that do not contain cholesterol-lowering plant compounds. These "in-betweens" would be better for kids and adults without high cholesterol. (For a listing, see "Sizing Up the Spreads" on the opposite page.)

SAY GOOD-BYE TO STICK MARGARINE

Some butter substitutes, especially the stick kind, are a major source of trans fat in the diet, supplying 1 to 3 grams per tablespoon. A Harvard University study of 85,000 nurses found that those who took in the most trans fat (about 5 grams daily) stood a 50 percent greater risk of heart disease than those who ate the least, even though their overall fat intake was the same.

"About 15,000 women die prematurely every year because of heart disease resulting from a high trans fat intake," explains study author Walter Willett, M.D., chairman of the nutrition department at the Harvard School of Public Health.

Chocolate Raspberry Thumbprint Cookies

The folks at Benecol passed along this recipe for cookies. They're really yummy—and contain much less unhealthy fat than most store-bought cookies.

½ cup sugar
1 egg
½ teaspoon vanilla extract
8 tablespoons Benecol Regular Spread
½ cup Dutch-process cocoa powder
1½ cups flour
½ cup dried cranberries, chopped
⅓ cup seedless raspberry jam

In a food processor, combine the sugar, egg, and vanilla extract. Process until pale, about 20 seconds. Add the Benecol. Process just until the mixture is creamy, about 10 seconds. Add the cocoa and 1¼ cups of the flour all at once. Pulse until a moist, soft dough forms, six to eight times. If the dough doesn't come together, add the remaining ¼ cup of flour and pulse three or four times. Mix the cranberries in by hand. Scoop out the dough, dividing it equally between two sheets of waxed paper. Form each portion of dough into a 1-by-12-inch log. At this point, you can bake the dough, refrigerate it for up to 24 hours, or freeze it for up to one month.

Preheat the oven to 350°F. With a sharp knife, cut one log into ½-inch slices. (Keep the other one chilled.) Roll each slice into a ball, and place on a baking sheet, arranging the cookies 1½ inches apart. Press your fingertip into the center of each. Bake until the cookies feel firm, about 13 minutes. While the cookies are baking, melt the jam in the microwave. Transfer the cookies to a rack. Spoon a dab of jam into the hollow in each cookie. Cool completely. Store in a tightly closed container for up to one week.

Yield: 48 cookies.

Nutritional data per cookie: Calories, 49; protein, 1 g; carbohydrates, 8 g; fiber, 1 g; fat, 2 g; saturated fat, 0 g; cholesterol, 4 mg; sodium, 20 mg; iron, 2% of Daily Value.

Simply Sweet Potatoes

Sweet potatoes are so scrumptious that they don't need much dressing up. So give yourself a break and keep things simple with this recipe.

4 medium sweet potatoes
2 tablespoons any trans fat–free margarine
1 teaspoon ground cinnamon
½ teaspoon ground nutmeg
¼ cup mini marshmallows (optional)

Bake the potatoes in the microwave or oven until done. Using a sharp knife, slit the center and open each potato. Season each with an equal amount of the margarine, cinnamon, nutmeg, and, if using, marshmallows.

Yield: Four servings.

Nutritional data per serving (using Promise Ultra): Calories, 138; protein, 2 g; carbohydrates, 28 g; fiber, 4 g; fat, 2 g; saturated fat, 0 g; cholesterol, 0 mg; sodium, 57 mg; calcium, 4% of Daily Value; iron, 4%.

Milk:
Nature's Nearly Perfect Food

BATTLES:
- cancer
- high blood pressure
- osteoporosis
- poison ivy
- premenstrual syndrome

BOLSTERS:
- bones
- weight control

Oh, baby, baby, baby. You started your life drinking milk. In fact, until you were six months old, milk, and milk alone, was the perfect healthy diet. Of course, milk had to make room for other important foods as you grew older. But it's still critical for maintaining a healthy body, no matter what your age.

Milk's image has suffered a little because of whole milk's high saturated fat content. But skim and 1 percent milk pack the same nutrition without the fat. Don't like the taste? Neither did Colleen when she was

Quick Fix:

Poison Ivy

If you have poison ivy and can't get to the calamine lotion, soak a washcloth in cold milk to make a compress for your itchy skin. It's an old-time remedy that really works, probably because the fat and proteins are soothing.

Vermont Country Milk

Fresh Premium Quality Milk from Vermont Dairy Farms

THINK YOU'RE INTOLERANT?

Many adults think they cannot digest lactose, the naturally occurring sugar in milk. But the calcium in milk is easier to absorb than the calcium in vegetables, and there's a lot more of it in milk. That's why a recent study found that adults who avoid dairy foods have an increased risk of osteoporosis. If that's you, here's what to do:

■ Drink milk in small portions. Many people can tolerate $\frac{1}{2}$ cup with no problem.

■ Gradually increase quantities to test and increase your tolerance.

■ Have your milk with meals. Food diminishes the lactose effect.

■ Try cultured buttermilk or Lactaid milk. Each contains less milk sugar than regular milk does.

■ Take a chewable lactase supplement with your milk. It provides the enzyme your body lacks to break down lactose.

little, so her dad added a little sweetener and vanilla and called it "skookie," and she was good to go!

BONE UP BETTER WITH MILK

When you consider the benefits of milk, you probably think of calcium, which is so beneficial in the fight against osteoporosis. And you're right. Milk and products made from milk, such as cheese and yogurt, supply about 300 milligrams of calcium per serving. That's about one-third of the daily value for folks under 50 and about one-fourth of what you need if you're older.

But only milk fortified with vitamin D will help prevent osteoporosis. Without the "sunshine" vitamin, you might as well take a bath in milk, for all the good it will do your bones. You

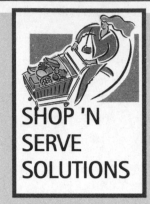

SHOP 'N SERVE SOLUTIONS

Need milk? Follow these simple, but important, guidelines to get the best.

WHEN SELECTING MILK:

■ Check the "sell-by" date on your milk to be sure it's fresh.

■ Always buy pasteurized milk. The brief, mild-heat treatment kills dangerous and deadly bacteria without changing the taste or nutrition.

WHEN STORING:

Heat and light are milk's enemies, destroying vitamins with exposure, so keep your milk in the refrigerator.

MILK IT

Here are some easy ways to keep milk in your life:

◆ **Flavor it.** Create a cocktail to fight premenstrual syndrome by adding fat-free chocolate syrup to a glass of calcium-rich skim milk. Or flavor sweetened skim milk with vanilla, almond, or peppermint. Or maybe make peppermint chocolate milk!

◆ **Warm it up.** Have a comforting cup of warm milk before bed. Or enjoy a cup of hot chocolate made with milk and a low-fat mix.

◆ **Swirl it.** For a real calcium jolt, add $1/3$ cup of nonfat dry milk to your next smoothie. It has all the nutrition of a full cup of liquid milk.

◆ **Lighten up with it.** Use evaporated skim milk to lighten your coffee. Half the water has been removed, so, measure for measure, it has twice the nutrition of regular milk.

◆ **Cook with it.** Use skim milk instead of water when you microwave your oatmeal or cook up creamed soups.

◆ **Snack on it.** Need some comfort food? Have a glass of milk and a couple of cookies or half a peanut butter sandwich.

Dueling Moo Juice

Cup for cup, skim milk has all the vitamins and minerals of whole milk, but fewer calories, less fat, and less cholesterol. See how the cow cartons (8 ounces each) stack up.

Milk	Calories	Fat (g)	Saturated Fat (g)	Cholesterol (mg)
Skim	85	0	0	4
1%	102	3	2	10
2%	121	5	3	18
Whole	150	8	5	33

simply cannot absorb calcium if you're D-ficient.

Most younger adults make enough vitamin D when the sun shines on their skin. Even so, a study at Harvard University found that 42 percent of adults under 65 years old were vitamin D–deficient. Worse, the study found that 99 percent of older adults who don't spend any time outdoors, or who live in northern areas where the sun's rays are too slanted to get the job done, are vitamin D–deficient. So baby yourself: Drink your milk.

DASH AWAY FROM HIGH BLOOD PRESSURE

Which do you think works better for lowering blood pressure—taking calcium supplements or drinking milk? You're correct if you guessed milk. All sorts of dietary supplements, including calcium and magnesium, have been tested for their ability to lower blood pressure. But what works best is real food.

In a study called Dietary Approaches to Stop Hypertension (DASH), researchers in several centers around the country found that when they switched people with moderately high blood pressure from a typical American high-fat diet to a low-fat diet rich in fruits and vegetables, the participants' blood pressure

Quick Fix:

Premenstrual Syndrome

Got PMS? Get milk. For women who suffer with PMS (and their partners!), boosting calcium intake to 1,200 milligrams daily can cut symptoms in half. It may take about three months before changes are really noticeable, but it just keeps getting better after that, according to Susan Thys-Jacobs, M.D. She notes, "I tell all my women to get two dairy foods and to take two Tums" to reach 1,200 milligrams. So don't be a cranky baby: Drink your milk!

started to come down. When they added three servings of dairy foods daily, even better things happened. In just two weeks, the participants' blood pressure dropped as much as if they had taken blood pressure medication. So be sure to drink up.

WEIGHT, WEIGHT, DON'T TELL ME

If you're struggling to control your weight (and who isn't?), milk could be a great ally. In research at Purdue University in West Lafayette, Indiana, scientists found that young women who averaged 1,900 calories or less daily, but who also consumed at least 1,000 milligrams of calcium per day, carried 6 pounds less body fat than similar women who consumed less than 500 milligrams of calcium daily. With only 85 calories in a cup of skim milk, you can't find a more nutrient-dense diet food.

Unfortunately, dieters often spurn milk while trying to lose weight, and that's a bad moooove. Carrying excess poundage is a weight-bearing activity that helps keep cal-

NUTRITION IN A NUTSHELL

Skim milk (1 cup)

Calories: 85

Fat: 0 g

Saturated fat: 0 g

Cholesterol: 4 mg

Sodium: 126 mg

Total carbohydrates: 12 g

Dietary fiber: 0 g

Protein: 8 g

Vitamin A: 10% of Daily Value

Vitamin B_2 (riboflavin): 20%

Vitamin C: 3%

Vitamin D: 25%

Calcium: 30%

cium in your bones. (It's one of the rare benefits of being over-weight.) When you lose weight, you start to lose calcium, even if you exercise. So, pretty baby, keep that low-calorie milk in your diet plan to minimize bone loss.

Amazing Instant White Sauce

Here's a rich-tasting way to get milk into your diet that's really good for your heart. Use this quick-to-fix white sauce over chicken, vegetables, rice, potatoes, or noodles, or in casseroles such as chicken potpie.

1 cup water
1 tablespoon olive oil
1 tablespoon flour
½ teaspoon chicken bouillon granules
⅓ cup nonfat dry milk
½ teaspoon dried thyme

Bring the water to a boil and set aside. In a small saucepan over medium heat, stir together the oil and flour until well blended. Gradually stir the water into the oil-flour mixture, stirring constantly with a wire whisk. Whisk in the dry milk and thyme. Stir until the sauce is thick and hot, but not boiling.

Yield: Two servings.

Nutritional data per serving: Calories, 118; protein, 5 g; carbohydrates, 9 g; fiber, 0 g; fat, 7 g; saturated fat, 1 g; cholesterol, 2 mg; sodium, 340 mg; vitamin B$_2$ (riboflavin), 13% of Daily Value; calcium, 14%.

Mint:

It Helps Keep You in Mint Condition

BATTLES:
- breast cancer
- upset stomach

BOLSTERS:
- digestion
- exercise performance

K now why Karen loves February so much? Nope—not because of Valentine's Day (although, if her husband is reading this, flowers would be nice). Or her father's birthday. Or the Founding Fathers' birthday, which gives her a long weekend. Okay, you can quit guessing.

February is the only month when Karen can get her hands on Girl Scout Thin Mint Cookies. She usually manages to devour a few before her husband finds the box and polishes off the rest.

Fortunately, Karen enjoys nutritious fresh mint (both peppermint and spearmint) the rest of the year in dishes that are almost as yummy as those cookies. We don't usually think of mint as some-

NUTRITION IN A NUTSHELL

Fresh spearmint (2 tablespoons)

Calories: 5

Fat: 0 g

Saturated fat: 0 g

Cholesterol: 0 mg

Sodium: 3 mg

Total carbohydrates: 1 g

Dietary fiber: 1 g

Protein: 0 g

Vitamin A: 9% of Daily Value

thing healthy to eat—or *un*healthy, for that matter—but it packs a wealth of benefits.

CANCER CRUSADER

"Mint contains limonene, a powerful anti-cancer agent that studies suggest can block the development of breast tumors and also can shrink them," points out Ritva Butrum, Ph.D., vice president of research at the American Institute for Cancer Research in Washington, D.C. Limonene hinders cancer cells from utilizing a protein that they need to survive. Mint also packs another breast cancer fighter—luteolin, which may inhibit the production of inflammatory compounds linked with the development of cancer.

At this point, scientists are testing these compounds to pinpoint the exact benefits they provide. In the meantime, Dr. Butrum says, "our best insurance is eating a wide variety of plant-based foods, including herbs such as mint."

Quick Fix:

Fatigue

The next time you need to crank up your workout—but don't really feel like it—take a whiff of peppermint. One study has shown that peppermint sniffing boosts exercise performance, making workouts seem easier to complete. And that's one illusion we could all use.

STOMACH SOOTHER

Your grandma probably told you that if you had stomach cramps, peppermint would take care of it. She's a smart lady. Peppermint contains menthol, a substance that helps prevent spasms in your digestive tract, lessening cramps.

What's more, a review of studies in the *Journal of Gastroenterology* suggests that peppermint oil (you can get this at a health food store) might even help people who suffer from irritable bowel syndrome, a condition that causes very frequent bowel movements.

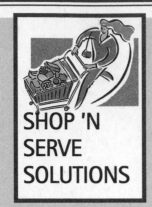

SHOP 'N SERVE SOLUTIONS

If you have peppermint or spearmint growing in your house or in your garden, you won't have to shop for it. But if you do need to buy some, don't sweat it. Mint isn't hard to find. Just head for the fresh herbs in the produce section of your local supermarket.

WHEN SELECTING MINT:

■ Look for a bunch that is evenly colored and shows no signs of wilting.

■ Peppermint has bright green leaves and purple-tinged stems, while spearmint has gray-green or plain green leaves. If you have trouble distinguishing between the two, your nose should be able to detect the difference: Peppermint is more pungent than spearmint. (And it's not used in as many recipes.)

WHEN STORING:

Once you have your mint home, shake it to remove grit and moisture, pack it loosely in paper towels, and keep it in your crisper or a special produce storage container, such as the type made by Tupperware. It should stay fresh for about a week.

Unfortunately, peppermint probably won't relieve heartburn—and, in fact, might even aggravate it—because it allows acid to flow more freely up into your esophagus. But two out of three isn't bad, huh?

SO COOL, IT'S HOT

Now here are some hot hints for using your cool mint:

◆ **Spice up a salad.** Toss in a couple of tablespoons of chopped spearmint to add zest to your favorite fruit salad. Spearmint works particularly well with melons and berries. Or add it to a cucumber salad. We like to mix diced cucumber, diced tomato, parsley, garlic, lemon juice, olive oil, feta cheese, and, last but not least, spearmint.

◆ **Electrify chicken.** Turn ordinary grilled chicken into fireworks for the taste buds simply by topping it with a creamy mint sauce. Don't worry—it only sounds fattening. Just mix $\frac{1}{2}$ cup of low-fat plain yogurt, 1 tablespoon each of chopped spearmint and parsley, 1 teaspoon of lemon juice, 2 minced garlic cloves (you can add more if you like), and $\frac{1}{4}$ teaspoon of ground black pepper. Refrigerate for at least a few hours so that the flavors blend together. The sauce will keep for about five days, so it's a good way to jazz up leftover chicken, too.

◆ **Play with pesto.** One of Karen's favorite restaurants makes a delicious mint pesto. The point: You can substitute spearmint for basil in your favorite pesto recipe.

◆ **Have a tea party for one.** Ditch the coffee, and soothe your nerves with a cup of peppermint tea. Simply steep a small handful of fresh peppermint in a cup of boiling water. If desired, sweeten with honey.

Fall Fruit Salad

It's fast. It's fun. And it's fall. There is no better dessert for your end-of-season cookout or picnic in the park to admire the foliage. Double the recipe if you like.

1 red or green apple, unpeeled and diced
1 pear, unpeeled and diced
1 banana, peeled and sliced
3 tablespoons lemon juice
¼ cup chopped fresh spearmint

In a medium bowl, combine the apple, pear, banana, lemon juice, and spearmint. Cover and chill for several hours before serving.

Yield: Four servings.

Nutritional data per serving: Calories, 74; protein, 1 g; carbohydrates, 19 g; fiber, 2 g; fat, 0 g; saturated fat, 0 g; cholesterol, 0 mg; sodium, 1 mg.

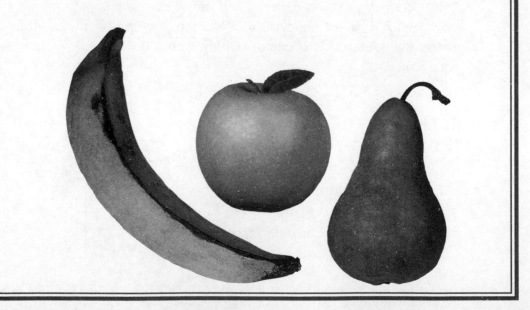

Mushrooms:

Fantastic Fungi

BATTLES:
- cancer
- high blood pressure

BOLSTERS:
- immune function
- metabolism
- weight control

Okay, we know that Alice's zany adventures in Wonderland were triggered by hallucinogenic mushrooms. Those are *not* the kind we're recommending! But we can recommend a growing variety of fabulous fungi, including the popular buttons, the meaty portobellos, the haute cuisine shiitakes, and more. Let's take a look at a few varieties—starting with the most familiar—and see just why they are so good for you.

BUTTON, BUTTON, WHO'S GOT THE BUTTON?

Childhood games aside, we're all most familiar with the white button mushrooms that spill out of grocery store bins. They're really low in calories, and despite their mild flavor, they're a powerful flavor enhancer

NUTRITION IN A NUTSHELL

Shiitake mushrooms (½ cup, cooked)

Calories: 40

Fat: 0 g

Saturated fat: 0 g

Cholesterol: 0 mg

Sodium: 0 mg

Total carbohydrates: 10 g

Dietary fiber: 2 g

Protein: 1 g

Vitamin B_2 (riboflavin): 7% of Daily Value

Vitamin B_3 (niacin): 5%

Vitamin B_6: 6%

Copper: 32%

Zinc: 6%

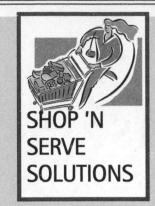

SHOP 'N SERVE SOLUTIONS

Mushrooms are available in all seasons. Regardless of which kind you choose, they should look pretty chipper.

WHEN SELECTING MUSHROOMS:

■ Look for mushrooms that are smooth, dry, and firm, without cuts or bruises.

■ Choose those that smell fresh and nutty, like bread.

■ Pass up mushrooms that look limp, dried out, wrinkled, leathery, or slimy.

■ Avoid those that smell moldy.

■ Also, check out the gills under the cap. Closed gills mean the mushroom is young; open gills are a sign of aging.

WHEN STORING:

Once you get your mushrooms home, put them in a paper bag, then put the paper bag in a plastic bag, says food physiologist Brian Patterson in his book *Fresh.* The paper bag will absorb moisture so the mushrooms don't get slimy, and the plastic bag will keep the mushrooms from drying out.

WHEN YOU'RE READY TO USE:

Don't wash your mushrooms! They're like sponges when they get wet.

for just about any food you mix them with.

Tastes great! Why do mushrooms turn a good meal into a great one? It's because they serve up a nice dose of glutamic acid, the good-for-you part of monosodium glutamate (MSG) that's also known as the fifth taste. Along with sweet, sour, salty, and bitter, experts now recognize the "umami," or "meaty," taste. You've probably noticed that when you cook mushrooms, they nearly vanish. That's because they're like little sacks full of water that leak when heated. And that's okay. It makes for tasty broth,

Instead, clean them gently by dusting them off with a fine, soft mushroom brush or a soft paper towel. Most mushrooms are grown in sterilized compost, so they're really very safe to eat when handled this way.

ADDING MUSHROOM MAGIC

Now make room for mushrooms in your meals. Here are some ideas:

◆ **Slim your sauce.** Substitute a can of sliced mushrooms for the usual meat in your spaghetti sauce. You'll cut calories while boosting flavor.

◆ **Spike your salmon.** Sauté sliced fresh shiitake mushrooms, 1 sliced yellow onion, and 2 cloves of finely diced fresh garlic in a few drops of olive oil. Season with a pinch of dried basil or oregano. Serve over grilled salmon.

◆ **Bump off that burger.** Instead of a burger, have a grilled portobello mushroom on your bun.

◆ **Stock up.** Save fresh mushroom stems to make stock for yummy mushroom soup.

◆ **Expect the unexpected.** Keep dehydrated exotic mushrooms on hand to create sensational dishes on a moment's notice.

and it concentrates the nutrients in the 'shrooms, so you get more per forkful.

More filling! And while mushrooms *will* increase flavor, they *won't* add to your waistline. Even though they have so few calories, mushrooms make a wonderful bulking agent for salads, soups, and sauces. They help you fill up without filling out! (Don't sauté them in butter, however. They'll soak up a ton of fat and calories!)

Good for you! Buttons are a good source of niacin and

Mushroom Mania

Once upon a time, there were only buttons. Now, fabulous fresh mushrooms abound. Check out the differences in these fantastic fungi.

Mushroom	Looks Like	Color	Taste
Button	Smooth, white button	White or off-white	Mild
Chanterelle	Frilly trumpet	Brown-gold to yellow-orange	Like apricots
Enoki	Long, skinny bouquet	Creamy white	Sweet
Oyster	Oyster clusters	Off-white or gray-brown	Meaty
Portobello	Burger patty	Dark brown	Meaty
Shiitake	Open umbrella	Brown-black	Rich
Wood ear	Flat plate	Grayish white	Mild

riboflavin, two of the B vitamins that act like converters as you metabolize your meals, turning your food into stuff your body uses for energy and to fight disease. They also are laced with copper, an important mineral for healthy blood and sturdy bones.

EXOTICA RUNNING WILD

The last few years have seen mushroom varieties, well, *mushroom*. And this is good news. The amazing array of shapes, colors, and sizes makes you wonder what Mother Nature was nibbling on when she invented mushrooms. (Way to go, Mom!) And the increasing variety sure makes dinner more interesting.

Better yet, these more exotic variations also appear to be sprouting natural chemicals with health-enhancing qualities. Shiitakes have a slight, but definite, ability to lower very low density lipoprotein (VLDL) cholesterol. (Eat them instead of a fatty burger for a double whammy!) And both shiitake and maitake mushrooms appear to boost immune system function, fight cancer, and lower blood pressure. Mushroom extracts are being studied for their cancer-curing potential.

Wild Creamy Mushroom Soup

No, we're not going to send you out to gather wild mushrooms. (Mistake their identity, and you could end up a missing person!) We'd just like you to go a little wild and pass up the button mushrooms for some that are just a tad unusual.

2 cups chopped fresh portobello mushrooms
1 cup chopped fresh shiitake mushrooms
1 cup chopped fresh cremini mushrooms
1 can (16 ounces) fat-free beef broth
¼ cup thinly sliced shallots
2 large cloves garlic, chopped
½ teaspoon paprika
½ cup reduced-fat ricotta cheese

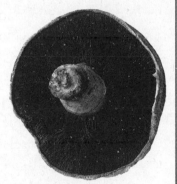

Place the mushrooms, broth, shallots, garlic, and paprika in the top of a double boiler. Cover, bring the water in the bottom to a boil, and then reduce the heat to simmer. Cook just until the mushrooms are tender and give up some of their liquid, about 10 minutes. Stir in the cheese. Heat until the soup is steaming hot, but not boiling.

Yield: Four servings.

Nutritional data per serving: Calories, 91; protein, 7 g; carbohydrates, 8 g; fiber, 2 g; fat, 3 g; saturated fat, 2 g; cholesterol, 15 mg; sodium, 473 mg; vitamin B_2 (riboflavin), 10% of Daily Value; vitamin B_3 (niacin), 10%; calcium, 11%; copper, 11%.

Nectarines:

Nectar of the Gods

BATTLES:
- cancer

BOLSTERS:
- immune function
- regularity
- vision

Luscious nectarines are in a class by themselves, although they are closely related to peaches (but sweeter). In fact, just one recessive gene, the "fuzz" gene, separates these two fruits on the tree of life.

That missing peach fuzz can be a bonus for itchy folks who can't stand peaches. They can eat the nectarine, skin and all, nudging themselves closer to the recommended 25 grams of fiber a day that will keep them moving regularly. (Most Americans get only halfway to their fiber goal each day.)

BETTER BETA

Like peaches, cantaloupe, carrots, and other orange-colored fruits and veggies, nectarines are packed with beta-carotene and beta-cryptoxanthin, two carotenoids that can turn into vitamin A in your body.

Fully formed vitamin A comes only from liver, fish liver oils, margarine, butter, milk, and eggs. And while small portions of those foods deliver needed nutrients, overdoing them can be a health hazard. So indulge in luscious nectarines on a hot summer day. While the juice is dripping off your chin, your body will make enough vitamin A from that fruit to bolster your skin and mucous membranes to defend against invading viruses and bacteria, and to boost your immune system to destroy invaders that breach the ramparts.

SHOOTING THE GAP

Endless studies make it clear that people who eat the most foods rich in beta-carotene have better protection against cancer. Exactly why is not clear. One possibility is that the beta-carotene boosts communication between cells. Basically, cells need to talk to each other across the spaces that separate them in order to coordinate their defenses. Two laboratory studies have shown that carotenoids improve this communication. They're like the string between the tin cans.

EYES BRIGHT!

Nectarines also carry small amounts of another carotenoid, lutein, which has been shown to defend against age-related macular degeneration, the leading cause of blindness in older adults.

Even though the amount of lutein in a nectarine is small, researchers have discovered that your body absorbs carotenoids twice as well from fruits as from dark green leafy vegetables, such as kale or spinach. So nectarines' visual impact may be greater than it first appears. Their vitamin A activity also fends off night blindness, and some studies suggest that beta-carotene battles cataracts, making nectarines the eye-deal fruit for your eyes.

NUTRITION IN A NUTSHELL

Nectarine (1 medium)

Calories: 67

Fat: Less than 1 g

Saturated fat: 0 g

Cholesterol: 0 mg

Sodium: 0 mg

Total carbohydrates: 16 g

Dietary fiber: 2 g

Protein: 1 g

Vitamin A: 13% of Daily Value

Vitamin C: 8%

Calcium: 1%

Iron: 1%

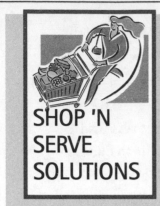

SHOP 'N SERVE SOLUTIONS

Most nectarines come from California's San Joaquin Valley, which produces 175 varieties. Nectarines from California are available all summer long, from mid-May through September. Chile also produces a nectarine crop that's on supermarket shelves during the winter.

WHEN SELECTING NECTARINES:

Each variety has its own flavor and color, ranging from a red-blushed golden yellow to almost entirely red. They'll be firm and a little underripe when you buy them.

WHEN STORING:

■ Once you get your nectarines home, put them in a paper bag on your kitchen counter for one to three days. Keep the bag out of the sun. They'll get sweeter and softer day by day. You'll know they're ripe when they smell heavenly and yield to gentle pressure.

■ Once they're ripe, put them in the refrigerator so that you'll have a nice supply at the peak of flavor.

SWEETEN YOUR SUMMER

Here's how to use nectarines to make your life sweeter:

◆ **Salsify 'em.** Finely chop a nectarine and toss the pieces into fiery salsa for a sweet-hot sensation.

◆ **Slice 'em.** Then use the slices to top frozen yogurt. Drizzle with chocolate syrup for a perfect dessert.

◆ **Smooth 'em.** Add chopped nectarines to your smoothie.

◆ **Pour 'em.** Finely chop ripe nectarines, mix with some cinnamon, and pour over your pancakes or waffles instead of using syrup.

◆ **Sliver 'em.** Then use the slivers to make our "Salmon with Nectarines" on the opposite page.

Salmon with Nectarines

When it's time to fire up the grill, enjoy this simple dish. It's a feast for your eyes, as well as your taste buds. And it's packed with nutrients for your brain, heart, and bones. Add a dinner roll and a glass of Beaujolais, and you're knocking on heaven's door.

4 cups torn red leaf lettuce, washed and spun dry
4 nectarines, washed, pitted, and slivered
2 avocados, peeled, pitted, and slivered
Juice of 3 limes
4 salmon filets (5–6 ounces each)
1 teaspoon salt
1 teaspoon freshly ground multicolored pepper
4 tablespoons chopped fresh chives

Preheat the grill and divide the lettuce among four dinner plates. In a medium bowl, combine the nectarines and avocados. Divide into fourths and arrange on half of the lettuce on each plate. Drizzle with the lime juice. Season the salmon with the salt and pepper. Grill over low heat until it flakes easily when tested with a fork, about 10 minutes. Place 1 filet on the lettuce on each plate, next to the nectarines and avocados. Sprinkle with the chives.

Yield: Four servings.

Nutritional data per serving: Calories, 462; protein, 33 g; carbohydrates, 32 g; fiber, 10 g; fat, 25 g; saturated fat, 4 g; cholesterol, 80 mg; sodium, 675 mg; vitamin A, 40% of Daily Value; vitamin B$_3$ (niacin), 74%; vitamin B$_6$, 70%; vitamin D, 159%; potassium, 49%.

Nuts:

A Heart-Smart Snack

BATTLES:
- heart disease
- high blood pressure
- stroke

BOLSTERS:
- bones
- weight control

Offer us a choice between anything plain versus nut-studded—muffins, breakfast cereal, salad—and you'll get an instant answer: "We're nuts about nuts!" From applesauce to zabaglione, those crunchy little nuggets make every dish taste better.

True, they've been in a dark period because of their high fat content, but through the marvels of modern science, we're beginning to see the light. Nuts are tiny power packets of heart-healthy fat, laced with trace minerals critical to health, but often missing from diets built on highly processed (read: white) foods.

HEART HEALTH IN A NUTSHELL

In 1992, researchers at Loma Linda University in California published a study showing that people who ate a handful of nuts five or more times a week cut their heart attack risk in half, compared with folks who never ate them.

Since then, one study after another has revealed the same

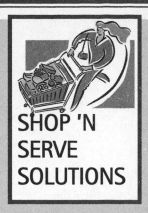

SHOP 'N SERVE SOLUTIONS

You can buy nuts fresh in the shell at most grocery stores, usually from early fall through late winter.

WHEN SELECTING NUTS IN THE SHELL:

■ Choose nuts that feel heavy for their size.

■ Pick those that appear clean, fresh, and free of mold.

The advantage of buying nuts in the shell is that they are unprocessed and unsalted. However, unsalted fresh nuts also are available already shelled and bagged, in the produce department of your grocery store. Smaller packages appear in the baking department.

We recommend these unsalted types. It's also a good idea to keep several varieties on hand so that you get a different taste each day.

WHEN STORING:

Keep shelled nuts in the refrigerator so that they don't become rancid.

LET'S GO NUTS!

Focus on using small servings of nuts in these delicious ways:

◆ **Sprinkle 'em on cereal.** Try a tablespoon or two of nuts on your hot or cold cereal in the morning. You'll be crazy about your breakfast. And that little bit of fat will help keep you satisfied until lunch.

◆ **Toss 'em into salad.** Especially good is a salad made with field greens, half a chopped apple, sliced dried figs, and toasted, chopped hazelnuts.

◆ **Grab 'em and go.** When you're starving, grab a bag of peanuts from the vending machine. For 170 calories, you'll be good to go until dinner.

◆ **Stash 'em in your desk drawer.** Use mini bathroom cups to measure out a serving.

◆ **Relish 'em on celery.** Stuff celery with reduced-fat ricotta cheese and top with chopped walnuts.

◆ **Stir 'em into yogurt.** Try sliced almonds—you'll love it!

protective effect of nuts, whether the nuts studied were walnuts, almonds, macadamias, mixed nuts, or peanuts. (Okay, peanuts are legumes, not nuts, but their fat, calorie, and nutrient profile is a very close match.)

How can all this fat be good for you? While it's true that eating lots of saturated fat from fatty meats, high-fat dairy foods, and baked goods can slam your arteries shut on a moment's notice, the kind of fat in nuts actually opens them up and makes them more pliable.

And walnuts offer something more. The kind of fat in walnuts, alpha-linolenic acid, turns into the same kind of fat you'd get from eating fish. It makes your blood less sticky and less likely to clot, so it reduces your chance of having a heart attack or stroke.

Other varieties of nuts pack big doses of monounsaturated fat, shown to lower bad low-density lipoprotein (LDL) cholesterol and triglycerides and to protect good high-density lipoprotein (HDL) cholesterol. And with nuts, this isn't just theory. Nut diets have been tested over and over again, and *they always work*.

DASH HIGH BLOOD PRESSURE

Health professionals have been so excited about this nutty good news that they've incorporated nuts in the Dietary Approaches to Stop Hypertension (DASH) diet. This incredibly powerful plan combines 8 to 11 servings of fruits and vegetables and 3 servings of dairy foods daily, plus a handful of nuts four or five times a week, along with some lean protein and a few whole grains every day.

NUTRITION IN A NUTSHELL

Pistachios (1 ounce, or 47 whole nuts)

Calories: 160

Fat: 13 g

Saturated fat: 1.5 g

Cholesterol: 0 mg

Sodium: 120 mg

Total carbohydrates: 8 g

Dietary fiber: 3 g

Protein: 6 g

Vitamin A: 4% of Daily Value

Calcium: 4%

Iron: 6%

Sometimes You Feel Like a Nut

And that's a good thing! They're all packed with protein, heart-healthy fat, vitamins, and the trace minerals often missing from American diets. Each one has its own unique nutrient profile. Pick your favorite from the list below and check its standout qualities. For best nutrition, mix and match. Nutritional values are based on a 1-ounce serving. (The number of nuts in an ounce is listed next to each type of nut.)

Almonds (24 whole nuts)
Vitamin E: 40% of Recommended Dietary Allowance (RDA)
Magnesium: 20%
Phosphorus: 15%
Calcium: 8%

Cashews (18 whole nuts)
Copper: 30% of RDA
Magnesium: 20%
Phosphorus: 15%
Iron: 10%
Zinc: 10%
Selenium: 6%

Macadamias (11 whole nuts)
Monounsaturated fat: 17 g
Vitamin B_1 (thiamin): 15% of RDA

Peanuts (30 whole nuts)
Protein: 7 g
Folate: 10% of RDA

Pecans (20 nut halves)
Monounsaturated fat: 13 g
Zinc: 10% of RDA

Pistachios (47 whole nuts)
Potassium: 290 mg
Vitamin B_6: 25% of RDA
Phosphorus: 15%
Vitamin B_1 (thiamin): 15%
Vitamin A: 4%

Walnuts (14 nut halves)
Polyunsaturated fat: 14 g
Copper: 25% of RDA
Vitamin B_6: 8%

The result: In just two weeks, people with moderately high blood pressure saw improvements as great as if they had been on blood pressure medication!

MIGHTY MINERALS

Beyond nuts' special fat, they're also packed with minerals, such as potassium (helps control blood pressure), copper (needed for healthy hemoglobin), and magnesium and phosphorus (great for bones). Plus, they're loaded with vitamins, such as thiamin, also known as vitamin B_1 (helps turn carbohydrates into energy), and vitamin B_6 (helps make serotonin, insulin, and antibodies that fight infection). In short, nuts are bursting with good stuff!

WHAT ABOUT WEIGHT?

But nuts are high in fat and calories. If you curl up in front of the TV every night with a can of nuts, you'll quickly pack on the pounds. And that's very bad for your heart and everything attached to it.

We're talking about eating a *handful*. One ounce. The light side of ¼ cup. But the good news is that working nuts into a healthy eating plan that gets 35 percent of its calories from fat can help you lose weight.

In an ongoing study at Brigham and Women's Hospital in Boston, people on this higher-fat diet were compared with a group on a diet containing only 20 percent fat. Although both groups lost the same amount of weight at the outset (an average of about 12 pounds), the nutty dieters kept the weight off for 18 months, while the low-fat dieters regained about half their weight. And twice as many low-fat dieters fell off the wagon and dropped out of the study as those who were enjoying the deliciously nutty plan.

Nuts Among the Berries

Looking for a quick dessert that's outwardly sinful but inwardly angelic? Try this simply nutty treat.

½ cup fresh raspberries
2 tablespoons chopped unsalted pecans
½ cup chocolate soy milk

Wash the raspberries and pat dry. Pile in a dessert dish. Roast the pecans in a toaster oven. Sprinkle over the raspberries. Pour the soy milk over all. Spoon it up and go nuts!

Yield: One serving.

Nutritional data per serving: Calories, 200; protein, 5 g; carbohydrates, 13 g; fiber, 6 g; fat, 12 g; saturated fat, 1 g; sodium, 0 mg; vitamin B_2 (riboflavin), 19% of Daily Value; vitamin B_{12}, 25%; calcium, 17%; copper, 11%; manganese, 65%.

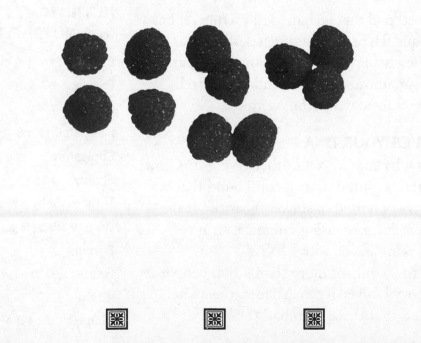

Okra:

Southern-Style Wellness

BATTLES:
- cancer

BOLSTERS:
- bones
- immune function

All you southerners are probably gonna laugh at us northern women trying to talk about okra. You most likely grew up on the stuff. But, for the benefit of the northern folks, give us a break and let us explain: Okra is a small, green (although some varieties are white), ribbed pod that is shaped like a tube. It has a unique flavor that has been described as somewhere between eggplant and asparagus, an unusual texture, and it goes well when mixed with other veggies.

SAVES YOUR DNA

But why should you bother trying it? Okra contains glutathione, a compound that shows potential to stave off cancer. It prevents cancer-causing chemicals from wreaking havoc with DNA.

In a study of more than 1,800 people at Emory University in Atlanta, researchers found that those who had the highest

NUTRITION IN A NUTSHELL

Cooked Okra (½ cup)

Calories: 27

Fat: 0 g

Saturated fat: 0 g

Cholesterol: 0 mg

Sodium: 4 mg

Total carbohydrates: 6 g

Dietary fiber: 2 g

Protein: 2 g

Folate: 9% of Daily Value

Vitamin C: 22%

Magnesium: 11%

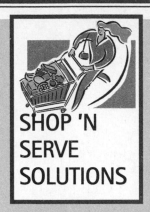

SHOP 'N SERVE SOLUTIONS

If you live in the South, you probably can buy fresh okra year-round. But most other folks will just have to settle for it in the spring and fall.

WHEN SELECTING OKRA:

■ Look for pods that are bruise-free.

■ Choose those that are tender, but not mushy.

■ Make sure they're no longer than 3 to 4 inches.

■ Avoid pods that are longer, blackish, or brownish, because they won't be as tender.

WHEN STORING:

■ Store okra in a plastic bag in the refrigerator. It'll keep for three to five days.

■ Don't wash it until you're ready to use it, or the pods will get slimy.

WHEN YOU'RE READY TO USE:

To prepare whole okra pods for cooking, just trim a teeny slice from both the stem end and the tip. You can also slice the pods before cooking. Either way, unless you're using okra in a soup or stew, you want to cook it quickly to prevent it from getting slimy.

DINNER, SOUTHERN-STYLE

Here are some suggestions for enjoying okra:

◆ **Sizzle it in stir-fries.** Toss okra into any of your favorite stir-fries—it makes a fine substitute for green beans.

◆ **Soup it up.** Gumbo soup is traditionally made with okra. We rarely whip up a batch from scratch, but we do like Healthy Choice Gumbo Soup. But you can stir okra into any soup, really—it'll even thicken the broth a bit.

◆ **Combine it with curry.** Okra and curries form a match made in heaven. In fact, this veggie goes especially well with Indian spices.

intake of foods rich in this compound were half as likely to develop oral and throat cancers as those who had the lowest intake.

Summertime Okra

Tomatoes and okra complement each other perfectly in this dish.

2 cloves garlic, minced
½ red onion, sliced
2 tablespoons olive oil
5 large tomatoes, chopped
¾ pound okra, cut into ½-inch-thick
pieces
¼ cup sliced fresh basil
¼ cup sliced olives
Salt to taste
Ground black pepper to taste

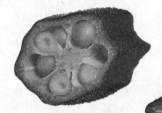

In a large wok, sauté the garlic and onion in the oil. Add the tomatoes and okra, and cook for 4 to 5 minutes, or until the okra is soft, but not limp. Add the basil and olives and cook for about 1 minute. Season with the salt and pepper.

Yield: Four servings.

Nutritional data per serving: Calories, 147; protein, 4 g; carbohydrates, 18 g; fiber, 5 g; fat, 9 g; saturated fat, 1 g; cholesterol, 0 mg; sodium, 212 mg; calcium, 9% of Daily Value; iron, 10%.

Olive Oil:
A Big Fat Difference

BATTLES:
- cancer
- dry nails
- heart disease
- high blood pressure

Years ago, way before meatless meals were cool, we discovered a recipe for Pesto Genovese. It was rich in olive oil and sweet basil—and it drove our husbands and kids wild. Now, we've discovered that all that olive oil was building a heart-protective shield around our families.

HEAD OFF HEART DISEASE

Researchers became interested in olive oil in the 1960s, when they realized that people in southern Italy, Greece, and on the Greek island of Crete ate whole vats of it, yet their life expectancy was the longest in the world. In addition, their rates of heart disease and some cancers were very low.

Americans were eating just as much fat—about 35 percent of our total calories

NUTRITION IN A NUTSHELL

Olive oil (1 tablespoon)

Calories: 120

Fat: 14 g

Saturated fat: 2 g

Monounsaturated fat: 11 g

Cholesterol: 0 mg

Sodium: 0 mg

Total carbohydrates: 0 g

Dietary fiber: 0 g

Protein: 0 g

Vitamin E: 22% of Daily Value

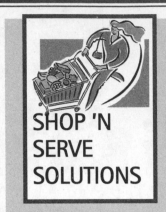

SHOP 'N SERVE SOLUTIONS

You might think that the color of olive oil tells you something about its taste. Not so, says the Olive Oil Source in Greenbrae, California. Greener oils are usually pressed from greener olives earlier in the season, and some olives are greener or more golden than others. But many of the oils on the market are blended from several varieties, so color is not the key.

The flavor of the oil really depends on when the olives were picked, how they were stored, how they were processed, the soil and weather conditions, and the age of the tree. (Olive trees reach maturity anywhere from 35 to 150 years of age and can live up to 600 years.) You'll just have to taste-test a few brands to find those you like best.

WHEN STORING OLIVE OIL:

"Olive oil does not age like fine wine," according to the Olive Oil Source. Light and heat are its enemies, so store it in a dark cupboard, a dark glass bottle, or a tin can in a cool location—not near the stove, where cooking heat will ruin it. In the fridge is okay, but the oil will turn almost solid, so you'll have to warm it before you use it.

BEYOND THE GREASE GUN APPROACH

Here are some ways to get the most benefit from olive oil:

◆ **Mist; don't fry.** Stop by a kitchenware store and invest in an oil mister. Fill it with olive oil, pump up the pressure, and then spray a light layer of body lube on broiled chicken or fish, oven-fried potatoes, or steamed vegetables.

◆ **Dip; don't spread.** Instead of butter for your bread, serve up small saucers of olive oil for dipping. Quality counts here, so choose an oil with a flavor that knocks your socks off. For added zing, season with crushed garlic and chopped fresh basil.

came from fat—but we were dropping like flies. The difference? We were eating cheeseburgers, hot dogs, and french fries—all of which are loaded with heart-trashing saturated fat.

Research by Penny Kris-Etherton, Ph.D., R.D., distinguished professor of nutrition at Pennsylvania State University in State College, explains the big fat difference. When 22 people were switched from a typical American diet to a diet high in the monounsaturated fat of olive oil, their total cholesterol dropped by 10 percent, their bad low-density lipoprotein (LDL) cholesterol plummeted by 14 percent, and their triglycerides fell by 13 percent. Yet their good high-density lipoprotein (HDL) cholesterol did not drop. All told, simply substituting olive oil for saturated fat lowered the chance of having a heart attack by *25 percent!* And that was twice as much of a reduction as the American Heart Association's very low fat Step II diet plan.

Quick Fix:

Dry, Brittle Nails

To rejuvenate dry, brittle nails, soak your hands in ½ cup of warm olive oil for 15 to 30 minutes. Your nails will slurp up the oil like a thirsty sponge!

RELIEVE THE PRESSURE

As Dr. Kris-Etherton was conducting her studies here in the United States, researchers in Naples, Italy, decided to see what effect olive oil might have on blood pressure. So they took 11 patients with high blood pressure and switched them to a diet rich in extra virgin olive oil. The result: Eight of the patients' blood pressure dropped enough so that they could give up their blood pressure medication. (Now, adding a teaspoon of olive oil to your salad sure beats the heck out of taking a pill—but don't stop your medication without talking to your doctor first. Discontinuing any blood pressure medication can be tricky.)

DEFINING AN OIL'S QUALITY

The Commission of the European Communities defines the titles on your olive oil label as follows:

■ **Extra virgin olive oil** is the highest-quality oil (less than 10 percent make the grade) from the first cold-press. It has perfect flavor and odor and less than 1 percent acidity, with great taste, mouth feel, and aroma. This is the best for using on salads, dipping, or adding to foods at the table.

■ **Fine virgin olive oil** has perfect flavor and odor and less than 2 percent acidity.

■ **Ordinary or semi-fine olive oil** has good flavor and odor and less than 3.3 percent acidity. This oil may have been refined to remove unwanted flavors or odors. It's fine for frying when flavor is not needed.

■ **Pure olive oil** is a low-cost blend of refined and virgin oils. It has less than 1.5 percent acidity.

SIDESTEP CANCER

Olive oil is made simply by squeezing (or in techno terms, *cold-pressing*) fresh olives, pits and all. Unlike other vegetable oils, it can be used fresh from the vat without heating or refining. This natural, unprocessed oil contains little bits of olive leftovers, such as phenols and squalene, that create its unique flavor, make it stable, and—best of all—may fight colon, breast, and prostate cancers.

Which is the best olive oil? Well, one market-basket analysis suggests that olive oils from the Mediterranean contain the most squalene, which preliminary studies suggest is the big gun that protects you.

Family-Party Pesto

Each September, Colleen harvests her basil leaves for an annual family pesto party. She happily admits that the sauce is incredibly rich, but a small serving satisfies.

1 cup extra virgin olive oil
2 large cloves garlic
3 tablespoons raw pine nuts (pignoli)
2 cups firmly packed fresh basil leaves, stems removed
1½ teaspoons salt
¼ teaspoon ground black pepper
1 cup freshly grated Parmesan cheese
1 pound spiral or small shell pasta
3 tablespoons toasted pine nuts (pignoli)

Place the oil and garlic in a food processor. Using the large blade, blend on high speed until smooth. With the blade spinning, open the shoot and gradually add the raw pine nuts. Process until smooth. Add the basil leaves a few at a time until well pulverized. Add the salt and pepper, then gradually add the cheese. (If necessary, stop the food processor and stir down the mixture with a stiff rubber spatula.) Continue processing until the sauce is smooth.

Cook the pasta according to package directions. Reserve ½ cup of the cooking liquid and drain off the remainder. Place the pasta in a large pasta serving dish and toss with the reserved cooking liquid. Top with the pesto sauce and toss with large salad servers until the pasta is well coated. Sprinkle with the toasted pine nuts.

Yield: Eight servings.

Nutritional data per serving: Calories, 555; protein, 15 g; carbohydrates, 44 g; fat, 35 g; saturated fat, 6 g; cholesterol, 10 mg; sodium, 596 mg; folate, 28% of Daily Value; vitamin E, 46%; calcium, 18%.

Olives:

Ripe for Health

BATTLES:
- ◼ cancer
- ◼ heart disease
- ◼ motion sickness

Quick Fix:

Motion Sickness

Sailing make you queasy? Flying turn you green? The next time you launch yourself into major motion, take along some olives. At the first sign of motion sickness, eat a couple. Olives contain tannins that dry your mouth, which reduces the excess saliva that can cause nausea.

Colleen's dad fondly remembers the highlight of every grade-school year: his class picnic. The best part was that, along with his lunch, his mother packed a skinny jar of pimiento-stuffed olives—and they were all for him!

Olives are still one of his favorite foods, and that turns out to be good news for him. It seems that because olives grow in searing sunlight, they produce an overload of anthocyanins, flavonoids, and phenols—all of which are naturally occurring plant chemicals that protect the fruit against sun damage. And once inside you, these same phytochemicals (*phyto* is from the Greek language and just means "plant") protect your cells from damage caused by pollution, illness, and even some of your own natural body processes that can throw off substances that cause disease. In fact, olives seem to protect you from everything but the sun!

GOOD FAT, BAD FAT

Like the oil they produce, olives contain heart-healthy monounsaturated fat that can do the following:

▶ Help lower your cholesterol and triglyceride levels.

▶ Reduce blood clotting.

▶ Possibly offer some protection against breast cancer.

But don't get carried away. A little bit of good fat goes a long way. Three super-colossal-size, canned ripe olives deliver nearly 40 calories. Eating too many olives can cause you to gain weight, and that, in turn, increases your risk of heart disease and cancer.

Those same three olives also pack more than 400 milligrams of sodium (about 17 percent of the Daily Value). As you already know, a high-sodium diet increases blood pressure in some people. But what you may not know is that lots of sodium also may drain calcium from your bones. So the trick is to use a few olives here and there to accent the flavors of other healthy foods.

VARIETY IS THE SPICE

You probably are most familiar with stuffed green Spanish olives or those jumbo ripe olives in the can. They will deliver the nutritional goods. But olive aficionados suggest that you broaden your horizons with other varieties, which are becoming more widely available.

One New York City restaurant boasts a complete olive menu, while some local groceries offer "olive bars," where you can pack

NUTRITION IN A NUTSHELL

Ripe olive (1 super-colossal)

Calories: 12

Fat: 1 g

Saturated fat: 0 g

Cholesterol: 0 mg

Sodium: 137 mg

Total carbohydrates: 1 g

Dietary fiber: Less than 1 g

Protein: 0 g

Vitamin E: 2% of Daily Value

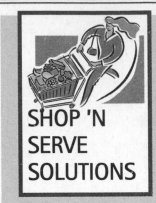

SHOP 'N SERVE SOLUTIONS

Your olive options are many—so experiment!

WHEN LOOKING FOR NEW OLIVE TREATS:

■ Check out either the deli or imported food section of your local grocery store, or try a natural food store.

■ Investigate Italian and Greek food stores, which usually carry ethnic varieties and may let you taste before you buy.

■ If you can't find olive novelties locally, check out the Santa Barbara Olive Company on-line at www.sbolive.com.

WHEN STORING OLIVES:

■ Store unopened canned or sealed-jar olives in a cool, dry pantry until you need them. Refrigerate after opening.

■ Refrigerate olives that are in unsealed deli containers, even though the olives have been both fermented and pickled.

OLIVE ACCENTS

With an interesting array of olives on hand, try a few of these tasty ways to add sparkle to your meals:

◆ **Have an olive-tasting party.** Use a little red wine or some thinly shaved fresh Parmesan cheese for palate cleansing between bites, but keep the focus on the fancy fruit. Display 5 to 10 varieties, and perhaps include slender green French Picholines, plump purple Italian Gaetas, and pea-size brown Spanish Arbequinas. Offer just enough so that each person eats about 10 olives. Follow with a light meal, such as a green

your own containers full of favorites such as Kalamatas, jumbo spiced green Italian olives, or even giant Cerignolas. Larger than a whole pecan in its shell, the ripe Cerignola is an inky black olive, with thick, meaty flesh and a mild, less salty, less tart taste. Another exotic treat is the pistachio-size ripe French Nicoise olive that is traditionally found in Salade Nicoise. These olives

salad and a dinner roll, with fresh berries and melon chunks for dessert.

◆ **Jazz up picnic salads.** Slice stuffed Spanish olives into potato salad, egg salad, or even tuna salad. To save a buck, buy the big jar of "salad" olives—the imperfect, beat-up kind that are fine when you're going to chop them up anyway. Cut back on the salt in your recipe to reduce sodium.

◆ **Go with the grain.** Rev up cold summer grain salads made with wheatberries, brown and wild rice, or tabbouleh with a few tangy chopped olives. Plump, smooth-flavored oil-cured olives make your taste buds sing.

◆ **Spice up old favorites.** Sliver a few Kalamata olives into that jar of store-bought spaghetti sauce for a piquant flavor that tastes homemade. *Molto bene!* Slice ripe Cerignolas into mashed potatoes, and replace the butter with a little olive oil. Top pizza with black and green olives. And turn tacos into heart-healthy treats: Wrap lettuce, chopped tomatoes, chopped onions, ground turkey, reduced-fat cheese, and sliced olives in a soft corn tortilla. *Ai, Chihuahua!*

◆ **Enliven lunch veggies.** Throw a few of your favorite olives into the raw veggie mix that you toss into your lunch bag. They'll give broccoli, cauliflower, and baby carrots some extra zip.

◆ **Tap into tapenade.** Whip out your blender and whirl up some tapenade, the Spanish olive spread. Served by little teaspoonfuls on thin crusts of toasted bread, it's an appetizer that makes your heart soar. (For a tapenade recipe, see "Crostini Trio" on page 304.)

also make a beautiful garnish scattered over grilled salmon.

And if you like your olives stuffed, you're in luck, because the creative juices are flowing at the olive-packing plant. Fabulous healthy fillings include almonds, garlic, mushrooms, onions, sun-dried tomatoes, jalapeño peppers, and for those who like it really hot, habanero chile peppers.

Crostini Trio

Stumped for healthy appetizers? This rainbow of Mediterranean spreads needs nothing more than a loaf of crusty bread—thinly sliced and lightly toasted—to soak up the delicious drippings.

TAPENADE
(SPANISH OLIVE SPREAD)

1 cup sliced black ripe olives

1 ounce anchovy paste

1 clove fresh garlic, pressed

1 tablespoon extra virgin olive oil

1 tablespoon fresh lemon juice

¼ teaspoon dried thyme

Place the large blade in a food processor bowl. Add the olives, anchovy paste, garlic, oil, lemon juice, and thyme. Pulse until the ingredients are evenly, but coarsely, chopped into a thick spread.

Yield: 16 servings.

Nutritional data per serving: Calories, 38; protein, 1 g; carbohydrates, 2 g; fiber, 0 g; fat, 4 g; saturated fat, 1 g; monounsaturated fat, 3 g; cholesterol, 1 mg; sodium, 419 mg; vitamin E, 9% of Daily Value.

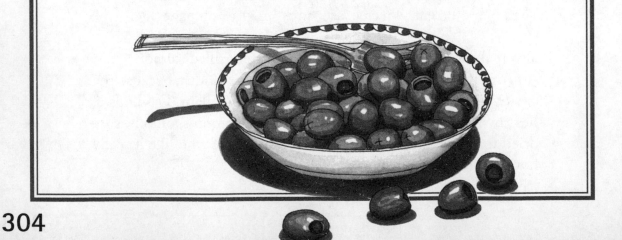

TUSCAN
TOMATO-BASIL SPREAD

4 very ripe plum tomatoes, seeded and diced
2 large fresh basil leaves, slivered
1 tablespoon extra virgin olive oil
Salt to taste
Ground black pepper to taste

In a medium bowl, combine the tomatoes, basil, and oil until well mixed. Season with the salt and pepper.

Yield: 16 servings.

Nutritional data per serving: Calories, 15; protein, 0 g; carbohydrates, 1 g; fiber, 0 g; fat, 1 g; saturated fat, 0 g; cholesterol, 0 mg; sodium, 3 mg.

MEDITERRANEAN
RADICCHIO TOPPING

2 heads radicchio, leaves separated and lightly chopped
1½ tablespoons extra virgin olive oil
1 tablespoon balsamic vinegar
½ teaspoon dried oregano
Salt to taste
Ground black pepper to taste

In a food processor, finely chop the radicchio. Remove to a mixing bowl. Add the oil and vinegar and mix well. Stir in the oregano, salt, and pepper.

Yield: 16 servings.

Nutritional data per serving: Calories, 15; protein, 0 g; carbohydrates, 0 g; fiber, 0 g; fat, 1 g; saturated fat, 0 g; cholesterol, 0 mg; sodium, 2 mg.

Onions:

Power-Packed Bulbs

BATTLES:
- allergies
- burns
- cancer
- cataracts
- diabetes
- heart disease
- infections
- stroke

BOLSTERS:
- bones
- vision

Onions make everything taste better, but Colleen didn't always think so when she was younger. Like many little kids, she fended them off with a screeching "Eeeeewww!" But her clever dad renamed them "mangles," and tricked her into eating them. Now, she willingly adds them to almost any savory dish—and that's a good thing. It seems the lowly onion is one of Mother Nature's truly power-packed veggies.

NUTRITION IN A NUTSHELL

Raw onion (½ cup chopped)

Calories: 30

Fat: 0 g

Saturated fat: 0 g

Cholesterol: 0 mg

Sodium: 2 mg

Total carbohydrates: 7 g

Dietary fiber: 1 g

Protein: 0 g

Vitamin C: 13% of Daily Value

Calcium: 4%

Iron: 2%

HEARTY VEGGIE

Onions are loaded with quercetin, a flavonoid also found in red wine, tea, and apples. Its benefit? Quercetin has an antioxidant punch more powerful than vitamin E's for preventing bad low-density lipoprotein (LDL) cholesterol from gunking up your arteries.

One study showed that drinking several cups of tea a day (a big quercetin provider) was associated with lower risk of cataracts. Since the amount of quercetin absorbed from onions is double that from tea, frequently eating onions may help protect against cataracts, too. And quercetin survives heat, so you can enjoy your onions cooked or raw.

Other compounds in onions—adenosine and paraffinic polysulfides—keep your platelets from clumping together, forming the clots that can trigger a heart attack or stroke. So eat your mangles!

A SLICE OF LIFE

Onions also boast several sulfur-containing compounds that are released when you slice into the bulb and break the cell walls. (Yes, they're also the tearjerkers, but more about that later.) These sulfur compounds appear to help fight dangerous blood clotting, as well as allergies, bacterial infections, and inflammation.

One study showed that students fed a high-fat diet actually had a drop in triglyceride levels (but not in cholesterol) when they added a big slice of onion to their burgers. So don't cry—just slice and dice!

Quick Fix:

Burns

Did you get a little kitchen burn? Run cold water over it, then apply a slice of onion. The same natural chemicals that usually make you cry also block the substances that make you feel pain. And here's a bonus: Onion juices have antibacterial properties that may help prevent infection.

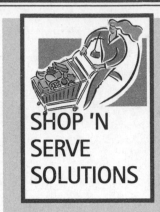

SHOP 'N SERVE SOLUTIONS

There are two kinds of bulb onions. One kind is called "fresh" onions. They're the sweet, mild type that folks love to eat raw. They're available in the market from March until August. These onions, which are grown in warmer climates, include Vidalias from Georgia, Walla Wallas from Washington, Mauis from Hawaii, and Super Sweets from Texas.

Fresh onions can be red, white, or yellow. All have thin, light-colored skin and a high water content that makes them tender and easily bruised. So handle them gently, and use them quickly.

The second kind of bulb onion is the "storage" onion. You'll find these in the market from August until the following April. They, too, are red, white, or yellow. Storage onions have several layers of papery skin, less water than fresh onions, and a more intense flavor.

Nothing is better for cooking. They turn a glorious brown when sautéed (with or without fat!), as their pungent components turn to sugar and caramelize to create a unique, sweet, cooked-onion flavor.

WHEN STORING ONIONS:

■ Store all your bulb onions in mesh bags or one of those cute multilevel hanging wire baskets. A nice dry cardboard box works well, too. The trick is to provide storage that allows air to circulate around the bulbs.

CANCER CRACKDOWN

A mound of evidence points to onions' elements as important cancer fighters. In one review, people who consumed the most quercetin had a 50 percent reduction in their risk of stomach and respiratory tract cancers.

■ Avoid the fridge like the plague. Cold, wet, stacked onions rot or grow mold. Dry storage onions keep all winter.

BRIGHT BULB IDEAS

Here are some hot ideas for cooking bulb onions:

◆ **Sweat the small stuff.** Instead of sautéing your onions in a glob of fat, try "sweating" them. Here's how: Lightly spray a nonstick skillet with cooking spray. Add sliced storage onions, and cook over medium heat, stirring occasionally, until they start to brown. Reduce the heat to low and cover. Cook until the onions sweat out their liquid and "melt down." If the onions start to stick or burn, add a little water. Serve over grilled chicken or pork tenderloin.

◆ **A slice is nice.** Use a serrated knife to shave thin slices of fresh red onions. Garnish your spinach salad with them, or stuff them in a veggie pita pocket.

◆ **A slab prevents flab.** Cut thick slices of fresh Vidalias or Walla Wallas for summer sandwiches. Try a thick slice on a grilled portobello mushroom sandwich with sprouts, cheese, and multigrain bread.

◆ **Soup up your onions.** Sauté sliced yellow onions in a little olive oil until soft. Add a tablespoon of flour and cook for 5 minutes. Stir in a can of beef broth to create instant onion soup. Top with melba rounds dusted with freshly grated Parmesan cheese. Too cool!

Other studies suggest that onions' sulfur compounds put the brakes on colon and renal cancers by causing cancer cells to die. Additional research shows that piling on the onions may reduce the risk of lung, bladder, ovarian, and brain cancers.

DIABETES DETERRENT

In one study, diabetic rats fed a diet high in onions managed their blood sugar as well as those taking insulin and other diabetes drugs. And they got a bonus! They created less cholesterol than the rats on drugs. (Warning: Don't try this at home. Always check with your doctor before adjusting your medication.)

Mesquite Onion Bloom

Avoiding those steak-house bloomin' onions, packed with calories and deep-fried fat, is a cool move. Instead, indulge in this foil-baked spicy blossom, compliments of Idaho–Eastern Oregon Onions. It goes great with grilled lean beef, pork, chicken, or shrimp. It's tops with beans and rice, too.

1 large onion
1 tablespoon dry mesquite-flavored marinade mix
2 teaspoons chopped cilantro
1 wedge lime

Preheat the oven to 425°F. Cut ½ inch off the onion top. Slightly trim the root end, but do not cut into the root base. Make the onion "blossom" with an onion-blooming tool (available at most kitchen equipment stores). Place the onion on a 10-inch-square sheet of aluminum foil. Sprinkle with the dry marinade mix. Wrap the onion in the foil, tightly sealing the edges. Place on a baking sheet or pie pan and bake for 20 to 30 minutes. Unwrap the onion and place on a dinner plate. Sprinkle with the cilantro and a squeeze of the lime.

Yield: One serving.

Nutritional data per serving: Calories, 84; protein, 2 g; carbohydrates, 20 g; fiber, 2 g; fat, 0 g; saturated fat, 0 g; cholesterol, 0 mg; sodium, 405 mg; magnesium, 5% of Daily Value; manganese, 13%; potassium, 8%.

Oranges:
Benefits beyond the C

BATTLES:
- birth defects
- cancer
- gallstones
- heart disease
- high cholesterol
- stroke
- wrinkles

BOLSTERS:
- bones and teeth
- circulation
- immune function
- wound healing

Of course you know that oranges are high in vitamin C. Your mother's been telling you that practically since the day you were born. Just one large orange or a 6-ounce glass of freshly squeezed orange juice feeds your need for C for the whole day. (Oh, and oranges are so refreshing!)

While vitamin C may not prevent the common cold, the C stands for "critical" when it comes to protecting the body in the following ways:

▶ Vitamin C creates collagen, the protein in connective tissue. Collagen forms the matrix

NUTRITION IN A NUTSHELL

Orange (1 large)

Calories: 86

Fat: 0 g

Saturated fat: 0 g

Cholesterol: 0 mg

Sodium: 0 mg

Total carbohydrates: 22 g

Dietary fiber: 4 g

Protein: 2 g

Folate: 14% of Daily Value

Vitamin C: 109%

that holds calcium in your bones and teeth.

▶ It forms scar tissue. From paper cuts to surgical incisions, it's vitamin C that helps knit your skin back together.

▶ It helps prevent wrinkles. So stay out of the sun, don't smoke (yes, smokers do need more C), and drink your orange juice.

▶ Vitamin C helps you absorb iron, making it a particularly important vitamin for vegetarians, teenagers, and women of child-bearing age. Each of these groups is at high risk for iron-deficiency anemia.

▶ It's an antioxidant that protects other vitamins and minerals from being ruined before they perform their normal tasks.

▶ Vitamin C also helps prevent gallstone formation.

ANATOMY OF AN ORANGE

Yes, an orange looks like a blazing little sun, and its various parts certainly offer some hot health benefits.

The skin. The benefits start when you peel an orange and get that pungent smell on your hands. The oil in an orange's skin is 90 to 95 percent limonene, a natural chemical that has been linked to preventing breast and cervical cancers, at least in test tubes. Limonene ends up in the orange juice you buy, because commercial machines squeeze the oranges so hard. And that's a good thing.

The pith. And then there's the white pith just under the skin. It's packed with pectin, a soluble fiber known for lowering cholesterol. And it's also higher in vitamin C than the juice is. So if you eat a little of the pith along with your orange, that, too, is a good thing.

The flesh and the juice. Oranges are a good source of cryptoxanthin, one of the beta-carotene cousins, which may fight cervical cancer. Canned mandarin oranges are loaded with it.

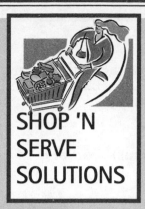

SHOP 'N SERVE SOLUTIONS

Consider trying the many different types of oranges. Part of the fun is to eat your way through the winter and spring, enjoying each variety at its peak.

WHEN SELECTING ORANGES:

■ Don't judge an orange by its color, because all oranges are picked when they're fully ripe. Some, especially those from Florida, remain slightly green even at their ripest. Others, such as those from California, turn completely, evenly orange.

■ Instead of focusing on color, choose oranges that are firm, heavy, and evenly shaped.

WHEN STORING:

■ There are some benefits to being thick-skinned. A heavy covering on the outside protects the fragile vitamins on the inside, such as vitamin C and folate. So, you can store thick-skinned oranges equally well at room temperature or in the refrigerator. In either location, they'll stay fresh for about two weeks.

■ But definitely keep your OJ in the fridge. If it's fresh-squeezed, it will begin to lose its vitamin C in 24 hours. Chilled juice will hang on to about 90 percent of its C for a week and 66 percent for two weeks.

USING ORANGE DELIGHTS

Here's what to do with your orange-arama:

◆ **Flavor with a peel.** Grate orange peel into vanilla yogurt to make the very best dressing for melon and berry salads. Also grate it into vegetable salads, muffins, and quick breads. You'll capitalize on the limonene in the peel.

◆ **Citrify a salad.** Use orange juice instead of vinegar to whip up a heart-healthy salad dressing. Or arrange thinly sliced, peeled navel oranges on greens for a different look.

Seasons in the Sun

Here's a mini schedule to help you find oranges at the peak of perfection.

Tangelos:	**November to February**
Navels and Clementines:	**November to April**
Jaffas:	**Mid-December to mid-February**
Temples:	**January to March**
Blood oranges:	**March to May**
Valencias:	**March to June**

Oranges also are an important source of folate, the B vitamin that is essential for preventing neural tube birth defects and for keeping blood levels of homocysteine under control. Minute increases in homocysteine can trigger a heart attack.

THE WHOLE FRUIT CATALOG

The orange's bountiful benefits haven't all been linked to specific nutrients or phytochemicals. In one small Canadian study, for instance, women who drank orange juice daily got a big surprise: Their levels of good high-density lipoprotein (HDL) cholesterol rose by 21 percent, a very unusual happening. Wine and chocolate are the only other foods known to raise HDL. Bigger studies will be needed to confirm these results.

But if you want big, there's the combined 100,000 nurses and professional men tracked by Harvard University researchers. The researchers found that eating cabbage family vegetables, green leafy vegetables, and citrus fruits and juices protected against ischemic stroke, the kind that comes from a blood clot in the brain. Each daily serving of these fruits and vegetables lowered stroke risk by 6 percent.

Oranges
to Beet the Band

Looking for a salad that's anything but green? Try this zingy side dish for a different taste and a big dose of health benefits.

1 can (15 ounces) whole baby beets, drained
½ cup canned mandarin orange segments, drained
½ teaspoon grated orange peel
¼ cup orange juice
⅛ teaspoon dried rosemary

Cut the beets in half and place in a small bowl. Add the orange segments, orange peel, orange juice, and rosemary, and stir. Chill well.

Yield: Three servings.

Nutritional data per serving: Calories, 80; protein, 2 g; carbohydrates, 18 g; fiber, 3 g; fat, 0 g; saturated fat, 0 g; cholesterol, 0 mg; sodium, 305 mg; vitamin A, 7% of Daily Value; vitamin C, 17%; iron, 8%.

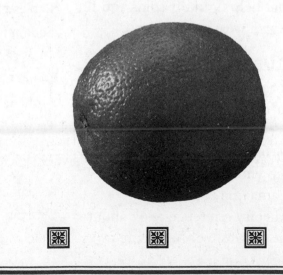

Papaya:
A Tropical Treasure

BATTLES:
- cancer
- heart disease
- high blood pressure

BOLSTERS:
- immune function
- vision
- wound healing

During the dark, cold days of February, nothing is finer than munching on a bit of papaya. Its sunny colors and sensuous flavor will brighten your days better than a trip to the Bahamas. (Well, maybe not that much, but it helps.) And papaya is packed with antioxidants that help fight off colds and flu until spring's warm weather returns.

TROPICAL ILLUSION

If you checked the stats and compared the amount of beta-carotene in a papaya (60 micrograms) versus the amount in a bowl of spinach (9,200 micrograms), you'd say, "No-brainer! Spinach wins hands down." But hold on for an amazing revelation.

In its new dietary reference book about carotenoids, the Institute of Medicine in

NUTRITION IN A NUTSHELL

Papaya (½ large)

Calories: 59

Fat: 0 g

Saturated fat: 0 g

Cholesterol: 0 mg

Sodium: 6 mg

Total carbohydrates: 19 g

Dietary fiber: 3 g

Protein: 1 g

Folate: 18% of Daily Value

Vitamin A: 11%

Vitamin C: 130%

Vitamin E: 14%

Calcium: 5%

Washington, D.C. (the group that publishes the Recommended Dietary Allowances, or RDAs) has disclosed that packaging matters. In fact, packaging is critical to how much beta-carotene your body can extract from the green and orange foods you eat, and how much is delivered to your blood.

And guess what? Fruits, *especially* papaya, lead the parade of foods that easily release their beta-carotene, while spinach and other green vegetables bring up the rear. So papaya is more potent than it first appears.

It's this simple: Carotenoids can boost your immune system and protect you from just about anything that can kill you, including cancer. But they work only when they're in your bloodstream, not when they're merely on your plate.

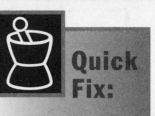

Quick Fix:

Hiccups

Suffering with the hiccups, belching, or bloating? Eat papaya. Its digestive enzymes may help relieve your distress.

A BONUS BETA

And here's a bonus: Papaya is also loaded with beta-cryptoxanthin, another carotenoid that can help beat vitamin A deficiency, along with its threats to your vision and skin.

AND A BETA BOOSTER

You'll get even more carotenoids if you serve your papaya (and your spinach, too) with a little fat. Nuts, olive oil, and canola oil are especially good choices. In fact, why not warm some papaya chunks and serve them on a bed of steamed spinach tossed with olive oil and sprinkled with toasted pine nuts? Talk about carotene heaven!

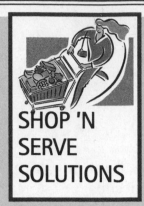

SHOP 'N SERVE SOLUTIONS

Papaya is a tropical treat that's available all year long, although you'll probably find the biggest piles of this fruit in late spring/early summer and then again in early fall. A papaya looks like a large, fat, greenish yellow pear.

WHEN SELECTING FRESH PAPAYA:

■ Choose papayas that are about half yellow. As they ripen, your papayas will begin to glow with a beautiful yellow-orange color.

■ Skip papayas that are all green, because they've been picked too early and may never ripen.

WHEN STORING:

■ Speed ripening by putting your papayas in a paper bag with a banana. (Yes, bananas produce ethylene gas just like apples!)

■ When your papayas are about three-quarters golden, they'll give slightly when pressed near the stem. (If they feel soft and mushy, you've waited too long.)

■ Once they're ripe, put them in the refrigerator (if you can wait!), where they'll last about a week. Better yet, eat them right away, before the flavor starts to fade.

WHEN YOU'RE READY TO USE:

Wash the outside under running water and pat dry. Place the papaya on a cutting board and slice in half lengthwise. You'll find a yellow-pink, fleshy interior, and a hollow filled with sparkling black seeds. Beautiful! Scoop out the seeds, and you're ready to eat!

TROPICAL DEPRESSION

If minimizing heart disease and reducing high blood pressure are on your list of things to do today, have a papaya. It's packed with these nutrients:

Other papaya products. You also can buy papaya dried, canned, and as nectar. These forms of papaya will all deliver beta-carotene and beta-cryptoxanthin, but the vitamin C will have dropped from a loud roar to a quiet whisper.

PAPAYA'S POTENT POETRY

Here's how to enjoy your papaya:

◆ **Blast winter's chill.** When you just can't take the snow anymore and need a bit of sunshine, grab a papaya. Stuff it with seafood salad made with crab, shrimp, and scallops. Sit by a sunny window and eat your fill.

◆ **Toss it on the grill.** Line up fresh papaya quarters alongside your chicken. Or skewer papaya cubes and shrimp for kebabs.

◆ **Drink it down at will.** Have a cup of papaya nectar for an afternoon snack.

◆ **Blend it for a thrill.** Add fresh papaya chunks, along with a banana, to your next smoothie.

◆ **Have a snack on the hill.** Stash chunks of dried papaya in your fanny pack when you go hiking. They're great for an energy boost along the way.

◆ **Lower your medical bill.** Replace high-fat gravy with pureed papaya. It works great on chicken, pork, or fish.

◆ **Avoid gelatin kill.** Don't put uncooked papaya in gelatin. Like fresh pineapple, it contains an enzyme called papain that disrupts protein and turns your gelatin to water.

▶ **Potassium.** This mineral is important for lowering blood pressure. (And there's more in a papaya than in a banana.)

▶ **Folate.** This is the B vitamin that tames homocysteine so it can't trigger a heart attack.

▶ **Vitamin C**. It may help prevent bad low-density lipoprotein (LDL) cholesterol from clogging your artery walls and may help your wounds heal if you need surgery. (A papaya offers more C than an 8-ounce glass of orange juice.)

So get happy. Have a papaya!

Crab-Stuffed Papaya

Sometimes the simplest things are best, especially if you're watching your weight and cutting down on rich sauces. This beautiful dish is as simple, and as good, as it gets.

1 large ripe papaya
2 cups torn red leaf lettuce
¼ lime
1 cup backfin crabmeat, chilled, shells and cartilage removed
2 teaspoons butter, melted

Wash the papaya under cool, running water and pat dry. Place on a cutting board, and with a sharp knife, slice in half lengthwise. Remove the seeds, rinse the papaya halves, and place on paper towels to dry. Cover two salad plates with the lettuce and place a papaya half on each. Squeeze the lime over the flesh. Fill each cavity with one-half of the crabmeat. Drizzle with the melted butter.

Yield: Two servings.

Nutritional data per serving: Calories, 180; protein, 14 g; carbohydrates, 22 g; fiber, 5 g; fat, 5 g; saturated fat, 3 g; cholesterol, 69 mg; sodium, 230 mg; folate, 26% of Daily Value; vitamin A, 40%; vitamin C, 138%; vitamin E, 19%; calcium, 14%; copper, 21%; potassium, 22%; zinc, 18%.

Parsley:
A Kiss of Health

BATTLES:
- bad breath
- cancer
- heart disease
- high cholesterol

BOLSTERS:
- bones

The next time someone garnishes your plate with parsley, don't just ask, "What's this green stuff?" and then push it aside. Instead, pop it into your mouth! Parsley squeezes so much good nutrition into such a small package that you shouldn't simply send it to the compost pile.

SAFE TO SMOOCH

Let's start with parsley's purely cosmetic benefit. This herb can de-funk your breath. The ancient Romans often ate parsley with bread for breakfast, probably to fight morning breath. Try it! It really is the herbal breath mint—and restaurants give it away for free!

NUTRITION IN A NUTSHELL

Fresh parsley
(2 tablespoons chopped)

Calories: 3

Fat: 0 g

Saturated fat: 0 g

Cholesterol: 0 mg

Sodium: 4 mg

Total carbohydrates: 0 g

Dietary fiber: 0 g

Protein: 0 g

Vitamin A: 8% of Daily Value

Vitamin C: 17%

MORE PARSLEY PERKS

Moving on to more serious health issues, a little bit of parsley offers quite a lot of the vitamins A, C, and K.

Vitamins A and C act as antioxidants, which destroy substances that can damage your cells before they trigger heart disease and cancer. Vitamin K, meanwhile, may help strengthen your bones. A recent study at Harvard University found that women who had the least amount of vitamin K in their diets were about 70 percent more likely to suffer a hip fracture than those who had the most in their diets.

Researchers also are reviewing certain plant compounds in parsley called terpenoids. Preliminary results suggest that terpenoids can reduce your level of bad low-density lipoprotein (LDL) cholesterol and also fight cancer.

Not too bad for a garnish, huh?

Quick Fix:

Garlic Breath

If you've just downed a bowlful of pasta in garlic sauce, but still want to get a smooch tonight, munch on a sprig of parsley. It'll help freshen your breath.

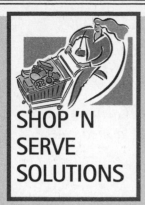

SHOP 'N SERVE SOLUTIONS

Picking fresh parsley is a breeze. Just decide whether you want the curly variety (the kind most often used as a garnish) or the Italian flat-leaf type (better used for cooking).

WHEN SELECTING PARSLEY:

No matter which type you choose, look for a bunch with bright green leaves and no signs of wilting.

WHEN STORING:

Rinse the parsley, shake off the excess water, wrap the parsley in paper towels, and then store it in a plastic bag in the refrigerator.

PARCEL OUT SOME PARSLEY

Now here are some suggestions to help you use every last sprig:

◆ **Brush off basil.** Substitute chopped fresh parsley for half the basil in your pesto recipe.

◆ **Season your spuds.** Add chopped fresh parsley to baked, roasted, or mashed potatoes.

◆ **Garnish your dessert.** Decorate your dessert plate with a small sprig of parsley, and use it as an after-dinner mint.

◆ **Tap into tabbouleh.** This traditional Middle Eastern side dish is mainly made with bulgur and parsley. Order it the next time it catches your eye on a restaurant menu.

Super Summer Pasta

In the heat of summer, when you don't feel like eating anything warm, pull out this recipe. It satisfies like a meal rather than a pasta salad, yet it's refreshingly light.

½ pound bow-tie pasta
3 tablespoons olive oil
1 cup chopped honeydew melon
½ cup seedless purple grapes, halved
½ cup finely chopped fresh flat-leaf parsley
2 tablespoons lemon juice

In a large pot, boil the pasta until al dente. Drain and toss with the oil. Cool completely. Toss with the melon, grapes, parsley, and lemon juice, and serve.

Yield: Four servings.

Nutritional data per serving: Calories, 340; protein, 8 g; carbohydrates, 53 g; fiber, 3 g; fat, 11 g; saturated fat, 2 g; cholesterol, 0 mg; sodium, 10 mg; calcium, 3% of Daily Value; iron, 18%.

Pasta:

Use Your Noodle

BATTLES:
- birth defects
- heart disease

BOLSTERS:
- energy
- mood

Every Sunday when Karen was growing up, she went to her grandparents' house for a huge pasta meal. Often it was just the usual spaghetti and meatballs, but sometimes it was gnocchi (potato dumplings) or manicotti (tubes filled with cheese or meat). Whatever her grandmother made, it tasted delicious.

These days, Karen doesn't limit pasta to Sundays. To hear her husband tell it, she'd make pasta every night of the week if she could. On Valentine's Day, he even cooks it for her. He must

(Continued on page 328)

THE FACTS ABOUT FLAVORED PASTA

Does that gorgeous red, green, or striped pasta pack more nutrients than the standard fare? The answer: Maybe.

Pasta flavored with tomatoes or red peppers may kick in some extra vitamin A and vitamin C, but the kind made with herbs or spinach doesn't usually offer any extras. Do, however, check the "Nutrition Facts" label on the package to be sure.

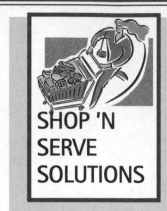

SHOP 'N SERVE SOLUTIONS

Pasta is available in a few different forms. Of course, there are the boxes of regular dried spaghetti, linguine, lasagna noodles, and so on found on supermarket shelves. Then, there is the "gourmet" fresh pasta found in the refrigerated case. If you're lucky enough to live near a good Italian market, you may also find homemade pasta, either dried or fresh. In addition, there is whole wheat pasta. And, finally, pasta comes in an array of cheery colors!

WHEN SELECTING PASTA:

Each of the two main types of pasta—regular and whole wheat—offers its own perks.

■ **Regular pasta.** Most regular pasta—even the refrigerated kind—is made with flour that has been enriched with extra nutrients, including, as of late, folic acid. To be certain, just look for the words "enriched flour" on the ingredients list. (Hate to break it to you, but the delicious pasta at Italian markets probably isn't enriched; to be sure, ask.)

■ **Whole wheat pasta.** This type, on the other hand, naturally contains small amounts of a wide range of vitamins and minerals. But while whole wheat pasta boasts three times the fiber of regular pasta, it's not required to carry the extra folic acid. Like regular pasta, it comes in dried and fresh varieties.

So which one's best? It's hard to say. We think that you should keep both on hand.

WHEN STORING:

■ Dried pasta maintains its flavor for up to a year when it's stored in a cool, dry place—such as your cupboard.

■ Fresh pasta lasts until the expiration date on the package.

Tightly cover opened unused portions to prevent drying. If you don't think you'll use it by the expiration date, you can freeze it for about a month. Don't thaw it before using. It'll take a minute or two longer to cook.

■ Frozen pasta can be stored for up to nine months if unopened. Tightly sealed leftover portions will keep for about three months.

PRESENTING PERFECT PASTA

Using either whole wheat or regular pasta, follow this step-by-step guide to building a great pasta dinner:

◆ **Select the right sauce.** Delicate pasta, such as angel hair or thin spaghetti, works best with thin sauces. Thicker pasta (we're thinking fettuccine) goes well with heavier sauces. And pasta shapes, such as bow ties or shells, are perfect for chunky sauces. In general, tomato sauce has the least fat and calories, while Alfredo (sorry) delivers the most.

◆ **Include veggies.** When you add veggies to spaghetti sauce, you can fill up your pasta bowl for fewer calories. Toss broccoli florets into tomato or marinara sauce; add green beans to pesto sauce; dice red bell peppers into garlic and olive oil sauce; or add a medley of colorful chopped veggies, such as carrots, squash, and green bell peppers, to white sauce.

◆ **Pump up with protein.** It'll help balance all the carbs you're consuming—and keep you full longer. Karen's husband thinks meatballs are a must, but she's of a different mind-set, preferring grilled chicken or shrimp.

◆ **Sprinkle on cheese.** A tablespoon of grated Parmesan or Romano will give your dish a calcium and flavor boost.

(Continued from page 325)

instinctively know that pasta is good for the heart. (Or it could be that pasta is all he knows how to make! Ah, to be kind, let's stick with the heart explanation.)

VALENTINE'S PASTA

Pasta pumps up your ticker in two ways. First, it's rich in complex carbohydrates—carbs, for short. When you eat more carbs and less fat in your diet, your cholesterol takes a nosedive.

Plus, most of the pasta that you pick up at the supermarket is enriched with folic acid, a B vitamin. In a Harvard University study of more than 80,000 women, researchers found that participants who had the highest intake of folic acid and vitamin B_6 were about 45 percent less likely to develop heart disease than those who had the lowest.

Folic acid also offers another important benefit—one that might come in handy on Valentine's Day. Getting the recommended 400 micrograms of the nutrient daily cuts the risk of neural tube birth defects in half. One cup of cooked pasta supplies about 25 percent of your daily requirement.

A SIDE OF ENERGY

The complex carbs in pasta aren't just good for your heart. They improve your stamina, too. Athletes often load up on pasta before a competition because it supplies time-released energy. In other

Quick Fix:

PMS

When you're plagued by premenstrual syndrome, sit down to a bowl of pasta. A diet rich in carbohydrates, such as pasta and whole wheat bread, helps increase your level of an amino acid that produces serotonin, a brain chemical that elevates your mood.

NUTRITION IN A NUTSHELL

Cooked spaghetti (1 cup)

Calories: 197

Fat: 1 g

Saturated fat: 0 g

Cholesterol: 0 mg

Sodium: 1 mg

Total carbohydrates: 40 g

Dietary fiber: 2 g

Protein: 7 g

Folic acid: 25% of Daily Value

Vitamin B_3 (niacin): 9%

Iron: 11%

DOES PASTA MAKE YOU FAT?

No! No! No! We've been dying to set the record straight: Despite what those diet books tell you, calories from pasta are not more likely to pack on the pounds than calories from any other food.

But portion sizes of pasta (especially in restaurants) have gotten out of control. For instance, when Karen ordered Linguini Pomodoro (that's just chopped tomatoes, garlic, basil, and olive oil) at an Italian restaurant recently, she received a mammoth bowlful—the equivalent of 5 pasta servings! If you clean your plate, you will gain weight.

So what's a serving? Not much, according to the USDA—just $\frac{1}{2}$ cup of cooked pasta. Our recommendation is to eat about 1 cup of cooked pasta and have it count as 2 of the 6 to 11 servings of grains that the USDA recommends you eat daily. Then top it off with about $\frac{1}{3}$ cup of sauce, $\frac{1}{3}$ cup of veggies, and 1 tablespoon of cheese.

words, you won't get a huge burst of energy at the beginning of your performance and tire out at the end.

Granted, you're probably not going for the Olympic Gold anytime soon, but this same concept can help you if you're taking a hike, walking a charity 5K, or even doing a lot of gardening.

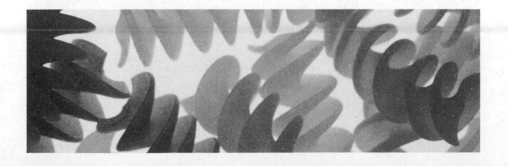

My Mother-in-Law's Lasagna

Karen's mother-in-law, Alyce, makes the best lasagna. The whole family begs her to whip up a pan for Christmas Eve dinner. It's almost as good as the presents.

2 cans (28 ounces each) crushed tomatoes
4 cans (8 ounces each) tomato sauce
1 can (6 ounces) tomato paste
1 pound ground beef, at least 93% lean
½ cup bread crumbs
1 egg
½ teaspoon dried basil
½ teaspoon dried oregano
1 pound lasagna noodles
12 ounces part-skim ricotta cheese
8 ounces part-skim mozzarella cheese, shredded

If you plan to bake your meatballs, preheat the oven to 350°F. In a large pot, mix the tomatoes, tomato sauce, and tomato paste, and cook over medium-low heat. Meanwhile, in a large bowl, combine the ground beef, bread crumbs, egg, basil, and oregano until well mixed. Form into mini meatballs. Fry in a nonstick skillet or bake until the insides are no longer pink. Drain well, removing the grease. Add the meatballs to the sauce, reduce the heat to low, and simmer. Meanwhile, in another large pot, cook the noodles according to package directions.

Increase the oven temperature to 375°F. Coat the bottom of a 13-by-9-inch baking pan with one-third of the sauce and meatballs. Top with one-third of the noodles and cheeses. Repeat the layers (sauce-meatballs, noodles, and cheeses) until you reach the top of the pan. Bake for 40 to 45 minutes, or until the cheeses are melted and the noodles are heated through. Allow to cool for a few minutes before cutting.

Variation: To reduce the sodium in this dish, use low-salt canned tomato products.

Yield: 12 servings.

Nutritional data per serving: Calories, 349; protein, 24 g; carbohydrates, 41 g; fiber, 5 g; fat, 10 g; saturated fat, 5 g; cholesterol, 33 mg; sodium, 979 mg; calcium, 29% of Daily Value; iron, 27%.

Last-Minute Pasta Salad

Ever invite some friends over for a cookout on short notice, and realize you have nothing except potato chips to serve with the burgers? Don't speed to the supermarket. Chances are, you already have all the ingredients for this easy-to-fix salad.

1 pound medium-size pasta, such as shells, rotini, or penne
1 green or red bell pepper, chopped
½ cup grated carrot
2 large tomatoes, chopped
4 ounces part-skim mozzarella cheese, cubed
1 bottle (8 ounces) low-fat salad dressing, preferably Italian or vinaigrette

Cook the pasta according to package directions. Drain in a large colander and run under cold water for a few minutes. Transfer to a large mixing bowl. Add the pepper, carrot, tomatoes, cheese, and dressing, and toss well. Refrigerate until ready to cat.

Yield: Eight servings.

Nutritional data per serving: Calories, 282; protein, 10 g; carbohydrates, 45 g; fiber, 3 g; fat, 6 g; saturated fat, 2 g; cholesterol, 10 mg; sodium, 297 mg; calcium, 11% of Daily Value; iron, 13%.

Peaches:
They're Keen for Your Health

BATTLES:
- cancer
- heart disease

BOLSTERS:
- immune function
- vision
- wound healing

During the dog days of summer, nothing beats the heat like the taste of a plump, juicy peach. Sliced, diced, or even straight from the tree, peaches are lip-smackin' good—and good for you, too! So don't be fooled by all that great taste. They have a whole lot more to offer than just their fantastic flavor.

WHAT'S ALL THE FUZZ ABOUT?

Peaches are packed with vitamins A and C. Vitamin A helps your eyes see normally in the dark and protects you from infection by keeping your skin and mucous membranes healthy. It also battles bad guys called free radicals that cause cell damage that may eventually lead to cancer and heart disease.

NUTRITION IN A NUTSHELL

Peaches (2 medium)

Calories: 70

Fat: 0 g

Saturated fat: 0 g

Cholesterol: 0 mg

Sodium: 0 mg

Total carbohydrates: 19 g

Dietary fiber: 1 g

Protein: 1 g

Vitamin A: 20% of Daily Value

Vitamin C: 20%

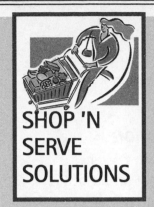

SHOP 'N SERVE SOLUTIONS

It's easy to pick a peck of perfect peaches!

WHEN SELECTING PEACHES:

Narrow your search to those with a deep yellow or creamy background.

■ Avoid those with a green hue—they probably won't ripen.

■ Then, depending on how quickly you'd like to eat them, choose peaches that are moderately hard (ready to eat in a few days) to slightly soft (ready now).

WHEN STORING:

■ Keep ripe peaches in the fridge, where they'll maintain their super flavor for about a week. That allows plenty of time for you and your family to dig in.

■ Place unripe peaches in a paper bag at room temperature for a day or two. Transfer them to the refrigerator when they're ripe.

WHEN YOU'RE READY TO USE:

◆ Wash peaches in cool water and dry them off with a paper towel.

◆ To peel peaches for a recipe, gently dip them in boiling water for 30 seconds, remove with a slotted spoon, and then immerse in cold water. The skin should come off easily.

◆ To ditch the pit in freestone peaches (the type most commonly found in supermarkets), carefully use a sharp knife to cut on the seam around the peach, all the way down to the pit. Then twist each half in opposite directions. With clingstone peaches, which have a pit that's even harder to remove, it's best to cut sections by slicing down to the pit and removing the desired amount.

Vitamin C has an equally impressive list of accomplishments. It helps produce the connective tissue collagen, which holds muscles, bones, and other groups of cells together. It also boosts

Quick Fix:

Sinusitis

If you've come down with sinusitis, pick up a peach. A recent small study found that sinusitis sufferers might not be getting enough glutathione, an antioxidant compound found in peaches and other delicious fruits such as watermelon and oranges.

your immune system, helps form and repair red blood cells, protects you from bruising, heals cuts and wounds, and even keeps your gums healthy.

MORE PEACHY PROTECTION

And that's not all that peaches offer. They're also a good source of glutathione, an antioxidant that may help prevent cancer, although it's still too early to tell for sure. A study in the British medical journal *Lancet* found that older adults have lower levels of this compound than younger folks do. Consider it just one more reason among dozens to eat your peaches.

Peach Trifle

We removed a lot of the calories, fat, and fuss—but not an ounce of the taste—from this traditional British dessert. Karen loves to make this summertime treat just to show off her trifle bowl.

8 ounces low-fat pound cake
1 package (3 ounces) vanilla instant pudding, prepared according to package directions
4 peaches, peeled and sliced
12 strawberries, sliced
¾ cup low-fat whipped topping
Chocolate shavings (garnish), optional

Cut the cake into small pieces. Place one-third of the pieces in the bottom of a trifle bowl or on a serving platter. Spoon one-third of the pudding over the cake. Top with one-third of the peaches. Add two more layers of the remaining cake, pudding, and peaches. Circle the top layer with the strawberries and top with the whipped topping. Garnish with a few chocolate shavings, if using.

Variation: Angel food cake can be used in place of the pound cake.

Yield: Eight servings.

Nutritional data per serving: Calories, 195; protein, 4 g; carbohydrates, 41 g; fiber, 3 g; fat, 2 g; saturated fat, 1 g; cholesterol, 4 mg; sodium, 451 mg; calcium, 8% of Daily Value; iron, 3%.

Peanut Butter:

Keeps You Young at Heart

BATTLES:
- cancer
- heart disease
- high cholesterol

BOLSTERS:
- weight control

One thing that makes you feel like a kid again is a peanut butter sandwich. And now, after years of bad press for being high-fat, peanut butter is back on the healthy foods list. Peanut-friendly researchers have clearly demonstrated that peanut butter's fat is mostly monounsaturated—the good kind of fat. And that's probably why clinical research shows that eating peanuts and peanut butter can lower bad low-density lipoprotein (LDL) cholesterol and triglycerides without lowering good high-density lipoprotein (HDL) cholesterol. That's a profile that's healthy for your heart.

Ounce for ounce, peanuts contain the same amount of monounsaturated fat as

NUTRITION IN A NUTSHELL

Creamy peanut butter (2 tablespoons)

Calories: 190

Fat: 16 g

Saturated fat: 3 g

Monounsaturated fat: 8 g

Cholesterol: 0 mg

Sodium: 150 mg

Total carbohydrates: 6 g

Dietary fiber: 2 g

Protein: 8 g

Vitamin B_3 (niacin): 21% of Daily Value

Vitamin E: 16%

Magnesium: 13%

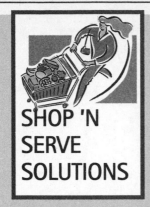

SHOP 'N SERVE SOLUTIONS

When it comes to peanut butter, buy what you like. Now, you may ask, "What about salt, sugar, and trans fat?" On average, a 2-tablespoon serving of unsalted peanut butter delivers about 5 milligrams of sodium, while the salted kind provides about 155 milligrams (about 6 percent of the recommended daily limit), an amount that doesn't make a huge difference. Some brands also contain a little sugar, but usually not very much.

Recently, the biggest flap was over trans fat, the Frankenstein fat created when hydrogen is forced into liquid oil to make it solid. Trans fat can push up your LDL cholesterol while dragging your HDL down, the worst possible scenario for your heart.

Indeed, some hydrogenated oils are added to peanut butter to keep the peanut oil from separating. But these amounts are so small that they rate a zero on the FDA's proposed labeling scale. Also reassuring is the fact that all the research showing how well peanut butter can lower your cholesterol was done with the hydrogenated kind. So breathe easy.

PLAY AROUND

Now try these simple ways to regain your lost youth:

◆ **Whip it.** Drop 2 tablespoons of peanut butter into your next fruit smoothie while it's whirling. A dollop of chocolate syrup is nice, too.

◆ **Berry it.** Forget the jelly. Make a grown-up sandwich with whole wheat bread, chunky peanut butter, and some fresh blueberries, raspberries, or sliced strawberries. Yum!

◆ **Crunch it.** Forget those neon orange peanut butter crackers from your wasted youth. To get a new lease on life, try some 100 percent stone-ground whole wheat Ak-Mak crackers spread with your favorite peanut butter.

◆ **Spread it.** Smooth your daily allotment of creamy goobers on celery stalks, carrot sticks, apple slices, or banana circles.

tree nuts such as walnuts, pecans, and almonds, which have also been shown to protect against heart disease. Serving for serving, peanuts contain almost as much protein as beans. Nature's whimsy has created so many delicious ways to grow a healthy heart!

WEIGHT A MINUTE

Of course, if you eat a ton of peanut butter, you'll gain weight, and that's bad for your heart. But if you eat peanut butter in moderation, you should have no problem. In an ongoing weight loss study at Brigham and Women's Hospital in Boston, the group eating peanut butter and other healthy fats is losing weight and keeping it off better than the guys and gals on the very low fat diet.

CRUSH CHOLESTEROL AND CANCER

But the latest nutrition news is that peanuts are packed with sterols, the plant version of cholesterol. Sure, that sounds like a potential problem, but it's not. Plant sterols, you see, are absorbed very slowly—so slowly that they actually get in the way of the cholesterol from your foods and prevent it from being absorbed.

And, at least in the laboratory, those sterols have been shown to stop the growth of colon, prostate, and breast cancer cells and to cause cancer cells to die. The bad news is that Americans average only 80 milligrams of phytosterols daily. Asians and vegetarians (who rarely get those cancers) get about 400 milligrams of phytosterols daily. Two tablespoons of peanut oil or peanut butter or $1/4$ cup of roasted peanuts delivers about 50 milligrams of phytosterols.

Warm Thai Beef Salad with Spicy Peanut Sauce

THAI BEEF SALAD

If you love the complex sweet-salty-spicy flavors and intriguing aromas of Thai food, you'll enjoy this hot-and-cold entrée.

4 cloves garlic
3 tablespoons minced fresh ginger
2 tablespoons fish sauce
2 tablespoons reduced-sodium soy sauce
1 tablespoon sugar
4 filet mignons (4 ounces each), trimmed of all fat
2 small heads butter lettuce
1 small red onion, thinly sliced (garnish)
1 green jalapeño pepper, thinly sliced (garnish)
½ cup chopped fresh cilantro (garnish)
½ cup chopped fresh mint leaves (garnish)

In a glass bowl, combine the garlic, ginger, fish sauce, soy sauce, and sugar. Add the filets and turn to coat well. Let stand for 30 to 60 minutes while you preheat the grill. Grill or broil to desired doneness. Cut each filet into ¼-inch-thick slices. Divide the lettuce among four small dinner plates. Top each with a sliced filet. Garnish with the onion, pepper, cilantro, and mint. Drizzle each with 2 tablespoons of "Spicy Peanut Sauce" (see page 340).

Yield: Four servings.

Nutritional data per serving (including peanut sauce): Calories, 350; protein, 30 g; carbohydrates, 14 g; fiber, 3 g; fat, 20 g; saturated fat, 6 g; cholesterol, 72 mg; sodium, 1,182 mg; vitamin A, 23% of Daily Value; vitamin B$_3$ (niacin), 30%; vitamin B$_6$, 29%; vitamin C, 14%; calcium, 8%; iron, 23%; zinc, 36%.

SPICY PEANUT SAUCE

We recently spent a couple of days with the chefs at the Culinary Institute of America at Greystone in Napa Valley, California, where we learned to make this savory sauce.

1 tablespoon peanut oil
1 teaspoon red curry paste
½ teaspoon ground turmeric
½ cup creamy peanut butter
½ cup unsweetened coconut milk
½ cup water
2 teaspoons fish sauce
1 teaspoon fresh lemon juice
Sugar to taste

Heat the oil in a nonstick saucepan over medium heat. Add the curry paste and turmeric, and cook, stirring often, until the mixture sizzles, about 1 minute. Add the peanut butter, milk, water, fish sauce, lemon juice, and sugar. Reduce the heat to low, and cook, stirring constantly with a whisk, for 3 minutes. When the mixture begins to bubble, remove from the heat and continue to stir until it reaches the desired consistency. If the sauce is too thick, thin with more water. Taste and adjust the seasonings to an interesting balance of sweet, salty, and spicy flavors.

Yield: 12 servings.

Nutritional data per serving: Calories, 77; protein, 3 g; carbohydrates, 3 g; fiber, 1 g; fat, 7 g; saturated fat, 1 g; cholesterol, 0 mg; sodium,127 mg; vitamin E, 6% of Daily Value.

Pears:
Healthy to the Core

BATTLES:
- cancer
- heart disease
- high cholesterol

BOLSTERS:
- regularity

Karen's parents had a lovely old pear tree in their yard when she was growing up. In late August, they'd harvest the pears, and her mom would use them in salads, sandwiches, and anything else that came to mind. Now, every August, Karen returns to her parents' house to pick up a big bag of pears. She knows for certain that pears pack a mighty health punch—and she'd be crazy to pass up this delicious (and free) treat!

FIBER FILL-UP

Hands down, the healthiest thing about pears is their high fiber content. A medium-size Bartlett pear boasts about 4 grams of fiber. And a study is underway to determine whether thicker-skinned varieties, such as Bosc pears, offer even more of this important compound.

DYNAMIC DUO

Better yet, pears pack a 50-50 blend of the two main types of fiber: soluble and insoluble.

(Continued on page 344)

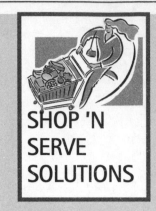

SHOP 'N SERVE SOLUTIONS

Pears were all the rage in France from the twelfth to the nineteenth century, and breeders continually developed new varieties. Eventually, 3,000 separate types came into existence. Fortunately, for those of us who have a hard time making up our minds, only a handful of pear varieties are grown commercially.

PICK A PEAR

Here are five of the most plentiful pears:

■ **Anjou.** The most popular pear, the Anjou is egg-shaped and remains green when ripe.

■ **Yellow Bartlett.** A sweet and most aromatic pear, the yellow Bartlett is usually green at the grocery store. It turns yellow while ripening in your kitchen.

■ **Red Bartlett.** This variety tastes and smells just as good as its yellow cousin. The red Bartlett will be dark red at the supermarket and will ripen to a bright red in your home.

■ **Bosc.** With a firm, dense flesh and super flavor, this variety is ideal for cooking and baking. You can easily spot a Bosc by its earthy brown color.

■ **Seckel.** This maroon-and-olive-green petite pear (about half the size of an Anjou) is the sweetest of all.

WHEN SELECTING PEARS:

Once you choose your variety, determine how ripe you'd like your pears to be. Do you want to eat them today? Or do you want to save them for a few days? Most supermarket pears are about one to three days from being ripe. Here's how to tell the degree of ripeness:

■ Ignore the color. Some pears do change colors when they're ripe, but other varieties remain the same hue.

■ Feel the flesh. With your thumb, gently press down near the base of the stem. If it yields slightly, it's ripe and ready to eat. If not, you'll have to ripen it at home.

WHEN STORING:

■ Refrigerate ripe pears immediately. Left at room temperature, they may turn brown inside. Ripe pears will last about a week in the refrigerator.

■ Place unripe pears in a brown paper bag along with a damp cotton ball (the moisture will help prevent shriveling), and store at 60° to 70°F. Check every day to see if the pears have ripened. If not, replace the cotton ball.

PEAR-FECT PEARS

Now try these unusual ways to enjoy this exceptional fruit:

◆ **Add crunch to your salads.** Forget croutons, and toss pear slices into your salad instead. If you're making the salad ahead of time, drizzle the pears with lemon juice to prevent browning.

◆ **Shake up your vegetable tray.** Bored with serving the same old broccoli pieces and carrot sticks with ranch dip at your parties? Try something new. Line a medium to large platter with romaine lettuce. On the right and left sides of the platter, horizontally place pear slices drizzled with lemon juice. In each corner, arrange a few purple grapes. Fill out the top and bottom with squash slices. And in the center? Toss on a mound of cooked shrimp. It'll look gorgeous—we promise!

◆ **Top your toast.** For a hint of sweetness (and extra fiber), top a piece of toasted whole wheat bread with peanut butter and pear slices.

◆ **Simplify your side dishes.** Bake pear halves with ham or pork during the last 15 minutes of cooking, basting them with the juices from the meat. Serve as a side dish. It's a lot easier than making mashed potatoes!

(Continued from page 341)

The soluble fiber in pears, called pectin, may help lower cholesterol levels, a critical way to reduce your risk of heart disease. Here's how it works:

▶ Soluble fiber helps bind together bile acids, enabling pectin to draw cholesterol out of your blood.

▶ It also helps block the fat and cholesterol in your foods from getting to the interior wall of the intestines, where it would be absorbed.

Researchers at Purdue University in West Lafayette, Indiana, found that eating about 9 grams of pectin daily reduced cholesterol by 10 percent. Pears have at least 2 grams of pectin in each fruit!

Lignin, the insoluble fiber in pears, is nothing to sneeze at, either. It helps bulk up the stools and makes them pass through the intestines faster, possibly reducing the risk of colon cancer. It also binds up the male hormone testosterone, and thus, may lower the chance of prostate cancer.

ONLY SKIN DEEP

Some people peel a pear before they eat it. Don't let them! According to a recent study at the University of California-Davis, almost all of the phytochemicals (healthy plant compounds) that pears have to offer lie in the skin. And red Bartletts pack about one-third more of these beneficial compounds—particularly the anticancer flavones and anthocyanins—than green varieties do.

NUTRITION IN A NUTSHELL

Bartlett pear (1 medium)

Calories: 100

Fat: 1 g

Saturated fat: 0 g

Cholesterol: 0 mg

Sodium: 0 mg

Total carbohydrates: 25 g

Dietary fiber: 4 g

Protein: 1 g

Vitamin C: 10% of Daily Value

Quick Fix:

Constipation

The next time your internal plumbing gets clogged, slice up a pear and mix it with a couple of prunes and a teaspoon of bran for a before-bed snack. Your plumbing will be fixed by morning—guaranteed!

While pears in general don't contribute as many of these compounds as some other fruits do (scientists consider their amount to be moderate), you'll want to hang on to every bit. So no peeling, okay?

Baked Pear-fection

End your fall or winter meal with this warm pear dessert. Don't feel guilty—it's fat-free!

2 pears, halved and cored
1–2 cups water
1 teaspoon ground cinnamon
½ teaspoon ground nutmeg
2 tablespoons honey
Raspberry or chocolate sauce (garnish), optional

Preheat the oven to 350°F. Place the pears in a baking dish. Fill the dish 1 to 2 inches with the water. Sprinkle with the cinnamon and nutmeg, then drizzle with the honey. Cover and bake for 35 to 40 minutes, or until the pears are tender. Put each pear half on a plate and, if desired, garnish with the raspberry or chocolate sauce. Serve warm.

Yield: Four servings.

Nutritional data per serving: Calories, 84; protein, 0 g; carbohydrates, 22 g; fiber, 2 g; fat, 0 g; saturated fat, 0 g; cholesterol, 0 mg; sodium, 1 mg; calcium, 2% of Daily Value; iron, 3%.

Waldorf Wrap

The Waldorf Salad was created in the 1890s at the Waldorf-Astoria Hotel in New York City, using just apples, celery, and mayonnaise. Since then, chefs have added nuts, and now they sometimes substitute pears for the apples. This wrap sandwich gives an old favorite an even more modern twist.

1 pear, sliced and cored
1 medium stalk celery, chopped
1 tablespoon chopped walnuts
3 tablespoons light mayonnaise
2 flour tortillas (8-inch diameter)
4 lean, low-sodium ham or turkey slices

In a medium bowl, combine the pear, celery, walnuts, and mayonnaise until well blended. Top each tortilla with 2 ham or turkey slices and half of the pear mixture. Wrap each tortilla and serve immediately.

Yield: Two servings.

Nutritional data per serving: Calories, 251; protein, 9 g; carbohydrates, 35 g; fiber, 3 g; fat, 8 g; saturated fat, 3 g; cholesterol, 24 mg; sodium, 517 mg; calcium, 6% of Daily Value; iron, 12%.

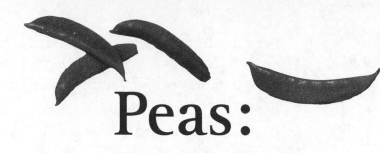

Peas:
Protein in a Pod

BATTLES:
- diabetes
- high cholesterol

BOLSTERS:
- energy
- regularity

When Colleen's kids were little, she liked to take them to "pick-your-own" farms so they'd know where food really comes from. It was a real eye-opener to find that milk didn't come from cartons or strawberries from jars. The thing that surprised them the most, however, was finding out that not only did early spring peas grow on a vine, but they also tasted completely different from their frozen or canned cousins at the supermarket. In fact, those fresh peas were so sweet and delicious that, on the way home, her family ate half of what they'd picked!

IT'S NOT EASY BEING GREEN

Sometimes it's hard to figure out just where peas fit in the overall scheme of nutrition. Technically, they're a green vegetable. But

Quick Fix:

High Cholesterol

Worried about high cholesterol? If you replace cold-cut sandwiches with pea soup for lunch, you'll get a double benefit. You'll cut out saturated fat that raises it and add the soluble fiber that lowers it!

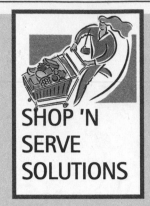

SHOP 'N SERVE SOLUTIONS

Peas are legumes—fleshy little seeds that grow in pods. Fresh peas are best, but they have a short season. Try the other forms, too, to enjoy peas year-round.

If you like fresh peas, be ready to rush to the farmers' markets or "pick-your-own" farms in April or May, the only time they're available. Then be ready to rush home and tenderly cook them as fast as you can. Like fresh corn, peas lose that incomparable sweetness quickly. In just 4 to 6 hours, you'll have old peas!

WHEN SELECTING FRESH PEAS:

Choose plump, bright green pods without blemishes, spots, or yellowing.

Frozen and canned peas. For everyday cooking, frozen peas are a good choice, although they have significantly less vitamin C than fresh. Canned peas can be used in a pinch, but they're not as flavorful or crisp.

Dried peas. Dried split green peas appear in 1-pound plastic bags in the rice and dried bean section of your grocery store. Always wash and check them before cooking up a pot of soup, because they sometimes contain small stones.

Glamorous peas. Snow peas are now available fresh in many large grocery stores. Look for crisp, clean, fresh, bright pods without cuts or blemishes. Avoid soggy or limp snow peas, because the vitamins

dietitians usually refer to *leafy* vegetables when they talk about greens. Peas are starchy little things—not fibrous veggies packed with vitamins A and C.

But what about snow peas? Yes! These are more like the traditional "greens" loved by nutritionists.

tend to exit along with the crispness. You might also find fresh sugar snap peas nearby. They're about halfway between a flat snow pea and a fully ripe green pea. You eat the peas and the pods. As you might expect, they're a nutritional cross, too, packing a little more protein than snow peas, but a little less vitamin C. You'll also find both kinds in the frozen food department.

Chickpeas. If you're relying on peas for protein, don't forget chickpeas, also known as garbanzo beans. You'll get an extra dose of folate along the way.

YOU'LL LIKE TWO PEAS AND THE POD

Now that your pantry's packed with peas, here's how to get all their benefits:

◆ **Pile 'em.** Pile peas and a sliced hard-boiled egg on your salad for complete protein along with your veggies.

◆ **Pack 'em.** Take along a can of pea soup for lunch, and heat it in the microwave. It counts as carbs, protein, and veggies, and it's so easy!

◆ **Pour 'em.** Pour frozen peas into any soup to provide protein.

◆ **Paste 'em.** Process a can of chickpeas into hummus. Just add a little lemon, garlic, and sesame oil, and whirl until smooth.

◆ **Prod 'em.** Stir snow peas into your stir-fry. Add them at the very last minute for crisp nutrition.

◆ **Pair 'em.** Perk up cooked carrots with a few sugar snap peas. They add color, texture, flavor, and fiber. And the combo is a feast for your eyes!

They're an immature version of peas in the pod, so you can eat the whole thing. Indeed, 1 cup of cooked snow peas packs a full day's worth of vitamin C—more than you'd get from a cup of cooked spinach or even from an orange. More fiber, too. And it provides a little vitamin A, about 4 percent of what you need for the day. So snow peas are great for building and protecting skin and for keeping your bowels working, too. Color snow peas green.

ANIMAL, VEGETABLE, OR MINERAL?

Okay, if peas aren't a green vegetable, then what are they? Try meat substitute, only better. Here's what they offer:

▶ **Powerful protein.** One cup of fresh, frozen, or canned green peas provides as much protein as an egg or an ounce of lean beef—without the fat!

In fact, 1 cup of peas, plus a cup of skim milk, provides more than one-third of your protein for the day. And the protein is complete, like the protein in meat, so it's great for building muscle, repairing tissue, boosting your immune system, and bolstering every cell, enzyme, and hormone in your body.

▶ **Fabulous fiber.** As if that weren't enough, here's an added bonus: Peas deliver one-third of your day's fiber—something you never get from meat!

▶ **Mighty meaty minerals and vitamins.** And except for zinc and vitamin B_{12}, peas match or exceed a full 3-ounce serving of lean beef for every mineral and vitamin you can think of.

Color peas powerful protein.

NUTRITION IN A NUTSHELL

Cooked chickpeas ($1/2$ cup)

Calories: 134

Fat: 2 g

Saturated fat: Less than 1 g

Cholesterol: 0 mg

Sodium: 6 mg

Total carbohydrates: 22 g

Dietary fiber: 6 g

Protein: 7 g

Folate: 35% of Daily Value

Calcium: 4%

Copper: 14%

Iron: 13%

Zinc: 8%

STARCH ON THE MARCH

Maybe you're thinking that, because peas are starchy, they'll make you fat. Think again. Peas make a great weapon against weight gain.

Here's why: While the starch in peas is pure carbohydrate, it's the slow-moving kind, with what's called a low glycemic index (GI). Unlike high-GI carbs (the kind found in white bread and potatoes) that get sucked into your bloodstream in a rush, the carbs in peas dillydally while being digested. Their energy is released slowly into your bloodstream, and that keeps you from getting hungry again too soon.

In fact, five out of five studies show that dieters eat fewer snacks after a low-GI meal, says Susan Roberts, Ph.D., director of the energy metabolism laboratory at Tufts University in Boston. If you have diabetes or insulin resistance, a modest portion of peas can also help control blood sugar's rise and allow time for insulin to work better.

Feeling fit as a fiddle and ready to work out? A bowl of pea soup before your run will fuel you steadily until you're done. Now that's powerful pottage!

Early Peas in Lettuce Cups

Nothing is sweeter than freshly gathered spring peas. They're so tender and flavorful that you'll want to eat them plain, so that nothing interferes with their natural flavor. Lettuce leaves provide just enough moisture for cooking without boiling away the vitamins.

2 large leaves iceberg lettuce
1½ cups freshly shelled green peas (about 1 pound in the shell)
1 tablespoon water
1 teaspoon butter

In a heavy nonstick skillet over low heat, balance 1 of the lettuce leaves so that it forms a cup. Fill it with the peas. Cover with the second lettuce leaf. Pour the water in the bottom of the skillet. Cover, and simmer for 10 to 15 minutes, or until the peas are barely tender. If necessary, add water by the teaspoon throughout the cooking to prevent the lettuce from burning. To serve, place the top lettuce cup on a plate, fill with one-half of the peas, and dot with one-half of the butter. Place the remaining pea-filled leaf on a plate, and dot with the remaining butter. Hurry up and eat!

Yield: Two servings.

Nutritional data per serving: Calories, 119; protein, 7 g; carbohydrates, 19 g; fiber, 7 g; fat, 2 g; saturated fat, 1 g; cholesterol, 5 mg; sodium, 24 mg; vitamin A, 17% of Daily Value; vitamin C, 20%; copper, 11%; iron, 11%; zinc, 11%.

 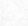

Pineapple:

Your Hawaiian Health Connection

BATTLES:
- cancer
- heart disease

BOLSTERS:
- digestion
- immune function

Pineapple conjures up visions of Hawaii—you know, glorious days filled with swimming, sightseeing, and, yes, eating lots of pineapple. In a word: paradise.

Well, if you can't make it over there, then do the next best thing—pick up some pineapple at your local supermarket. Sure, it isn't exactly the same, but you'll love it nonetheless. And pineapple is as good for you as it is good-tasting.

TROPICAL RELIEF

Depending on the variety of pineapple you select, one 4-ounce serving contains 25 to 150 percent of the vitamin C you need for the day. As you probably know, vitamin C is an antioxidant, gobbling up

NUTRITION IN A NUTSHELL

Pineapple (4 ounces, or two 3-inch slices)

Calories: 65

Fat: 0 g

Saturated fat: 0 g

Cholesterol: 0 mg

Sodium: 10 mg

Total carbohydrates: 16 g

Dietary fiber: 1 g

Protein: 1 g

Vitamin C: 25–150% of Daily Value

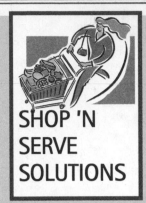

SHOP 'N SERVE SOLUTIONS

Buying pineapple is pretty much a no-brainer because you're rarely—if ever—going to see a pineapple that isn't ripe. That's because, unlike many other fruits, pineapple is picked only when it's ripe and then shipped to supermarkets.

WHEN SELECTING PINEAPPLE:

■ Look for fruits that have dark green leaves.

■ Avoid those that have bruises or soft spots. (Myth alert: The color of the pineapple's outer shell will give you no indication of its quality or ripeness.)

■ Check the variety. All pineapple varieties pack vitamin C, but the fairly new Del Monte Gold offers all the vitamin C (and then some) that you need for the day in just a single serving. The amount is four times greater than in traditional varieties.

WHEN STORING:

■ Wrap the pineapple loosely in plastic.

■ Refrigerate it for as long as five days.

WHEN YOU'RE READY TO USE:

■ Simply twist the crown off the pineapple.

■ Cut the shell away from the fruit.

■ Slice.

free radicals, bad guys that cause cell damage that can lead to heart disease and cancer. It also revs up your immune system so that it can ward off colds, flu, and other infections that make you feel miserable.

■ Or make chunks by cutting the pineapple in quarters lengthwise.

■ Trim each end, then cut away the center core strip.

■ Cut the quartered fruit into bite-size pieces, and that's it!

Sliced pineapple lasts up to three days in the fridge if you store it in a sealed container.

HAVE A HAWAIIAN HOLIDAY

To enjoy a taste of the tropics, try these simple suggestions:

◆ **Sweeten your breakfast.** Stir fresh or dried pineapple pieces into your morning yogurt. Warm fresh or canned pineapple slices and top your waffles with them. Or follow the Hawaiians' lead: Just slice 'em and eat 'em plain.

◆ **Light up the grill.** Grill pineapple slices on both sides just until warmed. Top with vanilla frozen yogurt for a decadent dessert.

◆ **Spark up a sandwich.** Tuck a pineapple slice into your next ham and cheese sandwich.

◆ **Set sail.** Here's how to make a pineapple "boat": Cut a pineapple in half lengthwise, leaving the crown attached to the shell. Remove the fruit by cutting close to the shell with a thin, sharp knife. Cut away the center core strip. Then cut the fruit into bite-size pieces. Mix with pieces of other fresh fruits (mangoes, melons, and strawberries are good choices), and serve in the boat.

OUTRIGGER ENZYMES

Besides vitamin C, pineapple is packed with additional compounds that may fend off cancer. Chief among them: bromelain, an enzyme that may help halt the spread of tumors.

Animal studies suggest that bromelain holds promise in fighting lung cancer and leukemia especially, but more tests need

Quick Fix:

Callus

To soften a callus, apply a piece of pineapple rind and cover it with adhesive bandages overnight, suggests James Duke, Ph.D., retired USDA researcher and author of THE GREEN PHARMACY. An enzyme in the rind does the trick.

to be done. In the meantime, however, it certainly won't hurt to add luscious pineapple to your list of anticancer foods.

Bromelain also gives you the more immediate benefit of aiding your digestion. So if a bowl of five-alarm chili has your stomach in knots, have a few chunks of pineapple or a glass of pineapple juice. It may supply the relief you need, without the side effects of antacids.

Tropical Fruit Salad

The next time someone asks you to bring potato or macaroni salad to a picnic, ask if you can make this fruit salad instead. Just one serving has nearly all the vitamin C you need for the day, and you won't have to turn on the stove.

2 cups pineapple chunks
2 cups mango chunks
2 cups cantaloupe chunks
½ cup sliced strawberries
¼ cup orange juice
¼ cup chopped fresh spearmint

In a large bowl, mix the pineapple, mango, cantaloupe, strawberries, orange juice, and spearmint. Serve immediately, or cover and refrigerate.

Yield: Six servings.

Nutritional data per serving: Calories, 89; protein, 1 g; carbohydrates, 22 g; fiber, 3 g; fat, 1 g; saturated fat, 0 g; cholesterol, 0 mg; sodium, 7 mg; calcium, 2% of Daily Value; iron, 2%.

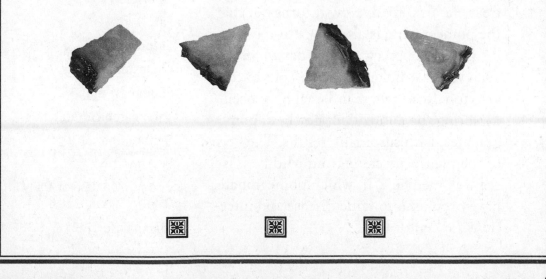

Pomegranates:

They're Sweet to Your Heart

BATTLES:
- aging
- cancer
- heart disease

BOLSTERS:
- enzyme activity

One of autumn's highlights is the arrival of pomegranates, those "jewels of autumn" that remind us of when we were young and shared the sparkling seeds with our friends. Back then, a pomegranate was a special treat—a "fun" food. Now it turns out that the pomegranate is also a health food.

In fact, a pomegranate a day might just keep your cardiologist at bay. Your oncologist, too. Researchers in Israel have been exploring the antioxidant power of pomegranates, with surprising results. The germ of their curiosity came from Middle Eastern folk medicine, in which pomegranates have been used to tame disease and infections for centuries.

NUTRITION IN A NUTSHELL

Pomegranate (1 fruit or ½ cup juice)

Calories: 105

Fat: 0 g

Saturated fat: 0 g

Cholesterol: 0 mg

Sodium: 4 mg

Total carbohydrates: 1 g

Dietary fiber: 1 g

Protein: 1 g

Vitamin C: 10% of Daily Value

Manganese: 44%

In the lab, researchers fermented the juice into wine and cold-pressed the oil from the seeds. They then extracted compounds called flavonoids from both of these liquids and tested their power against that of other known protective foods.

The researchers learned that pomegranate flavonoids were equal to green tea and even better than red wine at preventing the oxidation of low-density lipoprotein (LDL) cholesterol, the chemical change that allows plaque to clog and harden your arteries. They also found straight pomegranate juice to be more potent than red wine, which means you don't have to get tipsy to get healthy. Another likely benefit of pomegrante flavonoids is the slowing of cell aging.

OF MICE AND MEN

Going a step further, researchers found that pomegranate juice prevented plaque buildup in mice. And in a group of healthy men, drinking sparkling, sweet-tart pomegranate juice daily for two weeks increased production of an enzyme that can protect against cancerous changes in cells.

It turns out that pomegranates are packed with ellagic acid, a polyphenolic compound that prevents cancers from getting started. It has been shown to inhibit cancer start-up in the lungs, liver, skin, and esophagus of mice.

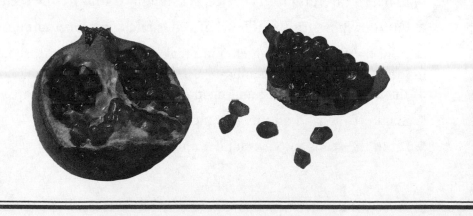

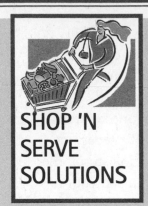

SHOP 'N SERVE SOLUTIONS

Pomegranates are available only from September to December, with peak supplies in October and November. During these months, pomegranates will arrive at your grocery store ripe and ready to eat.

WHEN SELECTING POMEGRANATES:

■ Pick those with thin, tough, unbroken skin.

■ Choose ones that are heavy for their size—a sign of juiciness.

WHEN STORING:

■ Even when fully ripe, pomegranates will keep well at room temperature for up to a month. So you could use a few in your Thanksgiving centerpiece and still be able to eat them later.

■ To keep them longer (up to two months), store them in the fridge.

GET TO THE GOOD STUFF

A pomegranate is a sort of leathery red pouch about the size of an apple, filled with sparkling, jewel-like seeds. The seeds are packed in a spongy white membrane that acts like a bubble wrap. You really can't eat the outer coating (the bubble wrap), so here's how to ditch the debris and get to the good stuff:

■ Cut off the crown.

■ With a sharp knife, score the leathery rind lightly from top to bottom, being careful not to cut deeply enough to rupture the seeds.

■ Put the whole fruit in a bowl of water and soak for 5 minutes.

■ Hold the fruit under water, and break the sections apart, separating the seeds from the membranes. The seeds will sink to the bottom of the bowl, and the rind and membranes will float to the top.

■ Skim off the rind and membranes and trash them.

■ Drain the seeds into a colander, then pat dry. Voilà!

USING POMEGRANATE SEEDS

Here are some tips for using pomegranate seeds:

◆ **Freeze them for later.** Yes, pomegranates are available only in the fall. But once you find out how good they are, with their sparkling, sweet-tart flavor, you'll want to eat them year-round. So just scatter the seeds in a single layer on a baking sheet and freeze until firm. Then pack them in freezer containers and store them for up to six months. (Okay, that won't get you through a full year, but half a year is better than nothing.)

◆ **Spin them into juicy juice.** Put $1\frac{1}{2}$ to 2 cups of seeds at a time into a blender or food processor, and whirl them around until liquefied. Pour the juice through a wire strainer lined with cheesecloth, draining it into a container. If you don't drink all of it right away, the juice will keep in the refrigerator for about five days or in the freezer for six months. You can use the juice to make lemonade, to color sliced pears and apples for salads, or as a stock for soups and stews. Nifty!

◆ **Bejewel your foods.** Just sprinkle the fresh or frozen seeds anywhere you need a brilliant red garnish—on salads, fruit desserts, even cakes and puddings. Toss them into rice or wheatberry salads, or stir them into applesauce. Or use them as a topping for waffles, pancakes, or frozen yogurt. Pretty!

◆ **Give them a big squeeze.** Pack a pomegranate in your lunch bag. At your desk, roll the fruit around with the palm of your hand to pop the seed sacs. Then just cut off the top and squeeze out the juice. Cool!

◆ **Simplest of all, eat them by the handful.** They'll be your sweet-tart.

Pomegranate, Clementine, and Kiwi Salad

If you're looking for a dash of color along with sparkling-fresh taste, add this spectacular salad to your next fancy feast.

6 cups mixed baby field greens, such as baby spinach, oak leaf lettuce, and frisée
⅛ teaspoon crushed red pepper flakes
4 tablespoons raspberry vinaigrette
3 Clementines, peeled and separated, or
1 cup juice-packed mandarin orange segments, well-drained
4 kiwifruits, peeled and thinly sliced
Seeds of 1 medium pomegranate (about ¾ cup)

In a large bowl, toss the greens, red pepper flakes, and 2 tablespoons of the vinaigrette until the greens are well coated. Arrange on six salad plates. Decoratively arrange the Clementine or mandarin orange segments and the kiwifruit slices on the greens. Drizzle with the remaining 2 tablespoons of vinaigrette. Sprinkle the pomegranate seeds on top.

Yield: Six servings.

Nutritional data per serving: Calories, 89; protein, 2 g; carbohydrates, 21 g; fiber, 4 g; fat, 0.5 g; saturated fat, 0 g; cholesterol, 0 mg; sodium, 29 mg; vitamin A, 39% of Daily Value; vitamin C, 68%; manganese, 26%.

Pork:

Fork It Over

BATTLES:
- heart disease
- high blood pressure
- high cholesterol

BOLSTERS:
- bones
- immune function

Last summer, we took a business trip to the Napa Valley—California wine country. We found that the chardonnay wasn't the only thing that tasted magnificent. On our first night in the Napa Valley, we dined at a winery that served a grilled Mediterranean-style pork chop. It was the best pork that either of us had eaten in a long time.

That single summer dinner (more so than any of those "other white meat" commercials) reminded us that pork, in the kitchen of the right person, can rival any gourmet food. And if you choose the right cut, it really can be as lean as chicken! (See "The Great Eight" on page 366.)

HOGGING ALL THE VITAMINS

When it comes to vitamins and minerals, pork is, well, a hog. It offers major amounts of 10 nutrients in just a 3-ounce cooked serving. Here are some of pork's nutritional highlights:

▶ **Vitamin B$_1$ (thiamin).** Pork packs 53 percent of your daily requirement for this vitamin, which is essential for metabolizing carbohydrates, protein, and fat.

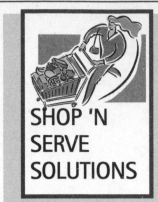

SHOP 'N SERVE SOLUTIONS

When it comes to pork, you can choose from a lot of cuts. But we recommend sticking to the "great eight" listed on page 366. More important, each has from 4 to 9 grams of fat in a 3-ounce cooked serving. Go one better by looking for Smithfield Lean Generation Pork, sold by a company that has specially bred its hogs to be leaner.

WHEN SELECTING PORK:

■ Make sure the meat is pink to pinkish gray, except for pork tenderloin, which should be deep red.

■ Check the "sell-by" date on pork products.

WHEN STORING:

Fresh pork will keep for a few days in the fridge.

WHEN YOU'RE READY TO USE:

■ Trim any external fat from the meat.

■ Use a meat thermometer to ensure that the internal temperature of your meat is 160°F. Food safety experts used to recommend cooking pork to 170°F, but now they've dropped that recommendation to 160°F. The reason? The parasite that causes trichinosis—a disease that pork could transport—is killed at 137°F. Cooking to 160°F gives you a big margin of error. At that temperature, your pork should still be juicy and a little pink in the center.

SWINE AND DINE

◆ **Fire up fajitas.** You don't have to limit yourself to beef or chicken. Pork tastes awesome in fajitas, too.

◆ **Triple your sauce.** One of Karen's favorite restaurants, The Apollo Grill in Bethlehem, Pennsylvania, serves a pork chop entrée made with a trio of barbeque sauces. Each part of the pork is brushed with a different kind of sauce. Try the same when grilling at home.

▶ **Vitamin B$_{12}$.** It helps build red blood cells. You soak up about 8 percent of your daily requirement when you eat a serving of pork.

▶ **Phosphorus.** Pork kicks in about one-quarter of your requirement for this mineral that helps strengthen bones.

▶ **Potassium.** You probably think that only fruits and veggies offer potassium, a mineral that helps maintain normal blood pressure. Pork offers 11 percent of your daily need.

HAVE A HEART

We know what you're thinking: "Sure, pork's leaner than it used to be, but can I substitute it for the chicken in my diet?" In a word: Yes. A study at Duke University Medical Center in Durham, North Carolina, found that substituting lean pork for fattier meats in the diets of people with high cholesterol dropped their levels about 7 percent—the same amount as for a group that ate skinless chicken instead of pork.

So if your family is complaining about having chicken again, add some pork to your weekly menu. The bottom line is that they're both healthy meats for your heart. Mix and match them in your diet to beat boredom.

NUTRITION IN A NUTSHELL

Pork tenderloin (3 ounces, cooked)

Calories: 139

Fat: 4 g

Saturated fat: 1 g

Cholesterol: 67 mg

Sodium: 48 mg

Total carbohydrates: 0 g

Dietary fiber: 0 g

Protein: 23 g

Vitamin B$_1$ (thiamin): 53% of Daily Value

Vitamin B$_2$ (riboflavin): 19%

Vitamin B$_3$ (niacin): 20%

Vitamin B$_6$: 30%

Vitamin B$_{12}$: 8%

Iron: 7%

Magnesium: 6%

Phosphorus: 22%

Potassium: 11%

Zinc: 15%

The Great Eight

These eight cuts of pork provide less than 190 calories and 4 to 9 grams of fat in a 3-ounce cooked serving.

Cut of Pork	Calories	Fat (g)	Saturated Fat (g)
Tenderloin	139	4	1
Boneless sirloin chop	164	6	2
Boneless loin roast	165	6	2
Boneless top loin chop	173	7	2
Loin chop	171	7	3
Boneless sirloin roast	168	7	3
Rib chop	186	8	3
Boneless rib roast	182	9	3

Tropical Marinade

This marinade makes pork taste like paradise.

½ cup orange juice
2 tablespoons lemon juice
2 cloves garlic, crushed
1 teaspoon dried oregano

In a large bowl, mix the orange juice, lemon juice, garlic, and oregano. Marinate pork for at least 30 minutes before cooking. Discard the marinade after using.

Apple-Cranberry Pork Chops

Karen has been making these pork chops ever since some folks from the National Pork Producers Council stopped by her office a couple of years ago with the recipe. Deeee-lish!

Canola oil cooking spray
4 boneless sirloin chops (¾ inch thick)
Salt to taste
Ground black pepper to taste
¼ cup apple cider or juice
½ cup cranberry sauce
2 tablespoons honey
2 tablespoons frozen orange juice concentrate, thawed
¼ teaspoon ground ginger
⅛ teaspoon ground nutmeg

Coat a large nonstick skillet with cooking spray. Heat over medium-high heat. Sprinkle both sides of the pork chops with the salt and pepper. Put the chops in the skillet and brown on each side. Add the apple cider. Cover tightly, and cook over low heat for 5 to 6 minutes, or until the chops reach an internal temperature of 160°F. In a small bowl, combine the cranberry sauce, honey, orange juice concentrate, ginger, and nutmeg. Pour over the chops. Cook for 1 to 2 minutes, or until heated through.

Yield: Four servings.

Nutritional data per serving: Calories, 278; protein, 26 g; carbohydrates, 28 g; fiber, 1 g; fat, 7 g; saturated fat, 3 g; cholesterol, 70 mg; sodium, 62 mg; calcium, 3% of Daily Value; iron, 5%.

Potatoes:

Simply Smashing Spuds

BATTLES:
- high blood pressure

BOLSTERS:
- bones
- energy
- mood
- wound healing

Athletes may start the day with Wheaties, but endurance specialists, such as marathon runners and triathletes, follow their exhaustive workouts with high-carbohydrate foods. And nothing refuels a jock better than potatoes—whether the jock is a Los Angeles Laker in California or a Milltown Midget in your backyard.

Here's why: As an athlete trains, his or her muscles learn to suck up carbohydrates from food, turn them into blood sugar, and then store the sugar in muscles as glycogen. That's the energy for tomorrow's workout.

But all carbs are not created equal. Some get digested and stashed faster than others. And potatoes lead the pack in the race to reenergize. Think that's just for kids

Quick Fix:

High Blood Pressure

Are you on a low-sodium diet to lower your blood pressure? Drop a peeled potato into your soup or stew, then discard. It will absorb some of the sodium.

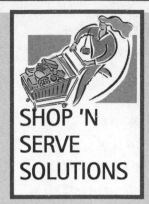

SHOP 'N SERVE SOLUTIONS

Potatoes come in two basic types. Idaho and russets are dry, mealy, and fluffy, so they have to soak up a ton of butter or sour cream to be palatable. Waxy potatoes, like red-skin, new, or Yukon Gold, have a higher water content and need little fat to make them delicious. (Guess which ones we prefer?)

WHEN SELECTING POTATOES:

■ Consider buying them loose so that you can handpick each one and get the size you prefer.

■ While you're at it, you can also check for cuts, bruises, and mold.

■ If you buy your potatoes already bagged, try to get a bag you can see through, or, if all else fails, use the "sniff test" to check for rotten stowaways.

■ You can also buy chilled potatoes already peeled, sliced, diced, or mashed, as well as canned and frozen.

EASY POTATO PREPARATION

Now try these various ways to enjoy potatoes:

◆ **Flavor with fish.** Top a baked potato with $\frac{1}{4}$ cup of canned salmon for a heart-healthy treat that's teeming with flavor. Or stuff your potato with shrimp salad, and let the mayo do double duty.

◆ **Season with salsa.** Dress your potato with salsa for a spicy side dish.

◆ **Opt for olives.** Spread your potato with olive spread, and do your arteries a favor.

◆ **Reach for the ranch.** Stir powdered ranch dressing seasoning into mashed potatoes for a ton of flavor without the fat. Or sprinkle some on a baked potato.

◆ **Serve speedy spuds.** Buy canned cubed or sliced potatoes for quick preparation and add to soups, stews, and other vegetable dishes.

or superstars? Not so. We've been checking out the Senior Olympics, and grown-up athletes are just as carbo-focused.

This ability to quickly turn carbs into blood sugar is often discussed as a problem for folks struggling with diabetes or insulin resistance. If that's you, you can still enjoy potatoes. Just eat them in small portions. Include the skins, season them with a little heart-healthy fat (such as olive oil), and have them as part of a meal. That will slow them down so you don't get a sugar jolt. Why not just avoid them? Because they're good for you in other ways.

MOOD SMOOTHER

Potatoes might be your best friend (second only to chocolate?). One medium baked potato delivers 24 grams of pure carbohydrate, known to soothe jangled nerves and elevate mood.

Not enough to chill you out? Your potato is studded with vitamin B_6, which is needed to boost serotonin, the natural brain chemical that makes you feel so happy.

Want more? Your potato is bursting with copper, magnesium, and manganese, which boost bone health.

And that's not all. That potato packs more potassium than a banana, so it will help you beat high blood pressure, too. And there's even some vitamin C in there to help heal those little shaving cuts. No wonder folks love potatoes!

NUTRITION IN A NUTSHELL

Plain baked potato with skin (1 medium)

Calories: 133

Fat: 0 g

Saturated fat: 0 g

Cholesterol: 0 mg

Sodium: 10 mg

Total carbohydrates: 31 g

Dietary fiber: 3 g

Protein: 3 g

Vitamin B_6: 21% of Daily Value

Vitamin C: 17%

Copper: 19%

Iron: 9%

Potassium: 14%

Garlic Crisp Potatoes

If you're like most Americans, you love fries! If you also hate the artery-clogging fat, don't fight. Switch to these crispy treats kissed with olive oil.

1 large baking potato, well scrubbed but unpeeled
2 teaspoons olive oil
½ teaspoon garlic powder
½ teaspoon dried dillweed
⅛ teaspoon finely ground multicolored pepper

Preheat the oven to 450°F. Thinly slice the potato crosswise, using a knife, a food processor, or Colleen's favorite oriental slicer, the Benriner (watch your fingers!). Brush the slices with the oil, or use a mister to thinly coat. Arrange in a single layer on a baking sheet. Sprinkle with the garlic, dillweed, and pepper. Bake for about 10 minutes, or until crispy. Using a thin spatula, transfer immediately to two dinner plates.

Yield: Two servings.

Nutritional data per serving: Calories, 143; protein, 2 g; carbohydrates, 24 g; fiber, 2 g; fat, 5 g; saturated fat, less than 1 g; cholesterol, 0 mg; sodium, 8 mg; vitamin B_6, 17% of Daily Value; vitamin C, 13%; vitamin E, 4%; copper, 14%; potassium, 11%.

Prunes:

They're Plum Good

BATTLES:
- cancer
- heart disease
- high cholesterol

BOLSTERS:
- energy
- mood
- regularity

No doubt about it: Prunes are the ugly duckling of the dried fruit family. To boost the image of prunes, the FDA recently agreed that their name could be changed to "dried plums." But as Shakespeare once asked, what's in a name? It's what's inside that counts—and there, prunes are plum beautiful!

LITTLE PACKAGES OF ANTIOXIDANTS

Ounce for ounce, prunes pack more than twice as many antioxidants as raisins do, according to a recent study at Tufts University in Boston. (And raisins are no lightweights themselves!) Antioxidants are valuable compounds because they help fight cancer and heart disease.

Additional research at the University of California-Davis suggests that one particu-

Quick Fix:

The Blues

Feeling a little blue? Have a glass of prune juice. It's rich in vitamin B_6, which research suggests may improve mood for some people.

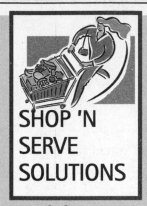

**SHOP 'N
SERVE
SOLUTIONS**

*There's a new wrinkle in picking prunes:
They're now called something different—
"dried plums." Despite the new name, what
you should look for remains the same.*

WHEN SELECTING PRUNES:

■ Look for packages that are tightly sealed.
Properly protected, the prunes will be moist
and clean.

■ If your diet falls a little short on iron, the B vitamins, and vitamin E,
consider picking up Mariani Prunes Plus, which offer 20 percent of the
Daily Value for each of these nutrients.

■ Living on a tight budget? Buy unpitted prunes and remove the
pits yourself, using a small knife.

WHEN STORING:

Once you open your package, tightly reseal it and stash it in the refrigerator, or transfer the prunes to an airtight container and store
them in a cool, dry place. They'll last for up to six months.

PERFECT PRUNES

Now check out all the ways that you can perk up foods with prunes:

◆ **Spread it on thick.** Add chopped pitted prunes to peanut butter
for an extra fiber boost.

◆ **Perk up pork.** Sauté pitted prunes with pears and red onion.
Serve this intriguing combination on the side with pork.

◆ **Make happy endings.** Soak pitted prunes overnight in orange juice.
Spoon them over sorbet or low-fat frozen yogurt for a healthy dessert.

◆ **Pour them into batter.** Whip up your baked goods using store-
bought prune puree. Simply use half the amount of butter or oil
called for in the recipe. Then replace only half the amount removed
with prune puree.

lar antioxidant in prunes, called neochloro-genic acid, protects the body by riding herd on low-density lipoprotein (LDL) choles-terol—the bad kind. It prevents LDL cho-lesterol from undergoing a process that eventually leads to clogged arteries. In one trial, for example, men with slightly high cholesterol who ate about a dozen prunes a day significantly lowered their bad choles-terol levels.

CONSTIPATION FIGHTERS

Antioxidants aside, prunes are famous (or maybe infamous) for something that you're probably familiar with: their laxative effect. Researchers still aren't exactly sure why prunes can relieve constipation, but they suspect that it's their un-usual combination of insoluble fiber and the sugar sorbitol, each of which bulks up the stool.

While most fruits offer very little sorbitol, prunes are com-posed of about 15 percent sorbitol. Eating about five prunes or drinking a cup of prune juice can help curb constipa-tion, although the fruit probably works a little better than the juice because it contains more fiber.

But prune juice has one advantage over the fruit: One cup kicks in about 17 percent of the energy-boosting iron you need for the day. Five prunes (oh yeah, dried plums) offer only about 4 percent.

If you'd rather drink prune juice than eat the dried fruit, look for brands without added sugar, to avoid packing on the pounds. One cup of unsweetened prune juice already has 70 more calories than the same amount of orange juice.

NUTRITION IN A NUTSHELL

Prunes (about 5)

Calories: 109

Fat: 0 g

Saturated fat: 0 g

Cholesterol: 0 mg

Sodium: 5 mg

Total carbohydrates: 26 g

Dietary fiber: 2 g

Protein: 1 g

Vitamin A: 17% of Daily Value

Iron: 4%

Oriental Chicken Salad

Prunes are a perfect fit in this sensational salad developed by the folks at the California Prune Board.

⅓ cup rice vinegar

¼ cup reduced-sodium soy sauce

2 tablespoons sugar

2 tablespoons chopped fresh cilantro

1 tablespoon minced fresh ginger

1 clove garlic, minced

½ teaspoon sesame oil

½ teaspoon red pepper flakes

4 boneless, skinless chicken breast halves (3 ounces each)

2 cups broccoli florets

2 carrots, cut into 1½-inch-long matchsticks

1 red bell pepper, cut into 1½-inch-long matchsticks

1 cup (6 ounces) pitted prunes, snipped into halves

3 green onions, sliced

4 lettuce leaves

In a medium bowl, whisk together the vinegar, soy sauce, sugar, cilantro, ginger, garlic, oil, and red pepper flakes. Remove ¼ cup of the dressing to a shallow 8-inch-square baking dish. Place the chicken in the baking dish. Turn to coat both sides. Marinate for 30 minutes. Place the broccoli, carrots, bell pepper, prunes, and onions in the bowl with the dressing. Toss until well coated. Let stand for 30 minutes.

Preheat the grill or broiler. Cook the chicken, basting with the marinade, for about 10 minutes, or until the meat juices run clear, turning once. Cut each breast into ¼-inch slices across the grain. Place 1 lettuce leaf on each of four plates. Top each leaf with one-quarter of the vegetable mixture. Place 1 sliced chicken breast on each plate, propped up against the veggies.

Yield: Four servings.

Nutritional data per serving: Calories, 293; protein, 25 g; carbohydrates, 46 g; fiber, 7 g; fat, 2 g; saturated fat, 0 g; cholesterol, 49 mg; sodium, 590 mg; calcium, 8% of Daily Value; iron, 21%.

Pumpkin:
Give Thanks for Its Potent Nutrients

BATTLES:
- cancer
- heart disease
- high blood pressure
- stroke

BOLSTERS:
- immune function
- vision

Early one Thanksgiving morning, just as the pumpkin pies were coming out of the oven, Colleen's mother-in-law called to remind her that her dinner contribution was to be celery and olives that year, not pie. Oooops! Now what?

Without a moment's hesitation, Colleen seized the day and called her family down to breakfast. She served them each a piece of warm pumpkin pie with an ice-cold glass of skim milk. Never before and never since has a piece of pie been so appreciated! The kitchen was still warm, and that heavenly spicy fragrance was wafting about. Everybody was hungry, and eating pie for breakfast was just so...decadent!

Fortunately, it was nutritious, too. That's because the canned pumpkin we all use to make pie is just packed with carotenes (three whole days' worth!), vitamin E, copper, iron, magnesium, and potassium.

Colleen uses evaporated skim milk instead of cream, so the filling is low in fat. And combined with the eggs she adds to the filling, each slice has as much protein as an ounce of meat.

Instead of lard or shortening in the crust, she uses heart-healthy canola oil, so they all started the day with an extra dose of vitamin E, plenty of B vitamins (including folate!), and half of their heart-healthy monounsaturated fat for the day.

Truly, not all pies are created equal. This one is head and shoulders above the crowd.

POWER VEGGIE

Pumpkin is as potent a vegetable as you'll find anywhere. Its deep orange color is a sure sign that it's just crazy with carotenes, which fight both heart disease and cancer. Cup for cup, pumpkin ranks with cantaloupe and cooked carrots as top beta-carotene carriers, and it delivers twice as much alpha-carotene as any other fruit or vegetable.

Both beta- and alpha-carotene can become vitamin A, with all its power to protect your night vision, rev up your immune system, and build skin and mucous lining barriers against bacteria and viruses.

But the beta-carotene itself can supercharge your immune system. It's been shown to jump-start natural killer cell activity in older men. It makes bacteria-munching monocytes work more effectively, and it highlights troublemaking antigens so that helper T cells can make the right antibodies to neutralize the antigens.

And pumpkin is the equal of yellow corn in the amount of

NUTRITION IN A NUTSHELL

Canned pumpkin (½ cup)

Calories: 42

Fat: 0 g

Saturated fat: 0 g

Cholesterol: 0 mg

Sodium: 6 mg

Total carbohydrates: 9 g

Dietary fiber: 3 g

Protein: 1 g

Vitamin A: 338% of Daily Value

Vitamin C: 6%

Vitamin E: 9%

Calcium: 3%

Iron: 9%

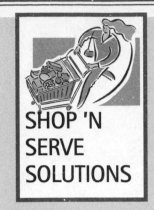

SHOP 'N SERVE SOLUTIONS

Beyond pie, when was the last time you ate pumpkin as a vegetable? You could be missing a lot, and using pumpkin in a meal is really pretty simple.

WHEN SELECTING PUMPKIN:

■ Check out farmers' markets and roadside stands.

■ Find one of those small, flat, red-orange pumpkins if you can. It'll be sweetest. Or select a nice little, bright orange jack-o'-lantern–type pumpkin

■ Pass up large pumpkins, which tend to be tough and stringy—and harder to work with. The last thing you need is a wrestling match!

■ No matter what kind of pumpkin you buy, get one that's unblemished, evenly shaped, and fresh-smelling.

WHEN YOU'RE READY TO USE:

Okay, you've picked the perfect pumpkin. Now how do you get it ready to eat? Follow these simple steps, and you'll have plenty of table-ready pumpkin for quick meals at a moment's notice:

■ Wash all the dirt off the pumpkin.

■ Place the pumpkin on a sturdy cutting board.

■ Using a large, sharp knife, cut the pumpkin in half.

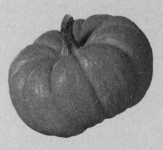

■ Scoop out the seeds and set them aside. (Toast them later if you like—they're yummy.)

lutein it can serve up. Lutein pumps up the macula of your eye (critical for reading, watching the speedometer, and noticing stop

Then use either of these methods to skin and cook:

Method 1: Cut your pumpkin into chunks and put the chunks on a well-greased baking sheet. Bake at 325°F for about an hour, or until the pulp is soft. Scrape the pulp from the shell, then toss it into your food processor to puree.

Method 2: Cut your pumpkin into chunks, peel the chunks, and place them in a saucepan. Add about $\frac{1}{2}$ cup of water, cover, and simmer until tender, about 25 minutes.

MAKE EVERY EVE A HALLOWED EVE

Now you're ready to enjoy your pumpkin in these smashing ways:

◆ **Make mashed pumpkin.** Warm pureed pumpkin with a little margarine, ground cinnamon, and skim milk. Serve like mashed sweet potatoes.

◆ **Serve saucy pumpkin.** Add a little salt and pepper to pureed pumpkin, then use as "gravy" with lean pot roast.

◆ **Choose chunky pumpkin.** Reheat pumpkin chunks in the microwave. Sprinkle with pumpkin pie spice and chopped toasted pecans. Serve as a side dish with pork tenderloin.

◆ **Slurp soupy pumpkin.** Stir pumpkin chunks into canned soup for a flavor and nutrient boost.

◆ **Savor smooth pumpkin.** Take the shortcut. Get your pumpkin from a can. Season with ground ginger, stir in some raisins or dried cherries, and microwave until warm. It's great with baked chicken.

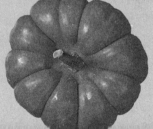

signs), protecting it against harmful blue light and thus fending off age-related macular degeneration.

Spicy Pumpkin Custard/Pie Filling

Sure, pumpkin pie is great for Thanksgiving. Put this recipe in your favorite piecrust (or ours), and you've got it. But who can afford the calories year-round? Bake the filling in custard cups for a power-packed dessert with half the calories!

2 cups canned pumpkin
1½ cups evaporated skim milk
½ cup packed brown sugar
¼ cup sugar
1 tablespoon blackstrap molasses
½ teaspoon salt
1 teaspoon ground cinnamon
¼ teaspoon ground nutmeg
⅛ teaspoon ground cloves
2 large eggs, lightly beaten

Preheat the oven to 300°F. In a large mixing bowl, combine the pumpkin, milk, sugars, molasses, salt, cinnamon, nutmeg, cloves, and eggs, and stir with a wire whisk until thoroughly blended. Ladle into six custard cups. Arrange on a rack set in a baking pan of hot water. (The water should not go more than halfway up the sides of the cups.) Bake for 50 to 60 minutes, or until a knife inserted in the custard comes out clean. Chill before serving.

Yield: Six servings.

Nutritional data per serving: Calories, 205; protein, 8 g; carbohydrates, 40 g; fiber, 3 g; fat, 2 g; saturated fat, less than 1 g; cholesterol, 73 mg; sodium, 296 mg; vitamin A, 238% of Daily Value; vitamin B$_2$ (riboflavin), 19%; vitamin D, 30%; vitamin E, 7%; calcium, 23%; iron, 10%; potassium, 12%.

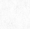

Canola Piecrust

Piecrust is a double whammy. It's packed with calories and artery-clogging saturated fat. But it's easy to switch to heart-healthy fat with this simple stir-and-roll pastry. We haven't been able to do much about the calories, though, so go easy.

1¾ cups enriched all-purpose flour
½ teaspoon salt
½ cup canola oil
3 tablespoons cold water

Preheat the oven to 425°F. In a small mixing bowl, combine the flour and salt. Add the oil and mix thoroughly with a fork. Sprinkle with the cold water and mix again. Roll out between two sheets of waxed paper until large enough to fit your pie pan. Peel off the top sheet of waxed paper. Holding on to the bottom sheet, invert and lay crust-side down over the pie pan. Gently peel off the second sheet of waxed paper, leaving the crust in place. Pat the crust into the pie pan, then trim the edge with a sharp knife. Prick in several places with the fork. Bake for 12 to 15 minutes, or until lightly browned, or proceed with recipes that don't require prebaking.

Yield: One piecrust, or six servings.

Nutritional data per serving: Calories, 293; protein, 4 g; carbohydrates, 28 g; fiber, 1 g; fat, 19 g; saturated fat, 1 g; cholesterol, 0 mg; sodium, 194 mg; folate, 14% of Daily Value; vitamin B₁ (thiamin), 19%; vitamin B₂ (riboflavin), 11%; vitamin B₃ (niacin), 11%; vitamin E, 26%; iron, 9%.

Quinoa:

It's Keen, Ma!

BATTLES:
- cancer
- diabetes
- heart disease
- stroke

BOLSTERS:
- immune function
- regularity

When Colleen was a little girl, she spent a lot of time with horses. Sure, she rode them, but she even loved cleaning their stalls and polishing their saddles and bridles. Best of all, she loved feeding them. In fact, she always savored the wonderful smells that wafted out of their grain bins. Now, when she cooks quinoa (pronounced keen-wah), her nose recognizes that familiar, grainy fragrance, and she gets nostalgic for her horses.

WE'RE NOT HORSIN' AROUND

Quinoa is not the same grain that she fed her horses, of course. But it does have a similar clean, fresh, earthy bouquet. And when it comes to whole grains, quinoa is as good as it gets.

It's a wee little grain that starts out about the size of a sesame seed, then quadruples as it cooks. So you put 1 cup of grains and some water in a saucepan, and when you take off the lid—presto!—you have a whole potful! (It's almost as amazing as popping corn, but without the noise.)

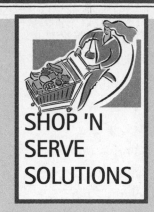

SHOP 'N SERVE SOLUTIONS

You'll find quinoa at your local health food store or natural food store, and maybe even at some larger grocery stores.

WHEN SELECTING QUINOA:

Look for small boxes that don't look as though they've been sitting on a shelf for 12 years.

WHEN YOU'RE READY TO USE:

To prepare quinoa, put it in a fine-mesh strainer and rinse it under running water to remove the fine powder you see there. Put 1 cup of quinoa and 2 cups of water in a $1\frac{1}{2}$-quart saucepan. Bring it to a boil. Reduce the heat to low, cover, and simmer for about 15 minutes, or until all the water is absorbed. You'll end up with a big potful, and that's good. Quinoa's gentle flavor is a great mate for sweet and savory dishes.

GETTING TO KNOW QUINOA

Here are some suggestions for adding quinoa to your weekly menu:

◆ **Stuff it.** Use cooked quinoa in place of rice when you make stuffed peppers or cabbage rolls.

◆ **Cook it.** Use cooked quinoa instead of rice to make "quinoa pudding."

◆ **Mix it.** Blend cooked quinoa with sautéed vegetables to make pilaf. Try our "Quinoa Pilaf" on page 382.

◆ **Toss it.** Mix cold cooked quinoa with chopped fresh vegetables and your favorite dressing for a cool summer salad.

◆ **Juice it.** Cook quinoa in fruit juice instead of water. Serve it with chopped nuts for breakfast.

◆ **Soup it up.** Stir a tablespoon or two of dry quinoa into soup a few minutes before serving.

Cooked, the grains turn into translucent mini pearls. Each has a tiny, yellowish "tail," formed when its outside germ spins away from the grain. The quinoa is amazingly light and fluffy, rather than heavy and starchy like rice or barley. (Think of the difference between regular cooked rice and puffed rice cereal.)

The flavor is very mild. Okay, maybe it's even bland. But that can be a plus for folks who are offended by the sturdy, slightly bitter taste of whole wheat.

A WAGONLOAD OF NUTRIENTS

What makes quinoa great is that it's just brimming with nutrients. It packs more protein than any other grain, and it stands out from the entire crowd of plant-based proteins because it delivers the full array of amino acids that make it as complete as meat. And its saddlebags are loaded with three times the vitamin E and twice the calcium, iron, magnesium, and potassium of other grains. It even has a little more zinc. It's also full of fiber, and its 2 grams of fat per ³/₄-cup serving are the heart-healthy mono- and polyunsaturated kind.

DELIVERING THE GOODS

Quinoa provides all the benefits that other whole grains do. An array of research shows that people who eat the most whole grain foods are less likely to have a heart attack or stroke, less likely to get cancer, and less likely to develop diabetes. The phytochemicals(natural plant chemicals) in whole grains appear to boost immune function, which not only fends off colds and flu, but also fights serious stuff such as cancer. And whole grains' insoluble fiber keeps your bowels running smoothly, staving off constipation and diverticulosis.

That's a lot of horsepower for such a tiny grain!

NUTRITION IN A NUTSHELL

Quinoa (³/₄ cup, cooked)

Calories: 127

Fat: 2 g

Saturated fat: 0 g

Cholesterol: 0 mg

Sodium: 7 mg

Total carbohydrates: 23 g

Dietary fiber: 2 g

Protein: 4 g

Vitamin E: 11% of Daily Value

Copper: 14%

Iron: 17%

Potassium: 18%

QUICK TO COOK

And now here's the best news for busy folks: Unlike other whole grains that take 45 to 60 minutes to cook, quinoa goes from package to table in just 15 minutes! So what are you waiting for? Saddle up your pony and hightail it down to your grocery store for a fresh supply!

Cozy Quinoa Breakfast

If you want warm whole grain cereal, but prefer a milder taste—such as cream of wheat—this is the bowl for you. Grab a spoon!

1 cup dry quinoa
2 cups water
¼ cup Sun-Maid tropical dried fruit medley
2 tablespoons chopped toasted pecans
2 tablespoons brown sugar
Dash of pumpkin pie spice
1 cup skim milk

Place the quinoa in a fine-mesh strainer and rinse under running water until the water runs clear. Put the quinoa in a saucepan, add the water, and bring to a boil. Reduce the heat to low, cover, and simmer for 15 minutes, or until all the water is absorbed. Stir in the dried fruit, pecans, brown sugar, and pumpkin pie spice. Ladle into two bowls. Top each with ½ cup of the milk.

Yield: Two servings.

Nutritional data per serving: Calories, 352; protein, 11 g; carbohydrates, 61 g; fiber, 4 g; fat, 8 g; saturated fat, less than 1 g; cholesterol, 2 mg; sodium, 76 mg; vitamin B$_2$ (riboflavin), 21% of Daily Value; vitamin D, 25%; vitamin E, 16%; calcium, 20%; zinc, 15%.

Quinoa Pilaf

Here's a side dish that's lighter than rice, yet packed with nutrients. And it's colorful, too!

¼ **cup diced carrot**
¼ **cup chopped red bell pepper**
¼ **cup chopped green bell pepper**
½ **cup diced onion**
1 **clove garlic, finely chopped**
1 **teaspoon olive oil**
½ **cup dry quinoa**
2 **cups fat-free chicken broth**
1 **teaspoon dried basil**
2 **tablespoons toasted sliced almonds**

In a large saucepan, sauté the carrot, peppers, onion, and garlic in the oil just until soft. Set aside. Place the quinoa in a fine-mesh strainer and rinse under running water until the water runs clear. Put the quinoa in a saucepan, add the broth and basil, and bring to a boil. Reduce the heat to low, cover, and simmer for 15 minutes, or until all the water is absorbed. Stir in the vegetables. Divide between two bowls. Top each with 1 tablespoon of the almonds.

Yield: Two servings.

Nutritional data per serving: Calories, 292; protein, 14 g; carbohydrates, 41 g; fiber, 6 g; fat, 8 g; saturated fat, less than 1 g; cholesterol, 0 mg; sodium, 195 mg; vitamin A, 118% of Daily Value; vitamin C, 51%; vitamin E, 27%; iron, 37%; magnesium, 30%; zinc, 12%.

Radishes:

Cancer-Fighting Crunch

BATTLES:
- cancer

BOLSTERS:
- weight control

When we throw a party (big or small, for friends or relatives), we always have a vegetable platter. To us, it's just as essential as buying a good bottle of wine or making a dessert that will be remembered. And what's on that platter? Usually carrot sticks, red bell pepper strips, celery slices, and slivers of radish. Most people think the radish is just for a little extra color, but we want our guests to really eat it. Its slightly peppery taste is a welcome contrast to the blander veggies—plus it's loaded with compounds that fight cancer. Is there a better gift we can give someone?

RADISHES RULE

Like broccoli, brussels sprouts, and cauliflower, radishes are a cruciferous vegetable. Compounds in this type of vegetable can reduce the risk of cancer—especially prostate, colon, bladder, and stomach. In a study of nearly 1,500 people, researchers in Germany found that radishes and onions

NUTRITION IN A NUTSHELL

Red radishes (8)

Calories: 6

Fat: 0 g

Saturated fat: 0 g

Cholesterol: 0 mg

Sodium: 9 mg

Total carbohydrates: 1 g

Dietary fiber: 1g

Protein: 0 g

Vitamin C: 14% of Daily Value

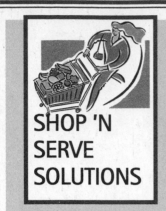

SHOP 'N SERVE SOLUTIONS

Some supermarkets carry a few different kinds of radishes. They'll offer red radishes (the kind you've seen all your life), daikons (large, carrot-shaped radishes), and black radishes (they have dark brown or dull black skin and a white interior). Chances are, you'll want to pick up the red radishes, but just in case you're feeling adventurous, we'll give you the lowdown on the other kinds, too.

WHEN SELECTING RED RADISHES:

■ Choose those that are smooth, firm, well formed, and brightly colored.

■ Skip any that are large (you won't like the taste), cracked, or spotted.

WHEN SELECTING DAIKONS:

Make sure that they're firm and evenly shaped, with glossy skin.

WHEN SELECTING BLACK RADISHES:

Choose those that are solid, heavy, and free of cracks.

Here's a rule that applies to all three: If you're buying radishes with the tops attached (they're sold with and without), make sure that the tops look fresh.

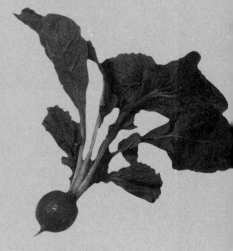

significantly lowered the chance of stomach cancer, while sausage, not surprisingly, increased it.

Sure, you're probably never going to eat as many radishes as you will broccoli florets and other members of the cruciferous clan. But every little bit helps. Just by sticking some slivered radishes in your sandwiches or salads, you can rack up an extra

WHEN STORING:

■ Remove any attached leaves.

■ Store the radishes in a plastic bag in the fridge. Red radishes and daikons will keep for about a week; black radishes may stay fresh for months. Just perforate the plastic bag so that they remain dry.

WHEN YOU'RE READY TO USE:

■ Trim off the stem ends and the tips.

■ Wash the radishes carefully.

■ You don't have to peel any type of radish—except black ones that have developed a thick skin.

GET RADICAL WITH RADISHES

Now use your radishes in these simply ravishing ways:

◆ **Color your crudités.** Slice red radishes, along with carrots, celery, and other veggies, and serve with a low-fat dip, such as ranch.

◆ **Spark your slaw.** Add ½ cup of slivered red or black radishes to your favorite coleslaw. What a color contrast!

◆ **Stuff your sandwiches.** Mix chopped radishes into egg, tuna, or chicken salad. Or tuck radish slices into your veggie pita pocket or turkey club.

◆ **Spice your stir-fry.** Slice strips of daikons and toss them into your wok with other veggies.

serving or two of veggies every week for barely any calories. And that may be just the edge you need to avoid cancer in the long run.

STAY-SLIM SECRETS

When you're trying to lose weight, you're probably always hungry. That's because your stomach is used to having a larger volume of food in it. You can trick your tummy into thinking that it's full by filling it with low-calorie, high-volume foods such as radishes. Eight radishes have just 6 (that's not a typo—just 6) calories. Crunch on them plain, or dunk them in a little low-fat yogurt dip. Or come to one of our houses for a party—we'll have some on the vegetable platter.

Pasta Chiller

When you make this salad for summer picnics, you'd better have extra copies of the recipe on hand.

½ pound medium pasta shells
2 cups chopped romaine lettuce
1 cup thinly sliced red radishes
¼ cup chopped fresh basil
½ cup olive oil vinaigrette dressing
4 ounces Asiago cheese, diced

Cook the pasta according to package directions. Drain well and rinse with cold water. Transfer to a large bowl. Add the lettuce, radishes, basil, vinaigrette, and cheese. Mix, then cover and chill for 1 hour before serving.

Yield: Six servings.

Nutritional data per serving: Calories, 157; protein, 8 g; carbohydrates, 13 g; fiber, 1 g; fat, 8 g; saturated fat, 3 g; cholesterol, 17 mg; sodium, 261 mg; calcium, 20% of Daily Value; iron, 5%.

Raisins:
Health through the Grapevine

BATTLES:
- cancer
- heart disease

BOLSTERS:
- energy
- memory
- regularity

What's not to like about raisins? You have to admit that their ad campaign is pretty cute—raisins rocking to "…Heard It through the Grapevine." But if that doesn't make you want to reach for a box and start munching, this will: Raisins are rife with the nutrients that will keep you groovin' for years and years!

BLAZIN' RAISINS

Just what exactly do raisins have to offer?

▶ **It's the antioxidants, bay-bee.** Abundant in raisins, antioxidants are substances that protect you from free radicals. Free radicals cause the cell damage that can lead to cancer, heart disease, and lots of other health problems. For optimal protection, researchers suggest that you get about 3,000 to 5,000 units of antioxidants daily. Just one itty-bitty 1½-ounce box of raisins kicks in 1,400 units!

Your memory benefits, too. A study on animals at Tufts University in Boston suggests that the antioxidants in grapes—which are fresh raisins—may help ward off memory loss and improve motor skills.

▶ **There's fiber to the finish.** And antioxidants aren't all that raisins have to offer. They also contain a hefty dose of inulin, a fiber that may reduce the risk of colon cancer. Studies suggest that inulin retards the growth of abnormal cells, which may lead to cancer.

The fiber in raisins, plus the tartaric acid (another unique compound found in high amounts in grapes), also helps prevent constipation. When researchers gave people who were eating low-fiber diets (that's most of us) three $1\frac{1}{2}$-ounce boxes of raisins daily, the average time that it took waste to move through their gastrointestinal tracts was cut in half.

Granted, three boxes of raisins are a lot, but the researchers speculate that substituting even one box of raisins for another food in your diet (such as potato chips) may keep you from singing those bathroom blues.

▶ **Plus, you get iron for energy.** Finally, raisins kick in a good deal of iron—considering that they're a nonmeat food. While most men get plenty of this nutrient, 15 percent of women under age 50 are either iron-deficient or anemic—two conditions that will sap your energy. So snacking on raisins really may help you dance—and not just to Marvin Gaye songs.

NUTRITION IN A NUTSHELL

Raisins (about ¼ cup)

Calories: 130

Fat: 0 g

Saturated fat: 0 g

Cholesterol: 0 mg

Sodium: 10 mg

Total carbohydrates: 8 g

Dietary fiber: 2 g

Protein: 1 g

Iron: 6% of Daily Value

Quick Fix:

Fatigue

Feeling exhausted all the time? Try a few days of raisin munching. If your fatigue is due to low iron levels—and if you're a menstruating woman, there's a good chance it is—then the iron in raisins will zip up your iron levels and reenergize your life.

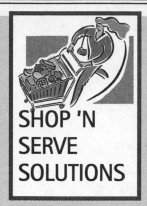

SHOP 'N SERVE SOLUTIONS

The different types of raisins don't vary much in nutrients, so sample all of them to see what you like best. One caveat: If you're allergic to sulfur, pass up golden raisins (sultanas), because they're usually treated with sulfur to preserve their color.

WHEN SELECTING RAISINS:

■ Look for a box or a bag that is tightly sealed. Squeeze the package to see if the fruit is soft.

■ If you purchase your raisins in bulk, look for covered bins. And make sure the raisins appear moist and clean.

WHEN STORING:

Once you return home with your raisins, store them in the fridge. That way, they'll retain their nutritional value and their great taste for up to five months. If you prefer eating your raisins at room temperature, just remove them from the fridge shortly before eating. They'll quickly warm up.

FOUR REASONS FOR RAISINS

Now you're ready to rock 'n roll with these raisin recipes:

◆ **Create a stir.** Most cereals that already come with raisins are also loaded with extra sugar. So, instead, stir a handful of raisins into your own favorite healthy brand of cereal.

◆ **Rais'n shine.** For another breakfast treat, stir raisins into your pancake or muffin batter.

◆ **Liven up your lunch bag.** Take a 1½-ounce box of plain raisins or the cinnamon-topped kind to work with you. Eat them when the vending machine calls.

◆ **Chip off the old block.** Whenever a recipe calls for chocolate chips, use half the chips and substitute raisins for the rest.

Cinnamon–Raisin French Toast

Sick of cereal? Bored with bagels? Give your breakfast a change of pace with this recipe that Karen adapted (read: made healthier) from the California Marketing Board.

Canola oil cooking spray
1 egg
2 egg whites
½ cup low-fat milk
½ teaspoon vanilla extract
8 slices cinnamon-raisin bread
½ cup light maple syrup
¼ cup honey
½ cup raisins
2 bananas, sliced

Preheat the oven to 450°F. Coat two baking sheets with cooking spray. In a shallow bowl, combine the egg, egg whites, milk, and vanilla extract until well blended. Dip the bread in the egg mixture to coat well. Arrange on the baking sheets. Bake for 10 minutes, or until the bottoms are golden brown. Meanwhile, in a small saucepan over low heat, warm the syrup, honey, and raisins. Top the toast with the banana slices and syrup mixture.

Yield: Four servings.

Nutritional data per serving: Calories, 435; protein, 12 g; carbohydrates, 90 g; fiber, 4 g; fat, 5 g; saturated fat, 1 g; cholesterol, 54 mg; sodium, 376 mg; calcium, 10% of Daily Value; iron, 30%.

Raspberries:
Take Your Pick of Health Benefits

BATTLES:
- allergies
- cancer
- heart disease
- high cholesterol

BOLSTERS:
- regularity

Karen loves raspberries. Her husband thinks she's crazy when she spends $5 to get a half-pint of them in the winter. But Karen thinks of raspberries as nutritional gems—rubies, really. They're sparkling with compounds that scientists believe may battle cancer, head off heart disease, and even ease allergies. Who would have thought that such tiny berries could be stuffed with so much?

CANCER ENEMY #1

Raspberries—specifically, the seeds—are chock-full of a compound called ellagic acid. Most produce contains this compound, but raspberries boast levels that are

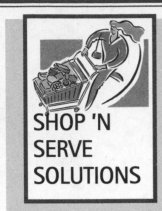

SHOP 'N SERVE SOLUTIONS

Karen's husband comes from New Jersey, which grows its fair share of raspberries. One day, back when they were still dating, Karen asked him to stop at half a dozen farm stands (he was still trying to woo her) before she finally found a pint of fresh-picked raspberries, which she intended to use in a dessert. But plans change, and Karen devoured every single berry herself—in less than an hour. The moral: Always pick up a pint to eat solo and another to use in cooking and baking!

WHEN SELECTING FRESH RASPBERRIES:

Choose berries that are in dry, unstained containers, because moisture speeds decay.

WHEN STORING:

■ Refrigerate your berries as soon as possible. Ideally, you should use them within three days from the time you bought them.

■ If you're lucky enough to have a bounty, freeze them. Simply wash them (as described below), carefully place them on baking sheets, and freeze them overnight. Then transfer the berries to a plastic container and refreeze. (Spreading the berries out on baking sheets and then refreezing them keeps them from clumping.)

WHEN YOU'RE READY TO USE:

■ Just before you're ready to use your fresh jewels, arrange them in a shallow pan and carefully wash them. Blot with paper towels.

five to six times greater than those found in other fruits such as plums and apples.

Ellagic acid does something really cool: It binds cancer-causing chemicals in your body, renders them inactive, and then destroys them. Most of the studies involving ellagic acid have

■ If you froze your berries, defrost them by putting them in the fridge for a day or by running them under cold water.

Frozen raspberries. Can't find fresh berries? Or they're too pricey for your wallet? Pick up frozen berries at your supermarket. But first, feel the bag or the box for ice crystals—a sign that the berries have been thawed and refrozen. In this condition, they won't be as tasty or last as long.

Other raspberry products. While you're at it, search your supermarket for products such as sorbet, jam (with the seeds, for more ellagic acid!), and vinaigrette made with raspberries.

MERRY BERRY PLANS

Once you have your stash, try these berry-good ideas:

◆ **Sweeten your salad.** Almost every night, Karen tosses a handful of fresh raspberries into a salad made with baby lettuces, crumbled Asiago or feta cheese, shredded carrots, and balsamic vinaigrette. It looks almost too pretty to eat!

◆ **Spread your bread.** Of course, you can top your bread with raspberry jam or jelly. But if you're worried about the extra sugar, smash very ripe raspberries as a spread for your toast, crackers, and bagels.

◆ **Season your chicken.** Marinate chicken breasts in low-fat raspberry vinaigrette. Then toss them on the grill.

◆ **Satisfy your sweet tooth.** Unwind from a long day with a bowl of raspberries topped with a tablespoon or two of light Cool Whip and drizzled with a little chocolate sauce.

been done in test tubes or on laboratory animals, but they have had very promising results. In these studies, researchers found that ellagic acid stopped cancer cell division within 48 hours and caused breast, prostate, skin, esophageal, pancreatic, and colon cancer cells to die within 72 hours.

To see whether ellagic acid will have the same dramatic effects on people, researchers at the American Health Foundation in New York City are conducting two major studies:

▶ One clinical trial is examining whether eating raspberries can reduce the number of colon polyps in people who are at risk for developing colon cancer.

▶ Another is determining whether raspberries can stave off cervical cancer in women at increased risk for the disease.

The results aren't expected for several years. But in the meantime, lead researcher Daniel Nixon, M.D., says he and his family are eating raspberries as often as they can.

CANCER ENEMY #2

As if that weren't plenty, raspberries also are rich in quercetin, an antioxidant. Like ellagic acid, quercetin seems to protect against cancer. Additionally, it may help do the following:

▶ Prevent bad low-density lipoprotein (LDL) cholesterol from causing blood vessel damage, which contributes to heart disease.

▶ Block the production of histamine, the substance that causes the runny nose, itchy eyes, and sneezing during allergy attacks.

Quick Fix:

Lazy Gut

Some older folks find that as they slow up a bit, their intestinal tracts seem to get lazy right along with the rest of them. The solution? Sprinkle ½ cup or more of raspberries on a high-fiber cereal every morning. Practiced every morning, this little trick should make everything come out right.

BLACK MAGIC

No doubt about it: Black raspberries are hard to find. But if you do run across them, by all means toss them into your cart! Black raspberries contain 10 to 20 times more anthocyanins than red raspberries do. Anthocyanins are powerful antioxidants that may help prevent heart disease and cancer.

FRUITFUL FIBER

Just 1 cup of raspberries packs about 6 grams of fiber—20 to 25 percent of what you need for the entire day! That's more than most other fruits provide, but not quite as much as the raspberry's cousin, the blackberry, has to offer. Better yet, raspberries have a mix of soluble and insoluble fiber. The soluble type lowers cholesterol—especially the bad kind—while the insoluble version wards off constipation.

Patriotic Breakfast Parfait

It doesn't have to be the Fourth of July for you to enjoy this creamy red, white, and blue breakfast. In fact, Karen likes to make it on a cold winter's day and then eat it by the fireplace and dream of summertime weather.

3 cups low-fat vanilla yogurt
⅔ cup fresh or frozen and thawed blueberries
½ cup whole grain cereal, such as Grape-Nuts
⅔ cup fresh or frozen and thawed raspberries
2 tablespoons chopped nuts

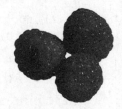

In each of two large sundae dishes or milk glasses, layer ½ cup of the yogurt, ⅓ cup of the blueberries, 2 tablespoons of the cereal, another ½ cup of the yogurt, ⅓ cup of the raspberries, another 2 tablespoons of the cereal, another ½ cup of the yogurt, and 1 tablespoon of the nuts.

Yield: Two servings.

Nutritional data per serving: Calories, 425; protein, 24 g; carbohydrates, 61 g; fiber, 6 g; fat, 11 g; saturated fat, 4 g; cholesterol, 22 mg; sodium, 451 mg; calcium, 70% of Daily Value; iron, 13%.

Rosemary:
Savor the Flavor

BATTLES:
- cancer
- food poisoning
- heart disease
- wrinkles

BOLSTERS:
- relaxation
- weight control

Last year, we were astonished to see a 3-foot-tall "Christmas tree" that was actually a large rosemary plant trimmed to shape. What a great kitchen gift for a favorite friend! When those postholiday blues strike, she'll still have pine-scented rosemary for comfort and cooking. It might even help keep her skin looking fresh and young as she heads to Florida to warm up after the winter chill.

LET THE SUN SHINE
While we're not advocating skipping your sunscreen, we are pretty excited about some face-saving research focused on rosemary. It turns out that your skin is just as vulnerable to oxygen damage as your heart is—

NUTRITION IN A NUTSHELL

Dried rosemary (1 tablespoon)

Calories: 2

Fat: 0 g

Saturated fat: 0 g

Cholesterol: 0 mg

Sodium: 0 mg

Total carbohydrates: Less than 1 g

Dietary fiber: Less than 1 g

Protein: 0 g

Vitamin A: 1% of Daily Value

Calcium: 1%

Iron: 1%

maybe even more so, because it's constantly exposed to air, sun, and pollution.

Preliminary laboratory and life studies have shown that consuming an extract of rosemary, packed with antioxidants, can help prevent damaging changes to skin by protecting the fat in your skin's cells. Much more study is needed, of course, but you'd better believe that we're cooking with rosemary!

BODY AND SOUL

Rosemary is packed with carnosol, a phenolic compound that fights cancer by interrupting inflammation so that those evil cells can't get a toehold and grow. Carnosol also appears to boost your liver's production of several cancer-fighting substances, including glutathione-S-transferase. In addition, rosemary may protect you against foodborne illness. Various studies suggest that it fights fungi, viruses, and bacteria. Still, to be really safe, keep cold foods cold (below 40°F) and hot foods hot (above 140°F).

As an added benefit, when you flavor with rosemary instead of lots of butter or sour cream, you protect your heart from saturated fat, and your waistline from excess pounds.

Rosemary also is being explored for its ability to relax you when inhaled. So always breathe deeply when cooking with rosemary.

Quick Fix:

Dizziness

Feeling a little dizzy? Make your own smelling salts. Place 1 to 4 drops of essential rosemary oil on a tissue and wave it under your nose. Rubbing the oil on your temples also helps.

How does this work? The oil stimulates both olfactory and trigeminal nerve endings, causing a reflex that improves breathing and circulation, according to RATIONAL PHYTOTHERAPY: A PHYSICIANS' GUIDE TO HERBAL MEDICINE.

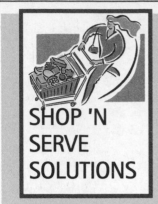

SHOP 'N SERVE SOLUTIONS

In some grocery stores, you'll find fresh rosemary tied in hand-size bunches. In others, you'll see a few little sprigs sealed in a tiny plastic container. Which size to buy depends on how much you need, although overabundance is rarely a problem.

WHEN SELECTING ROSEMARY:

This piney-looking herb should appear every bit as fresh as you'd want your Christmas tree to be. The needles should be deep green on top with whitish-looking undersides, without mold and without dark or wet spots.

WHEN STORING:

When you get your fresh rosemary home, wash it, pat it dry, wrap it in paper towels, and store it in a plastic bag. Or put it in a plastic container designed to allow air circulation.

WHEN YOU'RE READY TO USE:

If you're planning to actually eat the rosemary (and to get all its benefits, you should), you'll need to crush it, chop it, or grind it. (Those stickerlike little leaves are really *hard!*)

REALLY ROSY MEALS

Here are some fragrant ways to use your rosemary:

◆ **Branch out.** To infuse flavor in your meat, place a rosemary branch on your pork, chicken, or beef while it's cooking—and savor the smell!

◆ **Let it rain.** Sprinkle ground rosemary on salmon or tuna steaks before grilling.

◆ **Get grounded.** Stir ground rosemary into canned minestrone soup for authentic Italian flavor.

◆ **Shake things up.** Shake a little ground rosemary on your next pizza—it'll add some pizzazz.

Michael's
Rosemary Chicken

Colleen's hairdresser is an artist in all he does. He paints, he acts, and he loves to cook. He offered to share his simply delicious approach to cooking chicken. It fills the house with a heavenly pine scent. The big surprise? Cooking the chicken with the skin on keeps it moist and juicy. Just toss it before you eat, to keep the fat and calories under control.

2 chicken breast halves, bone in and skin on
2 small branches fresh rosemary
Salt to taste
Freshly ground black pepper to taste

In a heavy nonstick skillet, place the chicken breasts skin-side down. Lay a branch of rosemary on each. Cover, and cook on medium-high for 10 to 15 minutes, or until the chicken is no longer pink inside and the juices run clear. Remove the skin and rosemary. Lightly season with the salt and pepper.

Yield: Two servings.

Nutritional data per serving: Calories, 144; protein, 27 g; carbohydrates, 0 g; fiber, 0 g; fat, 3 g; saturated fat, 1 g; cholesterol, 73 mg; sodium, 64 mg; vitamin B_3 (niacin), 59% of Daily Value; vitamin B_6, 26%; iron, 6%; zinc, 6%.

Seeds:

Power Packets

BATTLES:
- heart disease

BOLSTERS:
- bones
- immune function

Baking fresh yeast rolls with her mom is one of Colleen's warmest memories. Before she was old enough to shape the dough, she got to sprinkle the poppy seeds or sesame seeds on top.

Turns out, those seeds were more than just tasty decorations. They're the storehouse of all the goodies a plant needs to reproduce itself. They're packed with proteins, vitamins, minerals, and good fat—just about everything it takes to get growing when the seed meets soil and water. And all those heart-thumping and bone-building nutrients can be yours when you start lightly scattering these nourishing nuggets over your meals and snacks.

SUNFLOWER SEEDS SHINE
Sunflower seeds are nature's powerhouse source of vitamin E. Unless you eat lots of whole wheat bread, dark green leafy

NUTRITION IN A NUTSHELL

Sunflower seeds
(1 ounce)

Calories: 165

Fat: 14 g

Saturated fat: 1 g

Cholesterol: 0 mg

Sodium: 1 mg

Total carbohydrates: 7 g

Dietary fiber: 3 g

Protein: 5 g

Vitamin E: 70% of Daily Value

Calcium: 20%

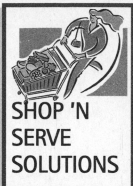

SHOP 'N SERVE SOLUTIONS

Fat is a major ingredient in seeds, putting them at risk for rancidity. So shop and store carefully.

WHEN SELECTING SEEDS:

■ Check the "sell-by" or "use-by" date on any cans or sealed jars of seeds you buy.

■ Take a good sniff if you're bargain hunting at the bulk bins, to be sure the odor of loose seeds is fresh. The nose knows!

WHEN STORING:

Store open packages in the refrigerator—at least until you get into the habit of using them. Once you get in the habit, they probably won't last long enough to spoil!

SEED STARTERS

Here's how to sow seeds into your daily life:

◆ **Mix 'em up.** Sunflower and pumpkin seeds make a crispy, crunchy addition to a power-packed trail mix. Start with dates, apricots, raisins, figs, and (a few!) pitted prunes. Add some seeds and, of course, a handful of M&M's for a heart-pounding treat. Go easy, though. This mix is really calorie-dense, so a little will take you a long way.

◆ **Stir 'em up.** Add seeds to hot or cold whole grain cereal to magnify your morning minerals. Keep all three kinds on hand, and then alternate from day to day for taste variety and optimal nutrition.

◆ **Whirl 'em up.** Toss a tablespoon or two into your next fruit smoothie as it spins away in your blender. It'll taste terrific, and the fat from the seeds will keep you from getting hungry too soon.

◆ **Scatter 'em.** Mix luscious summer melons and berries with plain or vanilla yogurt. Top the mix with pumpkin seeds and a dash of ground nutmeg.

vegetables, and high-calorie vegetable oil, you are probably not getting enough vitamin E from foods. So the addition of sunflower seeds to a normal diet is a big plus for just that reason. Just 1/4 cup of crunchy little, hulled sunflower seeds carries 70 percent of your daily requirement.

Numerous studies suggest that vitamin E may play an important role in preventing heart disease. In one 6-year study of 34,000 postmenopausal women, those who got the most vitamin E from foods had the lowest risk of heart disease. In that study, taking a vitamin E supplement appeared to have no benefit. Scientists speculate that the benefit may come from the vitamin E itself, or from some other element in the whole, natural food that is milled out of most processed foods or is not added to supplements.

SESAME SEEDS BUILD BONES

Sesame seeds will give you a surprising little calcium jolt where you least expect it. Just 1 ounce (about 1/4 cup) supplies 280 milligrams of calcium. That's more than one-fourth of the Daily Value! And those tiny little sesame seeds also pack a walloping dose of magnesium and manganese, now thought to protect against odd bone formations and bone calcium loss after menopause.

One of the most pleasant ways to eat lots of sesame seeds is when they have been ground into a paste called

HOW TO TOAST SESAME SEEDS

Sesame seeds are at their tastiest when toasted. Here's how to do it: Place a nonstick skillet over high heat. Sprinkle in a tablespoon or two of sesame seeds. As the pan begins to heat up, the kernels will start to pop. Begin shaking the pan like mad, just as you would when making popcorn the old-fashioned way.

Shake until the seeds are golden brown and smell too good to resist. Sprinkle over tossed salads, cooked vegetables, Asian stir-fries, or broiled chicken, fish, or shrimp.

Seeds of Distinction

Seeds pack all the nutrients needed to get a new plant started. But the details make the difference. Mix and match for best nutrition. Nutritional values are based on a 1-ounce serving.

Seed	Copper (% of Daily Value)	Iron (%)	Magnesium (%)	Manganese (%)	Zinc (%)
Pumpkin	10	5	19	7	19
Sesame	21	12	25	20	19
Sunflower	26	6	9	30	10

tahini, a standard ingredient in hummus. Tahini also delivers the goods.

PUMPKIN SEEDS OUT-ZINC CHICKEN

Pumpkin seeds are one of the best plant sources of zinc, a critical mineral in the maze of reactions that build immunity against invaders such as viruses and cancer. Just 1 ounce of pumpkin seeds delivers 3 milligrams of zinc. That's more than you'll get from 2 ounces of lean beef or 3 ounces of chicken breast.

CALORIES COUNT—BUMMER!

Seeds are packed with the unsaturated fat that your body needs for flexible arteries and healthy cell walls, but their calories do count in the battle of the bulge. Sunflower and sesame seeds weigh in at about 160 calories per ounce, while pumpkin seeds save you a few calories at 126. So don't curl up in front of the TV with a can of seeds and just munch away. Instead, use them to garnish or enhance the flavors of your foods. If you're crazy for trail mix, eat it for lunch *instead of* as a snack.

Sesame Chicken with Whole Wheat Linguine

Colleen first tasted this dish while she was on vacation in Florida, with the sun setting over Sanibel Island. Fortunately for us, she was able to talk its creator, Chef Marwan Kassem, into handing over the recipe. Here's her version.

8 ounces dry whole wheat pasta
3 tablespoons chili oil
4 boneless, skinless chicken breasts
1 bunch fresh cilantro, chopped
1 teaspoon wasabi mustard
1 cup low-sodium soy sauce
Hot sauce to taste (optional)
½ cup chunked papaya
1½ cups fat-free plain yogurt
Black and white sesame seeds

In a large pot over high heat, bring 4 quarts of water to a boil. Add the pasta, and cook until al dente, about 9 minutes. Heat the chili oil in a large skillet over medium-high heat. Add the chicken, and sauté, cooking until tender. Add the cilantro, mustard, soy sauce, and, if using, the hot sauce. Cook for 5 minutes. Add the pasta and papaya and mix well. Stir in the yogurt and heat through. Divide among four warm bowls, sprinkle with the sesame seeds, and serve immediately. Serve with additional soy sauce on the side.

Yield: Four servings.

Nutritional data per serving: Calories, 550; protein, 40 g; carbohydrates, 60 g; fiber, 8 g; fat, 14 g; saturated fat, 2 g; cholesterol, 67 mg; sodium, 2,265 mg; vitamin A, 17% of Daily Value; vitamin B$_3$ (niacin), 63%; vitamin C, 31%; calcium, 18%; iron, 75%; manganese, 91%.

Shellfish:

Health on the Half Shell

BATTLES:
- cancer
- heart disease
- osteoporosis
- overeating

BOLSTERS:
- bones
- immune function
- weight control

Kick off your shoes, roll up your pants, and let the surf tickle your toes while your clambake sizzles in the sand. Then stroll on over to a sumptuous feast of shellfish—clams, crabs, lobster, mussels, oysters, scallops, and shrimp—that will build your bones and rev up your immune system to fight everything from the sniffles to heart disease and cancer.

Shellfish are an outstanding low-calorie source of protein, which is needed to maintain every cell in your body and to keep your immune system in top fighting condition. Some research also suggests that protein satisfies your hunger, so you feel satisfied sooner and don't keep on eating. In other words, eating protein may help you control your weight.

NUTRITION IN A NUTSHELL

Cooked crabmeat (3 ounces)

Calories: 87

Fat: 1.5 g

Saturated fat: Less than 1 gm

Cholesterol: 85 mg

Sodium: 324 mg

Total carbohydrate: 0 g

Dietary fiber: 0 g

Protein: 17 g

Vitamin C: 5%

Calcium: 9%

Iron: 2%

And since shellfish contain almost no saturated fat, you don't have to worry about them raising your blood cholesterol level as you do with fatty meats. True, some shellfish, especially shrimp, pack more cholesterol than beef does, but research tells us that for most people, it's the saturated fat you eat, not the cholesterol in your food, that makes your blood cholesterol skyrocket. So relax and enjoy!

BETTER BONES WITH SHELLFISH

Shellfish can help strengthen your bones, too. But that's not because of their calcium, which is only in the shell! Their real secret is a treasure trove of trace minerals, such as magnesium and manganese, that your bones need in small but critical quantities. These same trace minerals may be missing from your diet if you eat a lot of processed foods, such as white bread, crackers, pretzels, and cookies.

But all shellfish are not created equal when it comes to minerals (and vitamins, too). So mix and match varieties for best nutrition. (See "Lean, Mean Protein Machines" on page 412, or try our "Quick Bouillabaisse" on page 414.) For bone strength, here are some noteworthy choices:

▶ Scallops are a good source of magnesium, which may prevent unusual formations that make bones brittle and more likely to break.

▶ Mussels are so loaded with manganese that only six steamed mussels pack a whole day's worth. This mineral is especially important to women because it may help reduce the loss of calcium in bone after menopause.

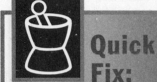

Quick Fix:

The Cold That Just Won't Go Away

Ever get one of those colds that seems to hang around forever? Well, once you've checked with your doctor to make sure that it's nothing serious, try adding a serving of shellfish to your diet once a day. The increased zinc may give your immune system enough of a boost to get it—and you—back on track.

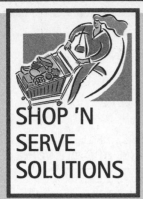

SHOP 'N SERVE SOLUTIONS

It's very important to buy shellfish that are fresh and healthy. Here are some guidelines.

WHEN SELECTING SHELLFISH:

■ Give them a sniff. One sign of freshness is their smell—which should be more like a fresh ocean breeze than a fishy odor.

■ Mollusks (clams, mussels, oysters, and scallops) in the shell should be alive, so choose only those that are tightly closed or that close quickly when you tap on the shell.

WHEN STORING:

Store live shellfish in a container covered loosely with a clean, damp cloth. Don't store them in airtight containers or in water.

COOKING TIPS

Using small pots, boil or steam mollusks in the shell, making sure that all are cooked thoroughly before serving. After boiling or steaming begins, the shells will open. Continue boiling for 3 to 5 minutes, or steaming for 4 to 9 minutes, to ensure that the shellfish are completely cooked. Throw away any that do not open during cooking. Shucked shellfish should be simmered for at least 3 minutes.

DON'T GET A RAW DEAL!

Prefer to eat your shellfish raw? Consider this: Raw mollusks may carry Norwalk viruses, which can cause severe diarrhea. Worse yet, they may harbor the bacterium *Vibrio vulnificus,* which, in up to half of all cases, triggers deadly blood poisoning in just two days.

People with diabetes, gastrointestinal problems, liver disease, or compromised immune systems due to AIDS, cancer, or other conditions are most at risk for getting sick from eating raw seafood—although even the healthiest person can fall victim. So cook your seafood to wipe out any bacteria. Remember: That raw seafood bar can be a raw deal!

Lean, Mean Protein Machines

Shellfish dish out plenty of low-fat protein and more concentrated vitamins and minerals than beef, chicken, or turkey. Catch up with them, and you'll improve your nutritional net worth! Nutritional values are based on a cooked 3-ounce portion.

Food	Calories	Fat (g)	Notable Nutrients (% of Daily Value)
Clams	125	2	Vitamin B_{12}: 3,505 Iron: 159 Copper: 23 Vitamin B_2 (riboflavin): 33 Manganese: 24
Lobster	98	3	Copper: 64 Zinc: 20 Vitamin E: 11
Mussels	146	4	Vitamin B_{12}: 851 Manganese: 165 Vitamin B_2 (riboflavin): 32 Vitamin B_1 (thiamin): 23

▶ Oysters are one of the few food sources of vitamin D, and without this nutrient, you just can't get calcium into your bones.

SWIM OR SINK WITH ZINC

Oysters may grow on river bottoms, but they're tops when it comes to delivering zinc. In fact, one little oyster delivers 15 milligrams of zinc—a whole day's worth!

Zinc is a mineral involved in at least 60 different enzymes that interact along complex pathways to affect your appetite, taste, and night vision, as well as your body's ability to fight invaders ranging from viruses that trigger colds and flu to carcino-

Food	Calories	Fat (g)	Notable Nutrients (% of Daily Value)
Oysters	117	4	Zinc: 1,290 Vitamin B_{12}: 1,240 Vitamin D: 273
Scallops	113	3	Vitamin B_{12}: 62 Vitamin E: 18
Shrimp	84	1	Iron: 18 Vitamin B_3 (niacin): 16 Zinc: 11
Beef round	169	4	Vitamin B_{12}: 96 Zinc: 32 Vitamin B_3 (niacin): 23 Iron: 19
Chicken breast	140	3	Vitamin B_3 (niacin): 83
Turkey breast	115	1	Vitamin B_3 (niacin): 46 Zinc: 12

gens that cause cancer. In the United States, half of all people over age 50 fail to get enough zinc from their diets.

So be sure to add more zinc-rich foods, such as chicken, fish, and of course, shellfish, to your diet. But don't overdo it. Over many months, getting an average of more than 15 milligrams daily can slow your immune system.

Quick Bouillabaisse

6 mussels in shells
1 tablespoon olive oil
1 medium onion, thinly sliced
1 large clove garlic, finely chopped or pressed
1 bottle (64 ounces) clam juice
1 can (15 ounces) stewed tomatoes with onions and green peppers
½ pint oysters, shucked
6 large scallops, shucked
1 can (6 ounces) minced clams
Salt to taste
Freshly ground black pepper to taste
Dash of Worcestershire sauce

Thoroughly scrub the mussel shells and rinse until the water is clear. Heat the oil in a wide-bottomed pot over medium heat. Add the onion and garlic, and sauté until softened, but not brown. Add the clam juice and tomatoes and bring to a boil over high heat. Add the mussels in shells and continue boiling until the shells open. After the shells open, add the oysters, scallops, and clams to the liquid, and continue boiling for 3 to 5 minutes, or until all the shellfish are thoroughly cooked.

With tongs or a slotted spoon, remove the mussels in shells to a bowl. Season the soup with the salt, pepper, and Worcestershire sauce. Ladle the soup into two soup bowls. Top each with 3 of the mussels in shells.

Yield: Two servings.

Nutritional data per serving: Calories, 336; protein, 30 g; carbohydrates, 32 g; fiber, 4 g; fat, 10 g; saturated fat, 1.5 g; cholesterol, 78 mg; sodium, 952 mg; vitamin C, 43% of Daily Value; calcium, 10%; iron, 50%.

Soy:
A Joy for Your Heart

BATTLES:
- cancer
- heart disease
- high cholesterol
- hot flashes

BOLSTERS:
- bones

For the longest time, Karen was dubious about the taste of soy foods. In a word: Yuck! But one day, a cookbook author came to her office and brought along a chocolate silk pie made with tofu. It changed Karen's attitude forever. Now she's a fan of soy—and her kitchen is often full of experiments that involve soy milk, soy burgers, tofu, or miso.

TICKER TALK

You probably know from watching the news that nutrition researchers like to hedge their bets—they're not certain about much of anything. Annoying, isn't it?

But one thing they'd put money on is that two to three servings of soy foods daily

(Continued on page 418)

NUTRITION IN A NUTSHELL

Tofu (3 ounces)

Calories: 64

Fat: 4 g

Saturated fat: 1 g

Cholesterol: 0 mg

Sodium: 6 mg

Total carbohydrates: 2 g

Dietary fiber: 1 g

Protein: 7 g

Calcium: 4–30% of Daily Value

Iron: 25%

Magnesium: 21%

Phosphorus: 8%

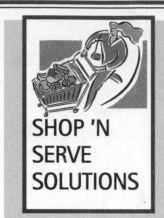

SHOP 'N SERVE SOLUTIONS

Have you looked around your supermarket lately? The selection of soy products has exploded in recent years. From soy staples such as soy milk, tofu, tempeh, and miso to products that use soy as an ingredient (we're thinking soy burgers, cereals, energy bars, cheese, and yogurt), there is a whole shopping cart of choices.

What's more, major food manufacturers are racing to bring dozens of additional lip-smackin' soy foods to your local grocery store as new processing techniques make them far superior in taste to the gritty brown soy milk or smelly cheese you choked down just a few years ago.

SELECT THE BEST

However, not all soy products are created nutritionally equal. Some of the new products are not-so-healthy foods with a little added dollop of soy. You want to select only the foods that have a reasonable amount of calories, fat (especially the saturated kind), and sodium.

For instance, one new soy cereal packs 200 calories and 440 milligrams of sodium per serving—more than many other cereals, even the kiddie kind.

Here's what to look for in the three soy products you'll probably use the most: soy milk, tofu, and soy burgers.

SOY MILK

You'll usually find a brand or two in the refrigerated dairy section near the cow's milk. You'll also find several varieties in aseptic containers in the cereal or baking aisle. No matter where the soy milk's located, the selection guidelines are the same.

WHEN SELECTING SOY MILK:

■ Make sure it contains no more than 3 grams of fat per cup (about the same as 1 percent cow's milk).

■ Choose a brand that's fortified with at least 30 percent of the Daily Value for calcium and vitamin D. Otherwise, if you replace cow's milk with soy milk, you won't be getting as much calcium as you normally would.

WHEN STORING:

Store leftover soy milk from aseptic containers in the refrigerator after opening. It'll keep for about five days.

TOFU

There are three main types of tofu: firm, soft, and silken.

WHEN SELECTING TOFU:

■ Choose firm tofu for stir-fries or whenever you want it to maintain its shape.

■ Choose soft tofu for dishes that require it to be blended.

■ Choose silken tofu for dishes that call for it to be pureed or blended.

■ Once you know which kind of tofu you need, compare the calcium content among several brands. Most tofu ranges from 4 to 30 percent of the Daily Value for calcium. Look for tofu that offers the most of this bone-building mineral.

WHEN STORING:

Keep tofu in the fridge. Use by the expiration date. If you have leftovers, rinse and cover them with fresh water before refrigerating. If you change the water every day, the leftovers will keep for about a week.

SOY BURGERS

Notice that we didn't say "veggie burgers." Some veggie burgers are made just from grains and, well, veggies. These don't have any soy at all. Even soy burgers can vary tremendously in the amount of isoflavones (beneficial compounds) they provide.

(Continued on page 418)

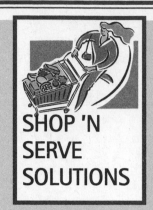

SHOP 'N SERVE SOLUTIONS

WHEN SELECTING SOY BURGERS:

Check the ingredients list for the words "soy protein isolate" and "soy protein concentrate." Soy burgers made with the isolate have all the isoflavones; those prepared with the concentrate offer just 5 percent, says soy researcher James Anderson, M.D., of the University of Kentucky in Lexington.

WHEN STORING:

Keep soy burgers in the freezer until you're ready to cook them.

SUPPLEMENTING WITH SOY

Once you get your goods, here's how to make the whole family love them:

◆ **Sub soy milk.** You can use soy milk in just about any recipe that calls for cow's milk—even cream sauces, puddings, and pancakes. Shop around for a brand you like. Our favorite: Silk.

◆ **Take a dip.** In a blender, mix your favorite dip packet (we like ranch) with a package of soft or silken tofu. Open up the low-fat nacho chips, and party!

(Continued from page 415)

lower your cholesterol, reducing your risk of heart disease by about 15 to 30 percent.

The reduction largely depends on your cholesterol level, but those numbers were good enough for the FDA to allow food manufacturers to claim heart health benefits on the label of any soy product that contains at least 6.25 grams of soy protein per serving. And the American Heart Association recently added soy to its list of ticker-friendly foods.

Researchers think that soy keeps your heart healthy in several ways:

▶ It acts as an antioxidant, gobbling up compounds called free radicals that can cause cell damage that leads to heart disease.

◆ **Dress up your burger.** We're not going to lie to you: Even the tastiest soy burger falls short of a mouthwatering real McCoy. But you can come pretty close if you—as Karen's mom always says—"doctor up" the burger. Here are five ways to spruce up a soy patty:

1. Marinate the patty in teriyaki sauce before cooking.

2. Melt on a thin slice of smoked cheddar cheese.

3. Toast the bun (and make sure you pick out a really delicious one).

4. Top with thin slices of avocado.

Spread on your favorite honey mustard.

◆ **Go stir-crazy.** Consider using firm tofu instead of beef, chicken, or pork the next time you fire up the wok.

◆ **Switch snacks.** Instead of noshing on chips and pretzels, curb your craving for crunch with soy nuts. Compared with regular nuts, they have about half the calories and one-third the fat per serving. You can buy them plain or seasoned. Or cook up some edamame, crunchy green soybean pods. Even kids think they're yummy—and you know how picky kids can be.

▶ It decreases blood clotting and inflammation.

▶ Perhaps most important, it promotes the expansion of blood vessels when they're under stress, so blood can continue its normal flow.

Many nutrition experts, such as Barry Goldin, Ph.D., professor of family medicine at Tufts University in Boston, encourage you to eat a serving of soy foods in place of something that isn't so healthy for your heart—such as fatty ground beef or whole milk.

IS IT WARM IN HERE?

You've probably heard that soy foods may help ease menopausal symptoms such as hot flashes and vaginal dryness. Research has shown that soy does help cool the midnight fire—but in many studies, a placebo (a fake pill) worked almost as well. Scientists are still trying to unravel the mysteries of hot flashes, and they concede that some women may get a lot of relief from soy, while others may see no benefit. To determine if you're one of the lucky ones, you'll just have to try it.

BUILDS YOUR BONES

But soy may help out with another pesky side effect of menopause: thinning bones. A new three-year study shows that a diet rich in soy lowers the rate at which you lose the bone mineral density that keeps your skeleton strong. Researchers still have to do more work to confirm the connection between soy and your bones, but at this point, it looks promising.

A CAUTION ABOUT CANCER

Now here's some news you've been waiting for: Scientists are fairly certain that soy lowers the risk of some types of cancer—especially prostate cancer. That's great news for guys.

Between the preventive effects of soy on heart disease and prostate cancer, "for men, eating soy foods should be a no-brainer," says Bill Helferich, Ph.D., associate professor of food science and human nutrition at the University of Illinois in Urbana.

But for women—especially those who are suffering from breast cancer or have a strong family history of the disease—soy becomes a little more complicated. Bear with us as we try to explain.

POSSIBLE PROBLEMS

Some types of breast cancer rely on the hormone estrogen to grow. Women make estrogen throughout their lives, although the amount significantly drops after menopause. Soy foods contain plant estrogens called isoflavones. Before entering menopause, about 60 milligrams daily of isoflavones (the amount in a serving or two of soy foods) seem to decrease your body's own estrogen

The Bean Counter

Use this handy guide to determine how much of your favorite soy product equals one serving.

Edamame (green soybeans): ½ cup

Miso: 2 tablespoons

Soy burger: 1 patty

Soy milk: 1 cup

Soy nuts: ¼ cup

Tempeh: ½ cup

Tofu: ½ cup

production by about 20 to 40 percent.

Less estrogen reduces your chance of developing breast cancer. So the under-50 crowd probably gains a lot of cancer protection from eating soy foods.

However, as you approach menopause and your body's production of estrogen plummets, the benefits of eating soy start to become iffy. Isoflavones have the potential to stimulate breast tissue, causing changes that may *speed up* growth of cancerous cells.

What's fueling a heated debate is how likely this scenario is to happen. Some experts think that it's a remote possibility; others have staked their careers on it. Studies currently underway should offer some insight into which theory is right.

But what do you do in the meantime?

▶ **If you have breast cancer** or are trying to prevent a reoccurrence, some researchers advise you to stay away from soy.

▶ **If you have a strong family history of the disease** and are postmenopausal, you probably want to limit yourself to no more than one serving a day.

▶ **Otherwise,** two to three servings daily seem to be fine.

Dreamy
Vanilla Pudding

Once you make this delicious and quick version from the Soy-foods Association of North America, you'll never buy instant mixes again.

½ **cup sugar**
2 **tablespoons cornstarch**
⅛ **teaspoon salt**
1½ **cups plain soy milk**
1 **teaspoon vanilla extract**

In a medium saucepan, stir together the sugar, cornstarch, and salt. Slowly add the soy milk, stirring frequently to prevent lumps. Bring to a boil, reduce the heat, and simmer, stirring constantly, for about 5 minutes, or until creamy and thick. Remove from the heat and stir in the vanilla extract. Pour into four dessert cups.

Yield: Four servings.

Nutritional data per serving: Calories, 144; protein, 2 g; carbohydrates, 30 g; fiber, 1 g; fat, 2 g; saturated fat, 0 g; cholesterol, 0 mg; sodium, 102 mg.

Stressful-Day Stir-Fry

This is a great dish to make after a tense day because, if you marinate the tofu ahead of time, it comes together in a flash.

10 ounces firm tofu, cut into cubes
½ cup teriyaki marinade
2 tablespoons canola oil
1 cup grated carrots
1 cup broccoli florets
1 small onion, chopped
2 cups cooked brown rice

Marinate the tofu in the teriyaki marinade for at least 30 minutes in the refrigerator. Heat the oil in a large nonstick wok. Add the tofu, carrots, broccoli, and onion, and stir-fry for 5 to 7 minutes. Stir in the rice just to heat through.

Yield: Four servings.

Nutritional data per serving: Calories, 261; protein, 10 g; carbohydrates, 32 g; fiber, 4 g; fat, 11 g; saturated fat, 1 g; cholesterol, 0 mg; sodium, 540 mg.

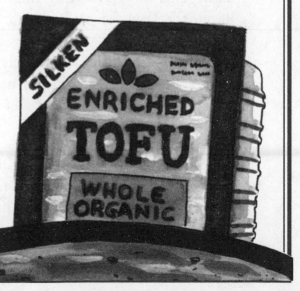

Spinach:

Sight-Savin' Goodness

BATTLES:
- age-related macular degeneration
- cancer
- cataracts
- fibroids
- night blindness

BOLSTERS:
- memory
- vision

Spinach is a very visionary vegetable. Nothing can beat it for fending off three major eye problems: cataracts, age-related macular degeneration (ARMD), and night blindness. True, carrots pack a little more beta-carotene. And yes, kale serves up more lutein and zeaxanthin. And surely oranges deliver a tad more vitamin C. But only spinach supplies big doses of all four.

SIGHT FOR SORE EYES

ARMD is a sight stealer—and the number one cause of incurable blindness in folks over 65 years old. The reason? The macula of the eye, a tiny spot on the retina, begins to fail. And along with it, goes central vi-

NUTRITION IN A NUTSHELL

Frozen spinach (1 cup)

Calories: 53

Fat: 0 g

Saturated fat: 0 g

Cholesterol: 0 mg

Sodium: 163 mg

Total carbohydrates: 10 g

Dietary fiber: 6 g

Protein: 6 g

Folate: 51% of Daily Value

Vitamin A: 296%

Vitamin C: 26%

Copper: 13%

Magnesium: 16%

Manganese: 89%

sion, the kind you need for reading or for seeing straight ahead.

Until recently, no treatment seemed to work. But now, there's the great green hope—spinach. The macula, it turns out, is packed with two sight-protecting carotenoids, lutein and zeaxanthin. And so is spinach.

In a small pilot study of 14 men with ARMD who ate ½ cup of cooked spinach four to seven times a week, 13 had improvements in night vision, contrast, and adjustment to bright light. Seven of 8 with distorted vision had improvements or complete remission of symptoms.

While nobody's quite sure how it all works, researchers think that lutein protects the macula by absorbing harmful blue light and defending against any light that does penetrate the macula. Other high-lutein greens include kale, collards, and turnip tops.

THE TIES THAT BIND

In nutritional analysis, spinach looks as though it's loaded with calcium and iron. And it is. Unfortunately, spinach also is overcome with oxalates that bind those minerals, so your body can't absorb them. But that's okay, because spinach is packed with plenty of other nutrients to recommend it.

EYE-DEAL FOR YOUR PEEPERS

And on the cataract scene, a Harvard University study of 36,000 male health professionals found that those who ate the most foods high in lutein and zeaxanthin had a 19 percent lower risk of cataracts that were severe enough for surgical removal. The men's top vegetable picks: spinach and broccoli.

In a parallel study of 50,000 female nurses, those who most frequently ate foods high in lutein and zeaxanthin had a 22 percent decreased risk of severe cataracts. The women's top veggie picks: spinach and kale. Is there an echo in here?

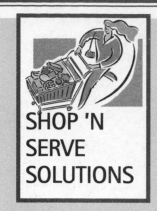

SHOP 'N SERVE SOLUTIONS

Fresh spinach is available all year long and comes in three styles. You'll find dark green, curly Savoy both loose and in 10-ounce bags. Flat, smooth-leaf spinach, which is the kind used in frozen and canned spinach, is now showing up in fresh bunches in health food stores. There is also a semi-Savoy, which is halfway between curly and flat.

WHEN SELECTING FRESH SPINACH:

■ Look for dark green, crisp spinach with no yellow spots.

■ Look for medium-size leaves with thin stems.

■ Avoid spinach that looks limp or pale.

WHEN STORING:

■ If you buy your spinach in a bag, just toss it in the vegetable crisper in your fridge until you're ready to use it.

■ Don't wash spinach until you're ready to use it. Wet spinach disintegrates faster than dry spinach, which should hold up well for three to four days when kept in the fridge.

WHEN YOU'RE READY TO USE:

■ Rinse, rinse, rinse your spinach until the water is free of superfine sand, no matter what the bag says about the spinach being pre-washed. The curlier the spinach, the harder it is to get the sand out.

■ Then remove the heavy stems, including the midribs running up the backs of the leaves, so that the leaves will be tender and delicious raw or will cook quickly and evenly.

A MEMORABLE VEGGIE

When spinach isn't working overtime for eye health, it's busy tuning up other body parts. Remember those blueberries that were so good for boosting memory in old rats? (See "Blueberries: They'll Keep You in the Pink" on page 68.) Well, a high-spinach

Frozen and canned spinach. Feel free to use convenient frozen spinach whenever the mood strikes. A food chemistry researcher found that after one year, frozen spinach retained more than twice the vitamin C of fresh spinach that had spent just seven days in refrigeration. And what about canned? Cup for cup, it's equal to or better than frozen in almost every vitamin and mineral. What could be easier?

SPINACH SENSE

Now you're ready to make spinach the highlight of your day. Try these ideas:

◆ **Sauté with Olive Oyl.** Popeye loves spinach *and* he loves Olive Oyl. And so will you. Simply sauté fresh spinach leaves in a little olive oil and some finely chopped garlic. Serve as a side dish or as a bed for grilled chicken or fish. You'll be infatuated.

◆ **Supersize soups.** Add leftover cooked or fresh spinach to any canned or homemade soup for a giant-size burst of nutrition.

◆ **Stuff it.** Use cooked spinach as a stuffing for rolled chicken breasts or appetizer pinwheels. Stuff fresh spinach and feta cheese into whole wheat pita pockets for a dazzling and delicious lunch.

◆ **Baby yourself.** Buy a bag of baby spinach. It's the hot new version that requires no stemming. Just rinse and eat. And keep an eye out for the microwaveable cellophane bag. Just slit the sack so that steam can escape, then toss the whole thing into the microwave. No dishes required!

diet works just as well for memory. What's more, it improves motor learning—a skill that's especially important for stroke recovery.

And women, now that you can remember to eat your spinach, here are some other benefits to reap:

▶ Researchers at the University of Minnesota found that women who ate the greatest amount of green leafy vegetables had the lowest risk of developing ovarian cancer. Wondering why? In German studies, spinach turned out to be one of the top veggies tested for their ability to prevent cells from turning cancerous.

▶ On the quality-of-life front, Italian researchers found that women who ate less meat and more green vegetables were the least likely to have painful benign uterine fibroids.

Spinach Pignoli

Is it possible for a vegetable to be considered the "nectar of the gods"? This spinach ambrosia is Colleen's version of a celebrated side dish at Baltimore's premier Spanish restaurant. After you try this, spinach will never be the same.

1 bag (10 ounces) fresh spinach, washed and heavy stems removed
½ cup Thompson seedless grapes, halved lengthwise
1 teaspoon butter
Dash of ground nutmeg
1 tablespoon pine nuts (pignoli), lightly toasted (garnish)

Place the spinach in a steamer basket, and cook for 5 minutes, or just until wilted. Drain thoroughly and return to a dry pot. Add the grapes, butter, and nutmeg, and toss until well mixed. Divide between two side dishes. Garnish with the pine nuts.

Yield: Two servings.

Nutritional data per serving: Calories, 101; protein, 5 g; carbohydrates, 13 g; fiber, 4 g; fat, 5 g; saturated fat, 2 g; cholesterol, 5 mg; sodium, 133 mg; folate, 70% of Daily Value; vitamin A, 192%; vitamin C, 49%; vitamin E, 16%; magnesium, 31%; manganese, 74%.

Squash:

Acorn-ucopia of Health

BATTLES:
- cancer
- heart disease
- high blood pressure
- stroke

BOLSTERS:
- bones
- immune function
- vision

Colleen did the impossible this past Thanksgiving: She got the kids (and the adults) to eat squash. And no one even said, "Yuck!"

The secret was in the presentation. She started with four different colors of acorn squash. One had the traditional green outer shell, and another was gold. The third was green with flecks of white and gold, and the fourth was green with gold stripes. She cut them crosswise into 1-inch-thick slices, re-moved the seeds, and—voilà!—squash flowers! Spritzed with olive oil spray, sprinkled with a little brown sugar and cinnamon, and then baked in the oven for 20 minutes, they were the surprise hit of the family gathering. Piled on a platter, they made a blooming garden of colors.

NUTRITION IN A NUTSHELL

Mashed butternut squash (½ cup)

Calories: 49

Fat: 0 g

Saturated fat: 0 g

Cholesterol: 0 mg

Sodium: 5 mg

Total carbohydrates: 13 g

Dietary fiber: 3 g

Protein: 1 g

Vitamin A: 172% of Daily Value

Vitamin C: 20%

Calcium: 5%

Iron: 4%

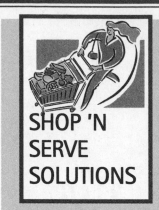

SHOP 'N SERVE SOLUTIONS

One especially nice thing about winter squash is that it shows up just when all those tender summer veggies, such as corn and tomatoes, begin to vanish. In September, you'll find winter squash in an array of colors, shapes, and sizes at supermarkets and roadside stands.

WHEN SELECTING WINTER SQUASH:

Choose squash that is firm, smooth, and evenly shaped.

WHEN STORING:

Scrub off the dirt, and you're done. With that hard outer shell, squash is tough enough to survive for months without refrigeration. Arrange an assortment in a spectacular autumn centerpiece, which will last until you serve the squash as a side dish with your Thanksgiving turkey.

SQUEEZE SQUASH INTO YOUR MENU

Here are some ways to liven up your weekly menu with squash:

◆ **Mini-mize it.** Choose a tiny acorn squash, split it lengthwise, and scoop out the seeds. Then microwave until fork-tender. (The amount of cooking time depends on the size.) Sprinkle with nutmeg and chopped walnuts. Makes two perfect ½-cup servings.

◆ **Soupersize it.** Use baked squash or the frozen pureed kind to make the silkiest soup. (Try our "Ginger Butternut Soup" on page 433.) Or add leftover chunks of baked squash to canned vegetable soup.

◆ **Idolize it.** Turn pureed golden squash into heavenly, healthy "gravy" for lean pork, pot roast, or chicken breasts by mixing it with onion flakes and garlic powder.

◆ **Fantasize it.** Turn squash into dinner. Split a small butternut squash and remove the seeds. Fill the cavity with a mixture of ground turkey breast, chopped celery, grated carrots, and cooked brown rice. Bake until tender.

THE COLOR OF HEALTH

It turns out that color is key for zeroing in on the healthiest foods from Mother Nature's garden. The very ingredients that produce the pretty colors are the same ingredients that enhance our vision, protect our cells against cancer, and defend our arteries against cholesterol buildup.

That beautiful deep orange color of winter squash is a sure sign that it's loaded with beta-carotene, a carotenoid that turns into vitamin A in your body. And just a tiny, $\frac{1}{2}$-cup serving of acorn squash delivers enough beta-carotene to meet half your vitamin A needs for a day. The same amount of Hubbard squash also delivers a whole day's worth. And get this—a small dollop of butternut squash is over the top, providing enough vitamin A for a day and a half!

JOBS WELL DONE

Dark green, deep orange, and bright red fruits and vegetables can deliver more than 400 carotenoids. About 50 of those carotenoids can create some vitamin A, but beta-carotene is, by far, the biggest supplier, and it has a lot of jobs to do:

▶ **Squashes cancer.** Beta-carotene helps prevent cancer by draining the energy out of singlet oxygen, an "excited" type of oxygen that otherwise can wreck cell membranes, destroy enzymes, and confuse your DNA into making cancer cells instead of normal cells.

▶ **Pumps up immunity.** Beta-carotene also appears to be a powerful stimulant for your immune system, keeping it alert to

Quick Fix:

Sunburn

Subject to sunburn? Eat a high-beta-carotene diet, including winter squash, carrots, apricots, and cantaloupe. It could boost the protective power of your sunscreen.

invading organisms and helping to remove potentially cancerous cells from your body.

▶ **Provides other protection.** Beta-carotene may help protect your skin against sunburn. In one study, women who got lots of beta-carotene and used sunscreen got more sunburn protection than those who used sunscreen alone.

Beta-carotene also may reduce night blindness. A study in Nepal showed that high beta-carotene intake reduced night blindness among pregnant women by 50 percent. In addition, beta-carotene can boost vitamin A's efforts to lengthen and strengthen bones.

POTS OF POTASSIUM

Maybe you've been eating lots of bananas for potassium, and that's a good thing. But if you'd like a change of routine, have squash sometimes instead (not for breakfast, of course). A mere ½-cup serving, enough to fill half a tennis ball, provides 20 percent more potassium than a banana does, for half the calories!

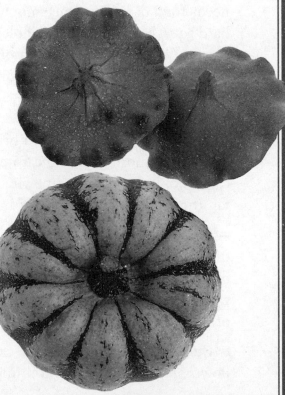

Potassium is especially important for heavy exercisers and anyone taking a diuretic, because this mineral regulates heartbeat and keeps blood pressure under control. And that reduces your risk of having a heart attack or stroke.

Ginger Butternut Soup

When autumn fades to winter and Jack Frost decorates the windowpanes, most folks cry out for soup. And this silky-smooth potful, with its soothing warmth and gingery bite, is all you'll need to chase away the winter chill. Best of all, it's on the table in 30 minutes!

1 medium onion, finely chopped
2 cloves garlic, minced
1 tablespoon ground coriander seeds
1 teaspoon ground allspice
2 tablespoons extra virgin olive oil
1 tablespoon butter
4 packages (12 ounces each) frozen pureed butternut squash
4-inch piece fresh ginger, finely minced
3 cans (14½ ounces each) reduced-sodium chicken broth
Salt to taste
Ground black pepper to taste
Reduced-fat sour cream (optional)

In a deep pot over medium heat, sauté the onion, garlic, coriander, and allspice in the oil and butter for about 15 minutes, stirring often. Add the squash, ginger, broth, salt, and pepper. Bring to a boil over high heat, reduce the heat, and simmer for 10 minutes. Top each serving with a small dollop of the sour cream, if using.

Yield: Six servings.

Nutritional data per serving: Calories, 240; protein, 8 g; carbohydrates, 39 g; fiber, 4 g; fat, 8 g; saturated fat, 3 g; cholesterol, 9 mg; sodium, 134 mg; folate, 14% of Daily Value; vitamin A, 219%; vitamin C, 19%; manganese, 30%; potassium, 15%.

Strawberries:

Antioxidants by the Pint

BATTLES:
- birth defects
- cancer
- constipation
- heart disease

BOLSTERS:
- memory
- regularity
- wound healing

Strawberries are a close runner-up to raspberries for our Fruit of the Planet award. That's because they're loaded with antioxidants—those amazingly powerful substances that gobble up free radicals, the bad guys that cause the damage to cells that may lead to heart disease, cancer, and other illnesses.

BERR-IFIC ANTIOXIDANTS!

Hands down, the most famous antioxidant in strawberries is none other than vitamin C. Consider this: A single medium-size strawberry boasts 19 milligrams of vitamin C—approximately 25 percent of the recommended daily dietary intake for women and 17 percent for men. And who can stop at eating just one? Not us!

Vitamin C is touted for boosting im-

NUTRITION IN A NUTSHELL

Strawberries (8 medium)

Calories: 50

Fat: 0 g

Saturated fat: 0 g

Cholesterol: 0 mg

Sodium: 0 mg

Total carbohydrates: 15 g

Dietary fiber: 4 g

Protein: 1 g

Folate: 20% of Daily Value

Vitamin C: 140%

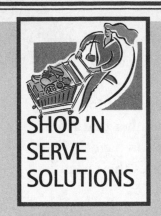

SHOP 'N SERVE SOLUTIONS

Picking strawberries is as easy as pie!

WHEN SELECTING STRAWBERRIES:

■ Look for berries that are dry, bright red, and fully ripe.

■ Choose those that are sporting their cute little green caps. (Removing the cap activates an enzyme that begins to destroy the vitamin C in the berry.)

WHEN STORING:

■ At home, carefully inspect the berries, discarding any smashed or moldy ones. You can return them to the original carton, but the California Strawberry Commission suggests that you transfer them to a large container lined with a paper towel. Layer the berries in the container, using additional paper towels between layers.

■ Store your berries in the fridge immediately, and use them within two to three days.

WHEN YOU'RE READY TO USE:

Wash the berries with the caps attached, so that they don't absorb a lot of extra water. Then remove the caps with a paring knife.

HAVE A BERRY-GOOD DAY!

Enjoy your berry bounty in these wonderful ways:

◆ **Brighten a salad.** Add strawberry slices to your spinach salad for a touch of sweetness. A side benefit: The vitamin C in the berries will help you better absorb the energy-boosting iron in the spinach.

◆ **Go European.** In Italy, cooks commonly drizzle some high-quality balsamic vinaigrette on a bowl of sliced strawberries.

◆ **Think tropical.** Even in the winter, you can whip up this refreshing drink, put a mini umbrella in it, and pretend you're on a sunny beach: In a blender, process 1 cup of sliced strawberries, 1 cup of sliced pineapple, 1 cup of pineapple juice, and 1 cup of low-fat strawberry yogurt until smooth. Sip away your worries.

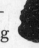

munity, making wounds heal faster (some dentists recommend it to their patients before gum surgery), and fending off heart disease and cancer.

And vitamin C isn't the only antioxidant do-gooder found in strawberries. They also contain ellagic acid (remember that from "Raspberries: Take Your Pick of Health Benefits" on page 395) and anthocyanin, the pigment that gives the berries their beautiful red hue.

When researchers at Tufts University in Boston measured the total amount of antioxidants in more than 50 fresh fruits and vegetables, strawberries ranked sixth, nudged out by blueberries, blackberries, kale, garlic, and cranberries. The point? Of these top 6 foods, strawberries are the easiest to eat every day.

A TEAM EFFORT

Eating a food that has a lot of antioxidants is one thing, but how well do they work together? Better than a Fortune 500 company. Here are the latest scientific findings:

▶ A recent study at Ohio State University in Columbus found that the antioxidants in strawberries might be able to inhibit cancer of the esophagus.

▶ A Harvard University study of more than 1,200 people concluded that strawberry lovers were 70 percent less likely to develop cancer than those who rarely ate the fruit.

▶ A project at Tufts suggests that eating strawberries may help slow down memory loss as you get older.

STRAWBERRIES AND THE STORK

If you're a mom-to-be or trying to conceive, think strawberries! One serving (about eight berries) supplies about 20 percent of the folate that expectant moms need to help ward off neural tube birth defects, such as spina bifida.

Because these birth defects occur early in the first trimester, the National Academy of Sciences in Washington, D.C., actually recommends that all women capable of having a child seek out plenty of folate from foods and take a folic acid supplement of 400 micrograms daily.

But why would you load up on folate if you were not planning a pregnancy? More than half of all pregnancies are—how shall we put it?—unscheduled.

After the first trimester, don't ditch the strawberries. They offer 4 grams of fiber per serving, plenty to help ward off the constipation that so often comes with pregnancy.

Strawberry-Spinach Salad

When you combine vitamin C–rich strawberries with spinach, it unlocks some of the iron in the greens.

4 cups spinach, stems removed, washed and shredded
8 strawberries, sliced
1 red onion, sliced
⅓ cup crumbled feta cheese
¼ cup low-fat raspberry vinaigrette

In a large bowl, toss the spinach, strawberries, onion, and cheese with the vinaigrette. Divide between two plates and serve.

Yield: Two servings.

Nutritional data per serving: Calories, 164; protein, 7 g; carbohydrates, 21 g; fiber, 6 g; fat, 7 g; saturated fat, 3 g; cholesterol, 13 mg; sodium, 576 mg; calcium, 22% of Daily Value; iron, 22%.

Sweet Potatoes:
Superstar Spuds

BATTLES:
- cancer
- heart disease
- leg cramps
- yeast infections

BOLSTERS:
- immune function

Thanksgiving dinner just wouldn't be the same without the warm, melt-in-your-mouth taste of sweet potatoes. Mmmmm, imagine them now. But if they taste so good, why do most people eat white potatoes all the time and reserve the sweet spuds for Thanksgiving? It's a mystery to us. Especially since, besides having remarkable flavor, sweet potatoes stuff our bodies with beta-carotene, a powerful antioxidant!

A VEGGIE ALL-STAR

When it comes to vitamins and minerals, sweet potatoes are all-stars. The Center for Science in the Public Interest, a nutrition advocacy group in Washington, D.C., recently ranked vegetables by adding up their percentages of daily requirements for six

NUTRITION IN A NUTSHELL

Sweet potato (1 medium)

Calories: 117

Fat: 0 g

Saturated fat: 0 g

Cholesterol: 0 mg

Sodium: 11 mg

Total carbohydrates: 28 g

Dietary fiber: 4 g

Protein: 2 g

Vitamin A: 498% of Daily Value

Vitamin C: 47%

important nutrients: folate, vitamin A, vitamin C, calcium, copper, and iron. Largely because of their vitamin A content, sweet potatoes came out on top, scoring 582 points. (Carrots, incidentally, ranked second, with 434 points.)

This contest, a Veggie Bowl of sorts, would mean nothing if the sweet potato's track record in research studies weren't so impressive. But here are some phenomenal findings:

▶ A Swedish study suggests that women who take in about 3.7 milligrams of beta-carotene each day from foods—the amount in about one-third of a single sweet potato—are up to 68 percent less likely to develop breast cancer than those who eat the least beta-carotene.

▶ A study from the Netherlands followed the diets and medical histories of nearly 5,000 people ages 55 to 95 for four years. The study found that those who ate the most beta-carotene had a 45 percent lower risk of heart disease than those who consumed the least beta-carotene.

▶ Closer to home, a study at Tufts University in Boston showed that older people who consumed at least 15 milligrams of beta-carotene daily—that's one sweet potato and ⅔ cup of baby carrots—bolstered their immune systems to ward off all kinds of bugs.

▶ Research from Albert Einstein College of Medicine in New York City suggests that a diet rich in beta-carotene may help prevent yeast infections.

The research just goes on and on. Dozens of studies have shown a link between beta-carotene and less risk of cancer, heart disease, and other heavyweight health problems.

Quick Fix:

Nighttime Leg Cramps

If you wake up in the middle of the night with painful leg cramps, you may not be eating enough foods rich in potassium. So add more sweet potatoes, bananas, or orange juice to your diet.

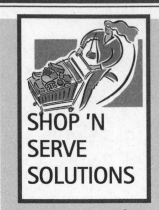

SHOP 'N SERVE SOLUTIONS

For the sweetest spuds, select and store with care.

WHEN SELECTING FRESH SWEET POTATOES:

■ Look for fresh tubers with tight, unwrinkled, and unblemished skin.

■ Avoid bruised sweet potatoes. They deteriorate quickly, and the flavor of the entire potato is compromised.

WHEN STORING:

■ Store your fresh spuds in a dark, cool, dry place. Don't put them in the fridge—unless they're cooked—because it'll sap their sweetness.

Canned sweet potatoes. When buying canned versions, compare the sodium and calorie contents among brands. Some may have added sugar.

SWEET TREATS

Now that you've selected your spuds, you could make candied sweet potatoes. But why not try one of these healthier, but equally delicious, options?

◆ **Make mashing smashing.** Substitute sweet potatoes for the white tubers in your mashed potato recipe. Season with ground cinnamon and nutmeg instead of salt and pepper.

◆ **Bake them to perfection.** Bake sweet potatoes at 400°F for 40 to 50 minutes. Top with a touch of maple syrup, ground ginger, and chopped pecans instead of butter or sour cream. Get your kids to eat them by tossing on a few mini marshmallows.

◆ **Start the day off right.** Try Bruce's Sweet Potato Pancake Mix. Check it out at www.brucefoods.com.

◆ **Slice 'n snack.** Just slice sweet potatoes into rounds and dunk them in applesauce.

PASS UP THE PILLS

But before you're tempted to take a supplement instead of a serving of sweet potatoes, consider this: Beta-carotene *from foods* seems to offer protection, but beta-carotene supplements are iffy at best. In fact, supplements may even increase the risk of lung cancer in smokers.

So here's some good advice: Have Thanksgiving—at least the sweet potato part of it—every Thursday of the year!

One Potato, Two Potato

What's in a name? Plenty, if you're trying to find sweet potatoes. Many supermarkets and canned-good manufacturers mislabel sweet potatoes—especially the darker-skin varieties—as yams. True yams are hard to find, and if you do run across them, they're usually sold in chunks sealed in plastic wrap. Here's a rundown of the differences between the two.

Characteristic	Sweet Potato	Yam
Beta-carotene content	Very high	None
Appearance	Smooth, thin skin	Rough, scaly skin
Skin color	Light yellow to dark orange	Brown or black
Flesh color	Pale yellow to bright orange	Off-white, purple, or red
Size	About ¼–½ pound each	Can grow up to 150 pounds each
Taste	Moist	Dry
Preparation	Can be used raw or cooked	Toxic if eaten raw
Where grown	In the United States	In the Caribbean

Sweet Potato Fries

The next time you hear french fries calling your name, hit the kitchen—not the Golden Arches. These homemade fries deliver more flavor—for far less fat and calories—than the fast-food variety.

Canola oil cooking spray
4 sweet potatoes, scrubbed, but not peeled
1 teaspoon ground cinnamon
½ teaspoon ground nutmeg
½ teaspoon ground black pepper
¼ teaspoon kosher salt
½ cup applesauce

Preheat the oven to 425°F. Spray two baking sheets with cooking spray. Cut the potatoes in half. Slice each half into several long wedges. Place on the baking sheets, mist with additional cooking spray, and sprinkle with the cinnamon, nutmeg, salt and pepper. Bake for 30 to 40 minutes, or until brown and soft, turning once. Serve with the applesauce for dipping.

Yield: Six servings.

Nutritional data per serving: Calories, 120; protein, 2 g; carbohydrates, 27 g; fiber, 6 g; fat, 1 g; saturated fat, 0 g; cholesterol, 0 mg; sodium, 149 mg; calcium, 5% of Daily Value; iron, 7%.

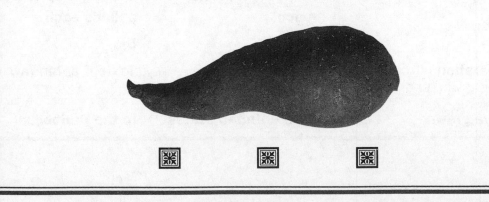

Tea:
A Party for Your Body

BATTLES:

- arthritis
- cancer
- cataracts
- heart disease
- stroke
- tooth decay
- ulcers

BOLSTERS:

- bones
- immune function
- vision
- weight control

NUTRITION IN A NUTSHELL

Hot tea (1 cup)

Calories: 2

Fat: 0 g

Saturated fat: 0 g

Cholesterol: 0 mg

Sodium: 7 mg

Total carbohydrates: Less than 1 g

Dietary fiber: 0 g

Protein: 0 g

Folate: 3% of Daily Value

Vitamin B$_2$ (riboflavin): 2%

Magnesium: 2%

Potassium: 2%

What could be better on a raw, rainy afternoon than sharing a pot of tea by a cozy fire? Tea has long been the great soother for Colleen and her daughters. It has been their balm for troubled times, the elixir of pain and worries. It has also been the libation of celebration in times of joy. Often it's simply the symbol of togetherness and family warmth, the "campfire" around which they gather.

And now, they're thrilled to discover that their lifelong family tradition also may be protecting their health. Although tea has

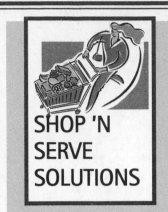

SHOP 'N SERVE SOLUTIONS

Many types of tea are available. Take your pick of these:

■ **Tea bags and loose leaves.** Whether you buy your tea in bags or loose, you'll get plenty of antioxidant punch, although (surprise!) the biggest boost comes from the tea bag. (And you thought that healthy eating would be harder!) That's because the crushed tea pieces offer more exposed surfaces during brewing.

■ **Caffeine-free tea.** And here's more good news: Decaffeinating tea doesn't disturb its antioxidants. So make it tea-sy on yourself. Choose the style and brand you like best, then drink up!

■ **Iced tea.** Bottled iced-tea drinks work, too. In tests of several brands and flavors, a few were as potent as a cup of brewed tea, while the rest delivered at least half the number of antioxidants as brewed tea—making any bottled tea more antioxidant-rich than any soft drink! But beware: Many bottled teas are loaded with up to 200 calories from sugar, which offers no health benefits, can raise your risk of weight gain, and can ruin your appetite for healthier foods. So read the label before you drink another drop.

ANY TIME IS TEA TIME

Here's how to become a tea-totaler:

◆ **Not a tea drinker?** Start small. Substitute a cup of tea for a cup of coffee in the morning. You'll still get a little wake-up call (tea delivers 47 milligrams of caffeine per cup, compared with brewed coffee's 140 milligrams), plus one-third of your day's worth of the cancer-fighting antioxidants your body craves.

◆ **Out to lunch?** Order iced tea. Ask if it's freshly brewed. If it's not, order hot tea and a glass of ice. Brew the tea in your cup, add a couple of ice cubes to tame the heat, and then pour the tea over the ice in your glass. (Pouring too-hot tea into your glass could shatter it!)

been soothing souls since prehistoric times, research into its possible benefits is only a few years old. But, oh, it looks promising!

OF MICE AND MEN

A while back, epidemiologists, the scientists who compare health risks from one big group of people to another, noticed that in countries where people drink lots of green tea (the kind you get at your local Chinese restaurant), folks rarely get certain kinds of cancer. So they started plying mice with green tea and found that it protected the mice against cancers of the skin, lung, esophagus, stomach, small intestine, colon, bladder, liver, pancreas, prostate, and mammary glands. Whew! That covers a lot of territory!

Mind you, their research doesn't *prove* that green tea can prevent cancer in humans. The researchers, after all, substituted green tea for every single drop of fluid that the mice usually drank. They were also able to control the mice's genetic backgrounds and other health habits. So, much is left to be done before we know for sure whether tea's benefits apply to people. But why might we think they would?

TEA IS TERRIFIC

It turns out that tea is packed with antioxidants—more so, in fact, than even the top fruits and veggies. One of its richest compounds, epigallocatechin-3gallate (EGCG, for short), has been shown in laboratory tests to block the action of urokinase, an enzyme needed by cancer cells so they can attack healthy ones. Without urokinase, cancer cells stop invading healthy cells and sometimes just fizzle out and disappear.

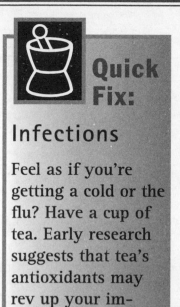

Quick Fix: Infections

Feel as if you're getting a cold or the flu? Have a cup of tea. Early research suggests that tea's antioxidants may rev up your immune system and help it fight back.

Recent research suggests that green tea and the black tea that most Americans drink have similar anticancer effects. (Green tea and black tea come from the same plant. Black tea is fermented; green tea is not.)

HALF THE RISK OF A HEART ATTACK!

Again, there is no *absolute* proof, but in a Dutch study, the top one-third of tea drinkers were the least likely to die from heart disease or have a stroke. And a Boston study found that people who drank 1 or more cups of black tea daily had half the risk of having a heart attack as those who were tea teetotalers. Scientists speculate that tea's powerful antioxidant package may help keep cholesterol in your blood from gunking up your arteries.

TAKE TEA AND SEE

Other preliminary studies suggest that tea is good for your body in additional ways. Both mice and men seem to get a metabolic boost from green tea, indicating that it might help with weight control.

Other research suggests that tea may help keep bones strong, perhaps because of its fluoride or phytoestrogens (estrogen-like plant compounds). In studies of rodents, tea also appeared to fight strep bacteria, heal ulcers, minimize arthritis, and protect teeth. Tea may also protect against cataracts.

So while you wait for more research and the final answers, sip some tea.

Mango Iced Tea

Looking for a cool summer treat? Brew up a pitcher of this exotic-tasting tea. Refreshing!

8 cups cold water, divided
4 tea bags
1 cup mango nectar

Bring 4 cups of the water to a boil. Pour over the tea bags in a heatproof pitcher. Let stand for 3 to 5 minutes. Remove the tea bags and discard. Stir in the remaining 4 cups of water and the mango nectar. Chill. To serve, pour over ice in tall glasses.

Yield: Six servings.

Nutritional data per serving: Calories, 26; protein, 0 g; carbohydrates, 7 g; fiber, less than 1 g; fat, 0 g; saturated fat, 0 g; cholesterol, 0 mg; sodium, 7 mg; folate, 2% of Daily Value; vitamin A, 10%; vitamin C, 4%.

Tomatoes:

A Man's Best Friend

BATTLES:
- cancer
- heart disease
- high cholesterol

Rover may be a guy's most faithful companion, but—believe this!—a gorgeous tomato is really his best friend. A growing pile of research shows that a compound found in tomatoes and tomato products, such as spaghetti sauce, can cut your risk of certain cancers by up to 40 percent. Ain't life sweet?

PROSTATE PROTECTION

Red tomatoes and all the yummy foods that you make with them—even pizza—are teeming with lycopene, an antioxidant that caught the attention of scientists in 1995. That's when Harvard University researchers released the results of a study involving 47,000 men ages 40 to 75.

During the six-year project, doctors diagnosed 812 cases of prostate cancer among the study participants. The researchers wanted to see if there were differences between the diets of the men who developed this all-too-common cancer and those who remained healthy.

Of the more than 40 foods examined, they found that only 4

protected against prostate cancer. Of those 4 foods, 3 were good sources of lycopene—tomato sauce, tomatoes, and pizza. (Strawberries, by the way, were the other beneficial food.) Eating tomatoes or tomato products twice a week, the researchers concluded, could lower the risk of prostate cancer by 20 to 40 percent.

HOPE FOR ALL CANCERS

Four years later, the Harvard researchers analyzed 72 studies regarding the relationship between lycopene and the prevention of *any* type of cancer. A whopping 57 of those studies found that frequently eating tomatoes and tomato products reduced the risk of cancer, especially cancers of the prostate, lung, and stomach. Lycopene also may help ward off breast, cervical, and colon cancers, the researchers found.

In fact, another group of researchers is now trying to determine whether eating more tomato products will improve the outcomes of breast cancer patients or those at high risk for the disease because they inherited a genetic susceptibility.

POSSIBLE HEART PROTECTION

The Harvard researchers are also examining whether having one to two servings of tomato products daily can keep heart disease at bay, since preliminary research suggests that lycopene may lower bad low-density lipoprotein (LDL) cholesterol.

A LARGE PEPPERONI, PLEASE

So how much lycopene do you need to consume to get these health benefits? "We're not exactly sure, but getting 30 milligrams

NUTRITION IN A NUTSHELL

Tomato (1 medium)

Calories: 35

Fat: 0.5 g

Saturated fat: 0 g

Cholesterol: 0 mg

Sodium: 5 mg

Total carbohydrates: 7 g

Dietary fiber: 1 g

Protein: 1 g

Vitamin A: 20% of Daily Value

Vitamin C: 40%

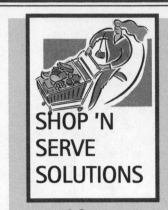

SHOP 'N SERVE SOLUTIONS

There's nothing like a tomato picked fresh from your garden. That's why we're counting the days until ours ripen! But if you don't have garden-grown tomatoes, be choosy about supermarket or farmers' market fare.

WHEN SELECTING TOMATOES:

■ Look for those that are smooth, plump, firm, and fragrant.

■ Avoid tomatoes with no aroma. If you can't smell a thing, they are immature and probably will never ripen.

■ If you want to use your tomatoes in the next day or two, select ripe fruits that yield to your touch.

■ Not planning on cooking your tomatoes until later in the week? Then opt for those that are partially ripe. They'll be light pink.

WHEN STORING:

■ Store ripe tomatoes at room temperature to preserve their flavor. Keep them out of direct sunlight.

■ Place partially ripe tomatoes in a paper bag, away from direct sunlight, with an apple or a banana to speed ripening.

■ Refrigerate tomatoes only when you need to stretch out their shelf life.

TOMATO TEMPTATIONS

Now try these tempting tomato treats:

Give them a starring role. Sure, you put tomatoes in your green salad. But then, they're just the supporting cast. Try these suggestions that give tomatoes top billing: tomato-cucumber salad (²/₃ cup of chopped tomatoes and ¹/₃ cup of chopped cucumbers tossed in Italian dressing) or tomato-basil salad (1 cup of chopped tomatoes and ¹/₄ cup of chopped basil leaves drizzled with balsamic vinaigrette).

Hit the Sauce

Some tomato products pack more cancer-fighting lycopene than the fruit itself does. Use this chart to calculate how to get your 30 milligrams of lycopene daily, the amount suggested by many researchers.

Tomato Treat	Lycopene (mg)
Tomato sauce (½ cup)	21.9
Tomato juice (¾ cup)	19.8
Tomato paste (2 tablespoons)	18.2
Vegetable juice cocktail (¾ cup)	17.6
Tomato puree (¼ cup)	10.4
Chopped raw tomato (½ cup)	8.3
Ketchup (2 tablespoons)	5.2

a day seems to offer protection," says A. V. Rao, Ph.D., professor of nutrition at the University of Toronto.

That's a cinch to do: Just consume ¾ cup of tomato juice and a single tomato, or a bowl of pasta with tomato sauce and a few tablespoons of ketchup.

For the lycopene contents of your favorite foods, see "Hit the Sauce" above. In the meantime, go ahead and order a pizza—with tomatoes on top!

A Midwinter Feast: Oven-Roasted Tomatoes

This recipe turns those run-of-the-mill tomatoes you find in winter into a warm, sweet, and extra juicy appetizer that your whole family will love.

Olive oil cooking spray
4 round tomatoes, cut crosswise into ¾-inch-thick slices
2 teaspoons sugar
1 teaspoon dried basil
½ teaspoon ground black pepper
2 teaspoons grated Parmesan cheese

Preheat the oven to 300°F. Line two baking sheets with foil. Generously spray the foil with cooking spray. Place the tomato slices on the baking sheets. Sprinkle with the sugar, basil, and pepper. Bake for 45 to 55 minutes, or until the tomatoes start to shrivel. Remove from the oven. Sprinkle with the cheese, and return to the oven for 1 to 2 minutes, or until the cheese melts. Serve warm.

Yield: Four servings.

Nutritional data per serving: Calories, 40; protein, 2 g; carbohydrates, 8 g; fiber, 2 g; fat, 1 g; saturated fat, 0 g; cholesterol, 1 mg; sodium, 30 mg; calcium, 3% of Daily Value; iron 5%.

Turkey:

A Nutritional Powerhouse

BATTLES:
- diabetes
- heart disease
- infections

BOLSTERS:
- energy
- immune function

Karen's mom invites her and her husband, John, over for "Thanksgiving dinner" at least a half-dozen times a year—even in July. Mom's got the right idea! Turkey is so healthy, why should you enjoy it only on Thanksgiving?

TALKIN' TURKEY

Turkey contributes generous portions of a half-dozen important nutrients. Here's the lowdown on the big six:

▶ **Vitamin B_3 (niacin).** This vitamin helps produce energy in all the cells of your body. If you don't get enough, you may become mentally disorientated or may suffer from diarrhea.

▶ **Vitamin B_6.** It helps convert an amino acid into serotonin, an important brain chemical that affects your mood. It also helps manufacture other crucial substances such as insulin and infection-fighting antibodies.

▶ **Vitamin B_{12}.** This nutrient works in conjunction with folate and folic acid to make red blood cells. They may also team up to fight heart disease.

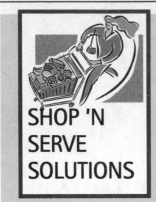

SHOP 'N SERVE SOLUTIONS

Fortunately, you no longer have to buy a whole turkey or even a turkey breast to enjoy this delicious and nutritious meat. Many manufacturers sell sliced turkey cutlets or ground turkey that's healthy and easy to incorporate in your meals.

WHEN SELECTING GROUND TURKEY:

■ Choose ground turkey that's made from skinless white meat.

■ Avoid ground turkey that contains dark meat and skin. Its fat content rivals that of ground beef.

WHEN SELECTING A FRESH OR FROZEN TURKEY:

■ Choose one with a tightly sealed package.

■ On frozen turkeys, you shouldn't spot any freezer burn or ice crystals, although the turkey should be very hard.

NEW WAYS TO GOBBLE IT UP

You know the most obvious way to serve your whole turkey, but what can you make with the leftovers, turkey cutlets, or ground turkey? We're glad you asked. Try these suggestions:

◆ **Case quesadillas.** One of Karen's friends makes quesadillas with leftover Thanksgiving turkey. She simply tucks small turkey pieces, vegetables, and cranberry relish into flour tortillas, and heats the whole shebang in the oven.

◆ **Make turkey noodle soup.** Skinless dark meat is a great addition to practically any noodle or vegetable soup.

◆ **Swap for chicken.** Did you already have chicken three nights this week? You can use turkey cutlets in many of the same recipes that call for chicken breasts.

◆ **Slim down your burgers.** Substitute white meat ground turkey for half of the ground beef you use for hamburgers.

▶ **Iron.** You know the deal on this one: If you don't meet your iron requirements, you may feel tired and lethargic. Eventually, you could develop iron-deficiency anemia, which would make your symptoms much worse.

▶ **Phosphorus.** This is one busy mineral. Next to calcium, phosphorus is the most abundant mineral in your bones and teeth. It also helps generate energy in your body's cells and helps regulate metabolism in your organs.

▶ **Zinc.** Several studies have shown that this mineral is essential for a strong immune system.

THE LIGHT-VERSUS-DARK DILEMMA

If you're really watching your fat intake, you should stick to white meat turkey without the skin—it has only 1 gram of fat per 3-ounce cooked serving. Otherwise, you can enjoy both white and dark meat—provided the skin is removed.

Dark meat isn't as fatty as you think, costing you just 30 extra calories and 3 additional grams of fat in a 3½-ounce cooked serving. On the plus side, dark meat turkey offers about twice as much zinc as white meat does. But don't be tempted to eat the dark meat with skin, because the fat content can jump up to 7 grams per serving, depending on the part of the turkey that you choose.

NUTRITION IN A NUTSHELL

White meat turkey, skin removed (3 ounces, roasted)

Calories: 119

Fat: 1 g

Saturated fat: 0 g

Cholesterol: 73 mg

Sodium: 48 mg

Total carbohydrates: 0 g

Dietary fiber: 0 g

Protein: 26 g

Vitamin B_3 (niacin): 30% of Daily Value

Vitamin B_6: 24%

Vitamin B_{12}: 6%

Iron: 7%

Phosphorus: 18%

Zinc: 12%

Terrific Turkey Salad Sandwiches

When Karen was a kid, her family used to take her to a restaurant that served awesome turkey salad sandwiches. What made them so good? A thin layer of cream cheese and the most delicious pumpernickel bread you've ever tasted. Although the restaurant is no longer in business, its legacy lives on in Karen's house with this recipe.

½ pound turkey breast, cooked
¼ cup low-fat mayonnaise
¼ cup finely chopped celery
¼ cup finely chopped red onion
¼ cup dried chopped cranberries
2 tablespoons low-fat cream cheese
8 slices pumpernickel bread

In a food processor, chop the turkey. In a medium bowl, mix the turkey, mayonnaise, celery, onion, and cranberries. Divide the cream cheese equally among 4 slices of the bread. Top each slice with one-quarter of the turkey salad and another slice of the bread.

Yield: Four servings.

Nutritional data per serving: Calories, 304; protein, 24 g; carbohydrates, 36 g; fiber, 5 g; fat, 7 g; saturated fat, 2 g; cholesterol, 57 mg; sodium, 568 mg; calcium, 7% of Daily Value; iron, 16%.

Watermelon:

The Summertime Health Saver

BATTLES:

- heart disease
- high blood pressure
- high cholesterol
- irregular heartbeat
- prostate cancer
- stroke

BOLSTERS:

- energy
- hydration

We believe that the very best way to eat watermelon is to sit with your legs dangling over the edge of a pier, and spit the seeds into the water. You should be wearing your bathing suit, and the juice should be dripping off your chin and elbows. There should be plenty of kids around to compete for who can spit the seeds the farthest. And when you're done, you should dive into the water to clean up and cool off. Barring that, second place goes to the more-civilized plate, knife, and fork routine, as you indulge in this sweetest of all cancer fighters.

NUTRITION IN A NUTSHELL

Watermelon (1 cup)

Calories: 49

Fat: 1 g

Saturated fat: 0 g

Cholesterol: 0 mg

Sodium: 3 mg

Total carbohydrates: 11 g

Dietary fiber: 1 g

Protein: 1 g

Vitamin A: 11% of Daily Value

Vitamin B_6: 11%

Vitamin C: 16%

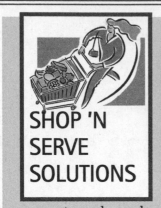

SHOP 'N SERVE SOLUTIONS

Want wonderful watermelon? Be choosy!

WHEN SELECTING WATERMELON:

A whole watermelon gives very few clues as to what's inside. Unlike with cantaloupe or honeydew, fragrance will not guide you. And the "thump" test turns out to be bogus (although it's still fun!). Fortunately, most places that sell whole watermelons also provide cut pieces, which may give clues to the quality of their whole melons. Colleen always checks out the cut pieces to be sure that most of them look red, ripe, and juicy and that the flesh looks dense and firm. If so, she figures it's safe to buy a whole watermelon, following these directions from the National Watermelon Promotion Board, who says choosing is as easy as 1, 2, 3:

1. Look over the watermelon. Choose one that's firm, symmetrical, and free of bruises, cuts, and dents.

2. Lift it up. The watermelon should be heavy for its size. Watermelon is 92 percent water, which accounts for most of its weight.

3. Turn it over. On the underside of the watermelon, there should be a creamy yellow spot from where it sat on the ground and ripened in the sun. That creamy yellow underbelly seems to be the key. If the melon is still green or white on the bottom, it is probably immature.

WHEN STORING:

Watermelon ripens on the vine, not on your kitchen counter. So basically, what you buy is what you get. To keep your melon at the

SEEING RED

Red watermelon is rich in lycopene, one of the six active carotenoids that create the red, orange, and yellow colors in foods and that are now being scrutinized for their power to prevent various cancers. (The others are alpha-carotene, beta-carotene,

peak of flavor, chill it promptly. A whole melon will keep for about a week in the refrigerator.

WHEN YOU'RE READY TO USE:

Wash any dirt off the rind before you cut it, so that you don't drag soil and bacteria through the melon with the first slice. Cover cut surfaces with plastic wrap, or store chunks in airtight containers. Once the melon is cut, its quality can deteriorate quickly, so go ahead and eat it.

BEYOND WATERMELON BASICS

Here are a few fun and festive ways to serve watermelon:

◆ **Pop your melon.** Cut watermelon into seedless chunks, puree it in your blender, and then freeze the juice in ice-cube trays. Add little sticks for tasty pops.

◆ **Get it in shape.** Thinly slice seedless watermelon or watermelon heart. Using cookie cutters, cut the slices into festive shapes to match the occasion.

◆ **Have a ball.** Get yourself a melon baller in two sizes. Scoop out a variety of big and little balls to add to fruit salad. Shape the empty rind into a disposable serving basket for the salad. Whirl the odd-shaped leftovers into "Watermelon Slush" (see page 457).

◆ **Ham it up.** Alternate thin slices of lean ham and watermelon on a bed of dark green lettuce for a cool, no-cook luncheon salad.

◆ **Say "Cheese!"** Surround a serving of calcium-added cottage cheese with watermelon cubes. Dust with ground cinnamon and garnish with a mint sprig.

cryptoxanthin, lutein, and zeaxanthin.)

At least two studies have shown that lycopene is tops when it comes to gobbling up dangerous singlet oxygen, before it can damage your cells and start them on the road to becoming cancer. And both studies found that men who ate the most lycopene and who had the most lycopene in their prostate glands had the least chance of developing prostate cancer. Although the men got most of their lycopene from tomatoes, analyses show that, cup for cup, watermelon delivers one-third more lycopene than fresh tomatoes do.

THE NATURAL SPORTS "DRINK"

Absolutely nothing tastes as good as a big chunk of ice-cold watermelon after a game of tennis or a long, hot afternoon of yard work. Watermelon is, after all, 90 percent water, so it goes a long way toward quenching your thirst.

And watermelon's natural sugars are so refreshing! They'll boost your energy and get your blood sugar (your brain's only food) back to normal, so you'll be physically coordinated and able to think straight. And like most fabricated sports drinks, watermelon packs potassium, which is especially important for maintaining a healthy heartbeat for people who take diuretics.

HEART-SMART

Scrimping on potassium can also open the door to rising blood pressure, a major risk factor for heart attack and stroke. Getting plenty of vegetables and fruits, such as watermelon, has been shown to lower high blood pressure. Also on the heart front, most of the fiber in watermelon is the soluble kind that ties up cholesterol in your intestinal tract, so you don't reabsorb it, and that helps lower your total blood cholesterol. What a sweet, wonderful way to a healthy heart!

Quick Fix:

Queasy Moms

Got morning sickness? Get watermelon. Although research has not yet been able to explain why, women who can't even keep water down do enjoy ice-cold chunks of watermelon without feeling queasy, according to Miriam Erick, R.D., director of the National Morning Sickness Nutrition Clinic at Brigham and Women's Hospital in Boston.

Watermelon Slush

In those lazy, hazy days of summer, when you lack the energy to spit out watermelon seeds, try a sippable slush, using this recipe from the National Watermelon Promotion Board. Freeze the watermelon cubes on a day when you're feeling more energetic, so that you'll be ready when indolence overcomes you.

1 can (10 ounces) frozen nonalcoholic margarita mix
3 cups cubed seeded watermelon
2 cups frozen cubed seeded watermelon* or ice cubes

In a blender or food processor, whirl the margarita mix and the unfrozen watermelon cubes until liquefied. Add the frozen watermelon cubes or ice cubes. Pulse until the mixture is slushy. Serve immediately.

*Cube seeded watermelon. Place the cubes on a baking sheet lined with waxed paper and freeze. When frozen, transfer to a plastic freezer bag and return to the freezer.

Yield: Six servings.

Nutritional data per serving: Calories, 61; protein, 1 g; carbohydratcs, 16 g; fiber, 1 g; fat, 0 g; saturated fat, 0 g; cholesterol, 1 mg; sodium, 3 mg.

Wheatberries:

Berry Good for You

BATTLES:
- constipation
- diabetes
- diverticulosis
- heart disease
- hemorrhoids

BOLSTERS:
- regularity
- weight control

Colleen struggled with wheatberries for a long time. It wasn't that she didn't like them. In fact, she *loved* them. Every time she found them on a salad bar, she took a healthy scoop. But she could never find wheatberries to cook at home.

She checked around the rice, barley, and pasta in every food store for a package labeled "wheatberries," to no avail. Finally, the clerk at a natural food store set her straight. She needed to buy "hard, red winter wheat."

Wheatberries, it turns out, are just whole little wheat kernels. When you cook them in lots of water for about an hour, they turn into chewy, nutty-tasting, plump little dark brown grains. Even when they're cooked without salt, they're delicious.

NUTRITION IN A NUTSHELL

Wheatberries (½ cup, cooked)

Calories: 158

Fat: 1 g

Saturated fat: 0 g

Cholesterol: 0 mg

Sodium: 1 mg

Total carbohydrates: 33 g

Dietary fiber: 6 g

Protein: 7 g

Copper: 10% of Daily Value

Iron: 10%

Magnesium: 15%

Manganese: 97%

Zinc: 9%

THE WHOLE STORY

Since the dawn of the Food Guide Pyramid, grains have been at its base. But as research continues to reveal the superior power of whole grains over processed white products, recommendations have shifted toward focusing on whole.

Why? Whole grains' vast array of vitamins, minerals, and phytochemicals appear to work synergistically to stave off all major lifestyle diseases.

Wheatberries, for instance, are packed with the following:

▶ **Insoluble fiber.** This is the type of fiber that's known to ward off digestive difficulties, such as constipation and diverticulosis—plus the hemorrhoids that can result.

▶ **Antioxidants (specifically, phenolic acids, lignans, and phytic acid).** Antioxidants mop up free radicals, the dangerous particles that form when body cells burn oxygen for energy. (Caution: Living is dangerous to your health!)

▶ **Vitamin E.** Wheatberries are a concentrated source of vitamin E, especially the tocotrienol isomer (one of the many subparts of vitamin E) that researchers think packs the most antioxidant benefits.

WHOLE FOR HEART AND DIABETES

Large scientific studies of many populations have found that whole grains offer great protection for your heart. The Iowa Women's Study, for instance, found that healthy postmenopausal

Quick Fix:

Constipation

Suffering from constipation? Add a serving of wheatberries and a couple of extra glasses of water to your diet. Just ½ cup of cooked wheatberries delivers one-fourth of your day's fiber, almost entirely the insoluble kind that keeps your bowels moving. Insoluble fiber soaks up lots of water in your digestive tract, so make plenty of water available.

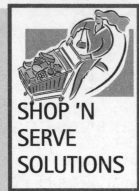

SHOP 'N SERVE SOLUTIONS

Wheatberries aren't very mainstream yet, so they're not available in most local supermarkets. You'll probably have to go to a health food or natural food store to buy your hard, red winter wheat.

WHEN SELECTING WHEATBERRIES:

You'll probably find them in a see-through package, and that's good. You'll be able to examine them for bugs.

WHEN STORING:

■ If you're not going to cook your wheatberries right away, put them in an airtight container and store them in your pantry for use within a couple of weeks.

■ For longer storage, keep them in the refrigerator to prevent their oils from becoming rancid. They'll keep for up to a year.

WHEN YOU'RE READY TO USE:

■ Put a cupful in a strainer and rinse with cold water to remove any dust or dirt.

■ Take this time to separate the wheat from the chaff and any other minor debris.

■ Put the wheatberries in a big pot, add 4 cups of water, and put a lid on the pot. Cook over high heat until the water comes to a boil. Reduce the heat to low and let the berries perk along for about an hour while you go do something else.

women who ate just one serving of whole grains daily had a 30 percent lower chance of having a heart attack than women who ate them once a week or less.

And two other studies, one of 43,000 men and the other of 65,000 women ages 40 to 65, showed that those who ate the most cereal fiber (such as wheatberries) were the least likely to develop type 2 diabetes, the kind that most adults get.

■ When you think they're done, take out a few, let them cool, and then give them the "bite" test. Continue to simmer them until they reach a consistency you like.

■ Pour off the excess water.

■ Use the berries right away, or store them in the fridge for later.

THEY'RE THE BERRIES!

If wheatberries are a new food for you, here are some introductory ideas on how to use them. (Pre-prepare the berries, and keep your cooked supply in the fridge.)

◆ **Heat for breakfast.** If Wheaties are the breakfast of champions, then wheatberries could lead to Olympic Gold! Warm them up in the microwave with a little honey, dried fruit, nuts, and milk.

◆ **Chill for salad.** Mix chilled cooked wheatberries with chopped raw veggies, such as celery, radishes, cucumbers, and carrots, and your favorite salad dressing.

◆ **Heat for soup.** Stir a big spoonful into canned bean, pea, or lentil soup for protein that's as complete as meat's.

◆ **Warm for dinner.** Replace pasta, rice, or potatoes with warm wheatberries dressed with olive oil, balsamic vinegar, and Italian herbs, such as basil, oregano, and thyme.

◆ **Blend for parties.** Combine cooked wheatberries with chopped ripe olives and toasted pine nuts for a fancy treat.

THE WHOLE WEIGHT PROBLEM

Weight control seems out of control in the United States, with one-third of all adults considered overweight or obese. But wheatberries and other whole grains can help those of us who need to shed a few pounds. While wheatberries are not "light," they contain no fat. And they are very filling. Some research even suggests that whole grain foods help you stay satisfied longer.

Wheatberry Breakfast

Chewy, yummy wheatberries mixed with fruit, nuts, and milk will jump-start your morning, providing one-third of your day's fiber, a bunch of B vitamins, and a truckload of minerals.

1 cup wheatberries (hard, red winter wheat)
4 cups water
2 whole dates, sliced
2 tablespoons chopped toasted pecans
Dash of allspice
½ cup evaporated skim milk

The night before, place the wheatberries in a heavy pot and cover with the water. Cover and bring to a boil over high heat. Reduce the heat to low, and simmer until the wheatberries are chewy, about 1 hour. Drain off the excess water and chill the wheatberries in the fridge overnight. In the morning, put ½ cup of the wheatberries in a microwaveable bowl. Cover and microwave on medium until piping hot. Stir in the dates, pecans, allspice, and milk. Your day's off to a powerful start!

Yield: One serving.

Nutritional data per serving: Calories, 407; protein, 19 g; carbohydrates, 62 g; fiber, 9 g; fat, 12 g; saturated fat, 1 g; cholesterol, 5 mg; sodium, 150 mg; vitamin A, 19% of Daily Value; vitamin B_1 (thiamin), 28%; vitamin B_2 (riboflavin), 28%; vitamin B_3 (niacin), 18%; vitamin B_6, 15%; calcium, 40%; copper, 22%; iron, 15%; zinc, 21%.

Wheatberries 'n Veggies

When you're bored with food and ready for something that ignites your taste buds, this is the way to go.

1 cup wheatberries (hard, red winter wheat)
¼ cup diced celery
¼ cup diced peeled cucumber
¼ cup chopped red bell pepper
¼ cup sliced ripe olives
2 tablespoons Ken's Light Caesar dressing
4 leaves lettuce

Cook the wheatberries the day before you plan to use them (see recipe on opposite page). The next night, when you're making dinner, place 2 cups of cooked wheatberries into a medium bowl. Add the celery, cucumber, pepper, olives, and dressing. Stir well. Divide the lettuce between two salad plates, then spoon equal amounts of the wheatberry mixture on top.

Yield: Two servings.

Nutritional data per serving: Calories, 221; protein, 8 g; carbohydrates, 37 g; fiber, 7 g; fat, 6 g; saturated fat, 1 g; cholesterol, 3 mg; sodium, 461 mg; vitamin A, 14% of Daily Value; vitamin C, 41%; vitamin E, 9%; calcium, 5%; iron, 14%.

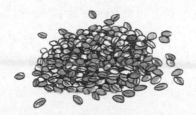

Wheat Germ:

Harvest the Goodness!

BATTLES:
- Alzheimer's disease
- birth defects
- heart disease
- high cholesterol
- stroke

BOLSTERS:
- bones

In her family, Colleen's mom led the way into the world of healthier food. One of her best-kept secrets was to add wheat germ in places where no one noticed, such as meat loaf. Now, it turns out, wheat germ may be the twinkle in Mother Nature's eye. Wheat germ is that tiny bit of the wheat kernel that gets left behind in making white flour for the puffy, white "balloon" bread that has overtaken most of America. And it's missing from all that other white stuff we're addicted to, such as pasta, most flake cereals, pastries, cakes, and cookies.

But the joke's on us. The germ is where the goodies are stored. And that just goes to show you why it's not smart to mess with Mother Nature—or Colleen's mother!

WHEAT BASICS

A kernel of wheat has three basic parts:

▶ **The endosperm.** This is the fluffy, white inside of the kernel, the part that is milled to make white flour. It's carbohydrate-rich

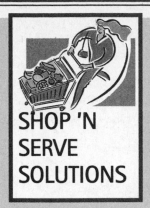

SHOP 'N SERVE SOLUTIONS

The rules for buying wheat germ are simple.

WHEN SELECTING WHEAT GERM:

■ You'll most likely buy your wheat germ in a vacuum-sealed jar. Look for the "best-used-before" date to make sure it's fresh.

■ If you buy your wheat germ in bulk, give the barrel a serious sniff. The heart of the grain should smell fresh. If it has a sour or musty odor, pass.

WHEN STORING:

■ Store unopened wheat germ in your pantry, away from heat, where it'll keep for about a year.

■ Once the jar has been opened, store it in the refrigerator, because the oil easily becomes rancid when exposed to air.

SPRINKLE IT EVERYWHERE

Now what do you do with your wheat germ? Here are some ideas:

◆ **Top off your salads.** After you've tossed your greens until they're glistening with dressing, sprinkle a tablespoon of wheat germ over the top. It will stick to the leaves instead of falling to the bottom of the bowl.

◆ **Bulk up your baked goods.** Just use your favorite muffin or quick-bread recipe, but replace up to ½ cup of the flour with wheat germ. You can add wheat germ to piecrust, too.

◆ **Revive your cereal.** Sprinkle wheat germ on your favorite hot or cold cereal for a toasty taste and a big boost of minor minerals.

◆ **Add velocity to your fruit.** For a speedy dose of vitamins, fold fresh fruit into blueberry yogurt, along with a tablespoon of wheat germ.

◆ **Be a turncoat.** Be loyal to your arteries! It isn't treason to trade wheat germ for white flour when you coat chicken or fish for oven frying. Try our recipe for "Crunchy Salsa Chicken" on page 472.

and also packs gluten, the protein that makes dough stretchy and elastic enough to capture and hold air while bread bakes.

▶ **The bran.** The outer coating, or bran, provides the "rough" in roughage. It's the insoluble fibrous part that keeps you regular. Just 2 tablespoons provide 10 percent of the fiber you need for the day, with no calories. What a bargain!

▶ **Then there's the germ.** It contains some unsaturated fat, vitamin E, the B vitamins niacin and thiamin, and the minerals copper, iron, magnesium, manganese, and zinc. Imagine all that in such a tiny little package. It's practically a miracle.

If you're a fat-a-phobic, you may fear that little bit of oil in wheat germ. But relax. It's key to carrying the fat-soluble vitamin E, so that your body can absorb it. Most of us get far too little vitamin E from foods.

Unless you've been living on another planet, you probably know at least a little about vitamin E. It has been implicated in fighting heart disease, stroke, and Alzheimer's disease. The oil is a good source of phytosterols. This plant version of cholesterol has been shown to lower human cholesterol levels and, at least in test tubes and lab animals, to fight cancer.

FORTIFIED FOLATE

Fortified wheat germ is also an excellent source of folic acid, a proven protector against neural tube birth defects. Experts at the National Centers for Disease Control and Prevention estimate that half of all neural tube defects could be prevented if women

NUTRITION IN A NUTSHELL

Wheat germ
(2 tablespoons)

Calories: 50

Fat: 1 g

Saturated fat: 0 g

Cholesterol: 0 mg

Sodium: 0 mg

Total carbohydrates: 6 g

Dietary fiber: 2 g

Protein: 4 g

Folate: 20% of Daily Value

Vitamin E: 20%

Magnesium: 10%

Manganese: 140%

would just get enough folic acid *before* they get pregnant. Folic acid is also known for managing out-of-control blood homocysteine levels, which can trigger a heart attack.

SYNERGY FOR BONES

Wheat germ delivers a truckload of minor minerals that now appear to be critical for bones. No, there's not much calcium in there. And you're right—calcium provides the bulk of bone matter. But bit players such as copper, iron, magnesium, manganese, and zinc play critical roles that make calcium look like a star. Their interaction seems to create a kind of synergy, where working together makes the total bigger than the sum of its parts—a sort of one-plus-one-equals-three, if you will.

Crunchy Salsa Chicken

Here's an incredibly zesty way to make "fried" chicken that's as good to your body as it is to your taste buds.

Canola or olive oil cooking spray
1 cup Kretschmer Toasted Wheat Germ
1 tablespoon pumpkin pie spice
1 tablespoon ground cumin
¼ teaspoon ground cayenne pepper
¾ teaspoon salt (optional)
2 egg whites
1 tablespoon water
4 boneless, skinless chicken breast halves (about 4 ounces each)
1 large orange, peeled and diced
¾ cup mild or medium salsa
1 tablespoon chopped fresh cilantro (optional)

Preheat the oven to 400°F. Coat a baking sheet with cooking spray. In a shallow dish, combine the wheat germ, pumpkin pie spice, cumin, pepper, and, if using, the salt. In a second shallow dish, beat the egg whites and water until frothy. Dip the chicken breasts in the egg-white mixture and then in the wheat germ mixture. Dip and coat again, covering thoroughly. Arrange on the baking sheet. Lightly spray the tops of the chicken breasts with cooking spray. Bake for 18 to 20 minutes, or until the chicken is no longer pink in the middle.

While the chicken bakes, combine the orange, salsa, and, if using, the cilantro in a small bowl. Serve with the chicken.

Yield: Four servings.

*Nutritional data per serving: Calories, 290; protein, 36 g; carbohydrates, 22 g; fiber, 5 g; fat, 7 g; saturated fat, 1 g; sodium, 430 mg; folate, 35% of Daily Value. * Recipe compliments of Kretschmer and the Quaker Oats Company.*

Whole Wheat Bread:

The Real Staff of Life

BATTLES:
- cancer
- diabetes
- heart disease

BOLSTERS:
- longevity
- regularity

You may not live as long as Methuselah, but there's a good chance that you'll increase your life span if you include a couple of pieces of whole wheat bread in your daily diet. That's the conclusion of the Iowa Women's Study that compared the diets of more than 40,000 women ages 55 to 69 to see how what they ate matched up with the chronic diseases they developed over a span of nine years.

The good news: Women who ate at least one serving of whole grain foods daily were 15 percent less likely to die from heart disease, cancer, or any other chronic disease than were women who blew off the whole grains and stuck with the starch.

A GRAIN OF TRUTH

Why is white flour so inferior, healthwise, to whole wheat? The process that turns whole wheat kernels into white flour hangs on

(Continued on page 476)

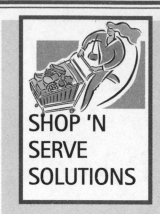

SHOP 'N SERVE SOLUTIONS

Be careful in your choice of wheat bread.

WHEN SELECTING WHOLE WHEAT BREAD:

■ Read the ingredients list, found in small print somewhere on the packaging. (If you're like us, you might have to take along a magnifying glass to get the scoop!) Ingredients are listed by weight, in order of predominance. That means there's the most of whatever ingredient is listed first and the least of the ingredient listed last. Choose bread made with whole wheat flour only, so that you get the biggest nutritional bang per calorie. Some whole wheat breads are only 51 percent whole wheat, with white enriched flour as the second ingredient.

■ Check the "Nutrition Facts" label for fiber. The more, the better.

WHEN STORING:

If you choose 100 percent stone-ground whole wheat bread, store it in the refrigerator to prevent the natural oils from turning rancid.

A WHOLE LOT OF HEALTH

Once you've found the staff of your life, lean on it like this:

◆ **Have breakfast on the run.** Spread two slices of whole wheat bread with peanut butter, slap them together, and take off.

◆ **Get a pocketful of fun.** Pita pockets count as bread! And yes, they come in whole wheat. Toast a pocket till it puffs, let it cool, and then slit the side. Fill it with tuna, shrimp, or chicken salad, leftover tossed salad and cheese chunks, or vegetarian refried beans and salsa.

◆ **Try a different angle.** Cut whole wheat pita pockets into wedges, toast them, and dip in salsa, olive spread, or veggie dip.

◆ **Be halfhearted if you must.** Having a hard time adjusting to the more full-bodied taste of real whole wheat bread? For a while, make your sandwiches with one slice of white and one slice of whole wheat. Bite your sandwich so that the white touches your tongue.

WHAT'S IN A NAME?

Plenty, if you're looking for the best bread. Here's a rundown geared to guide you toward the grainiest slices:

■ **Whole wheat bread** is made from flour that's been roller-milled. This process temporarily separates the bran and germ from the endosperm, which can then be ground to the best consistency. The three parts are then reunited to make whole wheat flour for bread. Legally, bread must contain at least 51 percent whole wheat flour to be called whole wheat. But 100 percent is better. When bread is made totally from whole wheat flour, it's nutritionally equal to 100 percent stone-ground whole wheat bread.

■ **One hundred percent stone-ground whole wheat bread** is made from flour created when wheat kernels are crushed between rolling stones without separating out the bran and germ. One possible drawback: It may turn rancid more quickly since the wheat germ oil is crushed in with the endosperm. But don't let that stop you from buying this bread. Just be sure to store it in the refrigerator.

■ **Enriched white bread** is made from roller-milled flour with the bran and germ removed and never returned. Four B vitamins (folic acid, niacin, thiamin, and riboflavin) and iron are added to restore natural levels, but at least 20 vitamins and minerals, as well as fiber, have gone permanently AWOL.

■ **Wheat bread** is made from a mix of mostly white flour and some whole wheat flour. This is a step up if you're stuck on white bread, but don't stop there. You haven't really arrived yet.

(Continued from page 473)

to the powdery endosperm, but dumps two important parts: the bran and the germ. (See "Wheat Germ: Harvest the Goodness!" on page 468.) And these two parts are loaded with vitamins, minerals, fiber, and functional bits and pieces such as phytic acid, phenols, and saponins that protect against destructive oxidation and keep your body in tip-top shape.

And it's not just a matter of life and death. Sure, wheat bran's insoluble fiber has been linked to protection against cancer. But comfort counts, too. And the rough stuff protects against embarrassing problems, usually unmentionable, such as constipation, hemorrhoids, and diverticulosis. So whole up, and get things moving!

NUTRITION IN A NUTSHELL

Whole wheat bread (1 slice)

Calories: 69

Fat: 1 g

Saturated fat: 0 g

Cholesterol: 0 mg

Sodium: 147 mg

Total carbohydrates: 13 g

Dietary fiber: 2 g

Protein: 3 g

Copper: 4% of Daily Value

Iron: 5%

Manganese: 32%

Zinc: 4%

BEATS DIABETES

Other information gleaned from the Iowa women focused on diabetes. It revealed that whole grains, cereal fiber, and dietary magnesium appear to protect older women from developing type 2 diabetes. So please pass the white and grab the wheat.

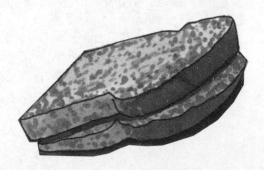

Whole Wheat Pita Wedges with Homemade Hummus

This hummus is the most intensely flavored we've ever eaten. Toasting the whole wheat pita chips brings out their slightly sweet taste, the perfect counterpoint to the savory dip.

1 can (16 ounces) chickpeas, drained
1 tablespoon freshly chopped or pressed garlic
2 tablespoons extra virgin olive oil
1 tablespoon tahini (sesame seed paste)
2 tablespoons fresh lemon juice
2 tablespoons chopped fresh parsley
½ teaspoon coarsely ground black pepper
¼ teaspoon salt
4 whole wheat pita pockets

Preheat the oven to 350°F. Meanwhile, in a blender or food processor, combine the chickpeas, garlic, oil, tahini, lemon juice, parsley, pepper, and salt until smooth. Remove to a serving dish. Cut each pita pocket into four triangles. Place on a baking sheet, and bake for 5 minutes, or until crisp. When cool, place in a napkin-lined basket and serve with hummus.

Yield: 16 servings.

Nutritional data per serving: Calories, 88; protein, 3 g; carbohydrates, 13 g; fiber, 3 g; fat, 3 g; saturated fat, 0 g; cholesterol, 0 mg; sodium, 175 mg; iron, 5% of Daily Value; manganese, 15%.

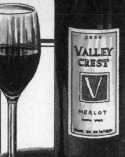

Wine:

Paradoxical Heart Health

BATTLES:
- cancer
- diabetes
- heart disease
- infections
- stroke

BOLSTERS:
- bones
- brain function

Quick Fix:

Cuts

Cut yourself? Pour some wine into the cut. Its polyphenols kill bacteria and prevent infection.

Several years ago, a family friend of Colleen's started making his own wine, and from time to time, he would invite her to get involved in the process. That's when she learned that the difference between red and white wines is how long the crushed grapes are allowed to "sit on the skins." White wine is removed quickly, while red wine is allowed to linger so that it can pick up the red color.

And now scientists have discovered that, along with the red color, the wine is also soaking up resveratrol, a natural compound that protects the grapes from fungi. Turns out, resveratrol also appears to protect the human heart from cholesterol and the vital organs from cancer.

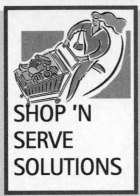

SHOP 'N SERVE SOLUTIONS

Remember the old rule: red wine with red meat, white wine with chicken and fish? Well, what do you serve with minestrone, crusty bread, and a salad? The "rules" for choosing wine are way too complicated to include in this book, so we'll keep it simple.

WHEN SELECTING WINE:

Some experts suggest that wines containing the most tannins (the chemicals that make wine "dry") also contain the most healthy ingredients. So enjoy the big reds: cabernet, merlot, and port.

ARE YOU IN THE SPIRIT?

Here are some tips for wine enjoyment:

◆ **Drink your wine with meals.** Food slows alcohol absorption, and wine may have greater benefits when it interacts with food. Wine also enhances the flavor of food, the very best reason to enjoy wine.

◆ **Make your wine a spritzer.** Mix it with seltzer water for a sparkling, light, refreshing drink.

◆ **Cook with wine.** When you simmer foods in wine long enough, all the alcohol evaporates, but the flavor lingers, enhancing and blending flavors. Wine also acts as a tenderizer for tough cuts of meat, such as stewing beef or round steak.

VIVE LA FRENCH PARADOX!

How could it be, researchers wondered a while back, that Americans stuffing down burgers, ribs, and fries keel over from heart disease, while the French get just as much fat dining on foie gras, creamy sauces, and pastry, but their hearts never skip a beat?

Could it be? *Mais oui!* The French, like the long-lived Italians and Spaniards, often drink wine in the normal course of dining. Scientists already knew that wine was a natural antioxidant, so the research was on.

It's also known that any kind of alcohol can have its benefits. But wine seems to be special. Take a look at this: The people of Belgium and Czechoslovakia drink as much alcohol as the French do, but they drink it in the form of beer—and they suffer more from heart disease.

TWO MAGIC INGREDIENTS

In searching for the heart answer, scientists stumbled onto resveratrol, as well as quercetin, the two compounds in wine that seem to work along with the alcohol to create a kind of synergy that prevents bad low-density lipoprotein (LDL) from turning into sludge on your artery walls and setting you up for a heart attack. And there's more.

Resveratrol also appears to be a potent cancer fighter. It can block an enzyme that cancer cells need in order to grow, and it appears able to detoxify mutagens—invaders that coax healthy cells to change into cancerous ones.

BONUS BENNIES

Health organizations are always reluctant to encourage people to drink alcohol, because it opens the door to so many other problems. But the more research they do, the more it becomes clear that, for adults who are not pregnant or do not suffer from alcoholism, enjoying red wine with meals adds to both the joy and length of life.

One study of Japanese-American men living in Hawaii, for instance, showed that those who had about one drink a day while in their 40s and 50s ended up 26 years later performing better on tests of thinking and reasoning than either those who didn't drink at all or those who drank more heavily.

Two other studies, one of male doctors in the United States and the other of female nurses, showed that moderate drinking (four to seven drinks per week) reduced their risk of developing type 2 diabetes, compared with people who never drank.

And a study of women over age 65 showed that those who drank moderately had greater bone density than women who didn't drink. Scientists think that the benefit accrues because alcohol affects parathyroid hormone levels in such a way that you don't lose as much bone.

MORE IS LESS

Now here's the bad news: Red wine's benefits arrive through a very small window of opportunity. Study after study has shown that moderate drinking (one drink a day for women, two drinks a day for men) is all it takes to get the goodies. More is not better.

In fact, it's much worse. Drinking more than one or two glasses of wine—or any other form of alcohol—a day actually increases the risk of some cancers, as well as high blood pressure, stroke, birth defects, alcoholism, violence, suicide, and automobile accidents. There is also a high level of concern about the fact that older adults are increasingly at risk for late-onset alcoholism.

So get this message straight: The benefits of red wine are *not* a green light for overindulgence.

WHO SHOULD NOT DRINK

The *2000 Dietary Guidelines for Americans* acknowledge that moderate alcohol intake may be beneficial for your heart, but they quickly point out that, if you don't want to drink, you can get similar benefits by eating a healthy diet, controlling your weight, exercising regularly, and not smoking.

NUTRITION IN A NUTSHELL

Red wine (5 fluid ounces)

Calories: 106

Fat: 0 g

Saturated fat: 0 g

Cholesterol: 0 mg

Sodium: 0 mg

Total carbohydrates: 3 g

Protein: Less than 1 g

Vitamin B_6: 3% of Daily Value

Iron: 4%

Magnesium: 5%

Potassium: 4%

The guidelines also point out that certain people should not drink at all:

▶ Children and teenagers.

▶ Pregnant women and those who could become pregnant.

▶ Problem drinkers, alcoholics, recovering alcoholics, and relatives of alcoholics.

▶ Anyone who plans to drive, operate machinery, or participate in any activity that requires attention, skill, or coordination. (Remnants of a single drink can remain in your blood for 2 to 3 hours.)

▶ Anyone taking prescription or over-the-counter drugs that can interact with alcohol. (Check with your pharmacist or health care provider.)

Sparkling Red Wine Cooler

Turn your glass of red wine into a refreshing summer cooler.

¼ lime
½ cup red wine
½ cup seltzer water

Half fill a tall glass with ice. Squeeze the lime over the ice. Pour in the wine, then the seltzer. Stir with a drinking straw. Cheers!

Yield: One serving.

Nutritional data per serving: Calories, 90; protein, less than 1 g; carbohydrates, 4 g; fiber, less than 1 g; fat, 0 g; saturated fat, 0 g; cholesterol, 0 mg; sodium, 6 mg; vitamin C, 6% of Daily Value; iron, 3%; magnesium, 4%; potassium, 4%.

Salmon Poached in Red Wine

Elegant and easy. Need we say more? Yes. By the time you finish simmering the salmon, it'll be rich with the wine's flavor and power-packed with its antioxidants.

½ **cup red wine**
2 **salmon filets (5 ounces each)**
⅛ **teaspoon salt**
Freshly ground black pepper to taste
2 **sprigs fresh dill**

Pour the wine into a skillet just large enough to hold the salmon. Add the salmon, season with the salt and pepper, and top with the dill. Bring the wine to a boil. Reduce the heat and gently simmer, uncovered, until the salmon flakes easily with a fork. If the wine dries up, add just a little water to prevent scorching. To serve, place a salmon filet on each of two dinner plates. Add a tablespoon or two of water to the skillet and deglaze. Pour the liquid over the salmon.

Yield: Two servings.

Nutritional data per serving: Calories, 250; protein, 29 g; carbohydrates, 1 g; fiber, 0 g; fat, 9 g; saturated fat, 1 g; cholesterol, 81 mg; sodium, 212 mg; vitamin B_3 (niacin), 56% of Daily Value; vitamin B_6, 55%; vitamin D, 159%; copper, 19%; potassium, 21%.

Yogurt:
The Benefits of Having Culture

BATTLES:
- ■ cancer
- ■ canker sores
- ■ diarrhea
- ■ high blood pressure
- ■ yeast infections

BOLSTERS:
- ■ bones
- ■ digestion
- ■ immune function
- ■ weight control

Yogurt is yummy—which is really why we like it so much. Thick and creamy, it's packed with calcium, that wonderful mineral that protects your bones and fights off osteoporosis. But even its bounty of calcium may not be the healthiest thing about yogurt. Instead, it's more likely to be its bugs.

BENEFICIAL BUGS

Yep, you read that right: Yogurt contains bugs. But they're not the kind you step on. They're microscopic forms of bacteria—and they're actually *friendly*. In fact,

Quick Fix:

Canker Sores

Constantly coming down with canker sores? Eat plain yogurt more often. Its helpful bacteria may fight off the ones that cause those painful sores.

THE SCOOP ON FROZEN YOGURT

Is "fro yo" as fabulous for you as regular yogurt? Sorry, but no, says Manfred Kroger, Ph.D., professor of food science at Pennsylvania State University in State College. The sweeteners and fruit added to frozen yogurt inhibit some of the beneficial yogurt cultures.

Even so, most frozen yogurts are still a better choice than ice cream. They usually offer more calcium (one of our favorites, Edy's/Dreyer's, packs 45 percent of your daily requirement in just half a cup), less fat, and at least some active cultures.

Next time you're shopping for frozen yogurt, pick up a brand that mentions "active cultures" on the label. The government requires manufacturers to supply enough of the good guys to meet a minimum standard.

studies suggest that they help destroy the bad guys that give us diarrhea, yeast infections, and—sit down for this—possibly cancer.

Here's what research has found:

► One study reported that eating 8 ounces of yogurt containing the bacterial culture *Lactobacillus acidophilus* reduced the risk of yeast infections threefold.

► Animal research suggests that this culture may decrease the risk of breast, colon, and liver tumors triggered by carcinogens.

"Although we have to conduct clinical human trials, the relationship between active cultures in yogurt and the reduced risk of breast and colon cancers looks very promising," says yogurt researcher Ian Rowland, Ph.D., of the University of Ulster in Ireland.

(Continued on page 488)

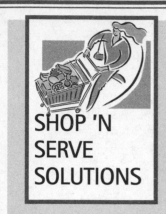

SHOP 'N SERVE SOLUTIONS

Yogurt with fruit on the bottom. Yogurt with fruit on the top. Yogurt topped with crushed nuts! Yogurt with a spoon included!! The yogurt section of your supermarket keeps growing larger and more confusing.

What kind of yogurt should you buy? We'll make it easy. Hands down, your best bet is plain yogurt, either low-fat or fat-free, with live and active cultures.

Why? Plain yogurt usually kicks in more calcium than the flavored fare. Plus, the fruit and sweeteners that manufacturers add to yogurt may, over time, inhibit the healthy bacteria.

If you like your yogurt flavored, customize it with all kinds of healthy goodies. Try fresh berries, chopped pineapple or peaches, raisins, cereal, chopped nuts, or even a few mini chocolate chips.

Beyond that, here are some tips for buying the very best yogurt.

WHEN SELECTING YOGURT:

■ Check the label to make sure the yogurt contains active cultures.

■ Look for yogurt that contains *Lactobacillus acidophilus* or *Bifidus*. These additional cultures may provide much of yogurt's stomach-soothing benefits.

■ Select yogurt with the best expiration date, because the amount of beneficial cultures declines with age.

■ Skip any yogurt that claims to be "heat-treated" or "pasteurized after culturing," because the beneficial cultures have been destroyed.

If you're wedded to flavored yogurt, all the rules for plain yogurt apply, plus these two:

■ Opt for fruit-on-the-bottom yogurt, which usually contains more beneficial cultures than yogurt with fruit mixed throughout the container.

■ Compare the calorie and calcium contents among brands since they vary widely. Select a yogurt that packs at least 30 percent of the Daily Value for calcium in a 6-ounce serving.

FIVE WAYS TO ADD HEALTH

Now that you've made your selection, see all the healthy ways that you can use your yogurt:

◆ **Slenderize your salads.** Substitute plain yogurt for one-third of the mayo that you typically use in tuna, chicken, or potato salad. You can also trade it for all of the sour cream called for in dip recipes. Try "A Dilly of a Dip" on page 489 at your next party.

◆ **Make a silky smoothie.** In a blender, combine ½ cup of strawberries, ½ cup of orange juice, ¼ teaspoon of vanilla extract, ¼ cup of skim or low-fat milk, and a few ice cubes until smooth. Stir in ¼ cup of plain yogurt.

◆ **Revitalize your rice.** Have leftover white or brown rice from your Chinese takeout? The next day, mix it with vanilla yogurt, ground cinnamon, nutmeg, and raisins for a quick, cold salad.

◆ **Make your waffles wild.** Instead of syrup, top your pancakes or waffles with yogurt and berries.

◆ **Remember your scouting days.** When your sweet tooth starts acting up, satisfy it with "S'Mores Yogurt": Just combine 1 cup of low-fat plain yogurt, 2 teaspoons of mini marshmallows, 2 teaspoons of mini chocolate chips, and 1 crushed graham cracker.

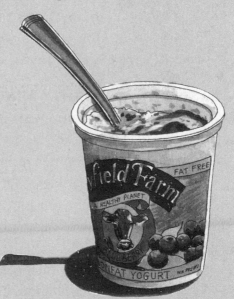

Quick Fix:

Body Fat

Researchers at the University of Tennessee recently studied the diets of more than 7,000 men and women. They found that those folks who consumed at least three servings of fat-free or low-fat dairy products every day had the lowest levels of body fat.

Why? "A diet high in low-fat dairy products causes fat cells to make less fat and turns on the machinery to break down fat," explains study author Michael Zemel, Ph.D. Now that's news we like to hear!

(Continued from page 485)

IMMUNITY BOOSTERS

Beyond bacteria, other compounds in yogurt may have anticancer benefits. "Certain lipids, acids, and peptides in yogurt may play a role in fighting cancer," says M. E. Sanders, Ph.D., of Dairy and Food Culture Technologies in Colorado.

In fact, yogurt may rev up the entire immune system. A recent review of studies at Tufts University in Boston suggests that people with compromised immune systems, especially older folks, may increase their resistance to certain diseases by eating yogurt. Researchers point out, however, that more studies are still needed to make the connection for sure.

MIGHTY MINERALS

The minerals in yogurt deserve some special attention, too. A 1-cup serving of low-fat plain yogurt offers 100 milligrams more potassium than a banana does. Getting plenty of potassium, may help keep your blood pressure in check, reducing the risk of heart disease and stroke.

And then, of course, there's calcium. One cup of low-fat plain yogurt delivers about 150 milligrams more calcium than a glass of milk does. That's good news for your bones!

NUTRITION IN A NUTSHELL

Low-fat plain yogurt (1 cup)

Calories: 155

Fat: 4 g

Saturated fat: 2 g

Cholesterol: 15 mg

Sodium: 172 mg

Total carbohydrates: 17 g

Dietary fiber: 0 g

Protein: 13 g

Vitamin B_2 (riboflavin): 30% of Daily Value

Calcium: 45%

Phosphorus: 35%

Zinc: 15%

A Dilly of a Dip

The next time you want to perk up raw veggies, dunk them in this dressing for a flavor and calcium boost.

1 cup low-fat plain yogurt
¼ cup minced fresh dill
¾ teaspoon Dijon mustard
¼ teaspoon onion powder
½ teaspoon ground black pepper
Salt to taste

In a medium bowl, combine the yogurt, dill, mustard, onion powder, pepper, and salt. Eat immediately, or cover and chill.

Yield: Six servings.

Nutritional data per serving: Calories, 27; protein, 2 g; carbohydrates, 3 g; fiber, 0 g; fat, 1 g; saturated fat, 0 g; cholesterol, 2 mg; sodium, 45 mg; calcium, 8% of Daily Value.

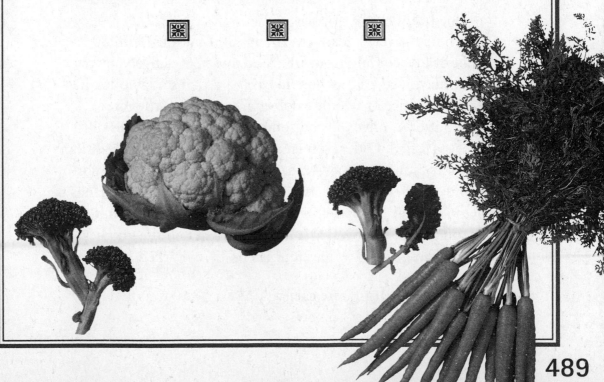

Super-charged Menus

Yes, you can have it all! Once you've found out how easy and delicious power-packed foods can be, you'll want to start using our recipes as building blocks for daily menus. So we've stacked up a few for you, to demonstrate the beauty of balance.

Each day's array adds up to about 2000 calories, with 30 percent or less coming from fat. Men and very active younger women may need a little more to eat. And that's easy to fix. Just add an extra slice or two of whole grain bread, a little more peanut butter or olive oil, and some fruit and raw veggies until you feel satisfied. Older women may need to eat a little less than 2000 calories daily. If that's you, just shave a little off each portion, buy smaller pieces of fruit (use clementines, baby bananas, gala apples) and use half-size dinner rolls. But don't cut out any one food group. That way you'll be sure to get all the goodies!

Page numbers for recipes in this book are marked in parenthesis.

Here's what healthy looks like.

Day One

Fending off autumn's chill?
Help is at hand!

BREAKFAST
1 cup Orange Juice
2 Van's Whole Grain Waffles
topped with
1/4 cup Part-Skim Ricotta Cheese
and
Chunky French Applesauce (p. 4)
Green Tea with Lemon

LUNCH
Ginger Butternut Soup (p. 433)
Egg Salad Sandwich (p. 187)
1 cup Skim Milk
Fresh Pear

DINNER
Michael's Rosemary Chicken (p. 403)
Italian Braised Celery (p. 126)
Small Crusty Roll
with
2 teaspoons Olive Oil
5 ounces Red Wine

DESSERT
Nuts Among the Berries (p. 291)
Black Tea with Skim Milk

Day Two

Got the Moody Blues?
Here's a transitional day
in late summer or early fall.

BREAKFAST
Breakfast Danish
1 cup Fat Free Hot Cocoa

LUNCH
2 Southwestern Sprout Wraps
(p. 85)
Sweet Potato Fries (p. 442)
Watermelon Slush (p. 461)

AFTERNOON SNACK
Dannon Light Yogurt
Mini Box of Raisins
Iced Green Tea

DINNER
Perfect Red Salad (p. 254)
Family-Party Pesto (p. 299)
2 Dinner Rolls
5 ounces Red Wine

491

Day Three

Beat July's heat!
(Firecrackers not withstanding!)

BREAKFAST
Patriotic Parfait (p. 399)
Tea with lime

LUNCH
Summer Pasta (p. 324)
on
2 cups Romaine Lettuce
2 Whole Grain Rolls
Hearty Purple Cow (p. 222)

AFTERNOON SNACK
1 ounce Bag of Peanuts
Fresh Peach
Iced Tea with Lemon

DINNER
Crab-Stuffed Papaya (p. 320)
Hazelnut Asparagus (p. 19)
Garlic Crisp Potatoes (p. 371)
Mango Iced Tea (p. 447)
Colleen's Famous Gingerbread
(p. 214)

Day Four

Bust the blahs any time of year
with ever-ready ingredients!

BREAKFAST
2 Amazing Apricot Waffles (p. 10)
1 cup Skim Milk
Hot Tea

LUNCH
Wild Creamy Mushroom Soup
(p. 281)
Tuna Tucks (p. 234)
Five-Minute Asian Slaw (p.100)
Bunch of Grapes
Iced Tea with Lime

DINNER
2 Portions Stressful Day Stir Fry
(p. 423)
Whole Wheat Dinner Roll
Wedge of Melon
1 cup Fat Free Frozen Yogurt
Hot Tea

Day Five

Sail through a hot August
morning, noon, and night—as
cool as a cucumber!

BREAKFAST
Cranberry Muffin (p. 172)
Blueberry Breeze (p. 71)

LUNCH
Chill-a-Melon Soup (p. 111)
Super Summer Quesadillas (p. 167)
Aunt Shirley's Three-Bean Salad
(p. 46)
Iced Green Tea

DINNER
Grilled Salmon Primavera
(p. 201)
Wheatberries 'n Veggies (p. 467)
Spinach Pignoli (p. 428)
Grainy Dinner Roll
5 ounces Red Wine
Hot Tea

Day Six

Get the most out of spring fever.
Dine al fresco all
day long.

BREAKFAST
Whole Wheat English Muffin
2 tablespoons Peanut Butter
2 tablespoons Raspberry All-Fruit
Preserves
1 cup Vanilla Soy Milk

LUNCH
Waldorf Wrap (p. 346)
Cheery Chocolate Slush (p. 159)
Banana

AFTERNOON SNACK
Whole Wheat Pita Wedges with
Homemade Hummus (p. 477)
(3 servings)
Iced Tea with Mint

DINNER
Mediterranean Salad (p. 27)
Pasta Primavera Marinara
(p. 62)
Crusty Dinner Roll

DESSERT
Blackberry Peach Crisp (p. 67)
Hot Tea with Skim Milk

Day Seven

Beat post-Thanksgiving Stress Syndrome with a little leftover turkey and a lot of other goodies!

BREAKFAST
Fresh Start Breakfast (p. 131)
Hot Tea with Skim Milk

LUNCH
Chilly Beet Soup (p. 57)
Terrific Turkey Salad Sandwich (p. 456)
Fall Fruit Salad
Hot Tea

AFTERNOON SNACK
4 Whole Wheat Crackers
1 tablespoon Almond Butter

DINNER
Apple-Cranberry Pork Chops (p. 367)
No-Fail Kale (p. 239)
Quinoa Pilaf (p. 386)
Multi-Grain Dinner Roll
5 ounces Red Wine

DESSERT
Dreamy Vanilla Pudding (p. 422)
Hot Tea with Mint

Index

A

Age-related macular degeneration (ARMD), 59, 166
    eggs, 181, 185
    greens, 227, 229
    kale, 235–236
    kiwifruit, 241
    pumpkin, 379
    spinach, 424–425
Aging, 150, 155, 156, 358, 359
Alcohol, 82, 114, 480, 481–482. *See also* Wine
Allergies
    blackberries, 63, 66
    cranberries, 168, 170
    cucumbers, 174
    kale, 235
    onions, 306, 307
    raspberries, 395
All-Occasion Vegetable Platter, 122
Alzheimer's disease, 468, 470
Amazing Apricot Waffles, 10, 492
Amazing Instant White Sauce, 271
Anemia, 49, 312, 392, 455
Appetizers
    All-Occasion Vegetable Platter, 122
    Artichoke Appetizer with Fresh Gazpacho Dip, 15
    with grapes, 220
    with pear, 343
    with peppers, 149
    with wheatberries, 465
Apple-Cranberry Pork Chops, 367, 494
Apples, 1–4, 140
    in Curry Rice Pilaf, 180
    in Fall Fruit Salad, 276
    with peanut butter and chocolate, 158
    stored with other foods, 18, 113
    in Sweet Potato Fries, 442
Applesauce, 4, 491
Apricots, 5–10, 35, 492
Arthritis, 139, 140, 443, 447. *See also* Rheumatoid arthritis
Artichoke Appetizer with Fresh Gazpacho Dip, 15
Artichokes, 11–15
Asparagus, 16–19
Asthma, 41, 45, 215
Athlete's foot, 207, 208
Aunt Shirley's Three-Bean Salad, 46, 493
Avocados, 20–27, 285

B

Bacteria. *See also* Food poisoning; Infection
    E. coli in bagged lettuce, 251
    H. pylori. See Ulcers
    Lactobacillus acidophilus in yogurt, 484–485, 486
    on produce. *See* Washing produce
    and salmon, 198–199
    salmonella, 108, 144, 182, 184, 186
    Vibrio vulnificus in shellfish, 411
    yogurt and canker sores, 484
Bad breath, 190, 209, 321, 322
Baked Brussels Sprouts, 95
Baked Pear-fection, 345
Banana Breakfast Danish, 32
Banana-Peanut "Pudding," 31
Bananas, 28–32, 439
Barley, 33–36
Barley-Feta Toss, 36

Basil, 37–40
　in Basil Balsamic Vinaigrette, 106
　in Cherry Pork Wrap, 142
　in Family-Party Pesto, 299
　in Five-Ingredient Cucumber Toss, 176
　in Grilled Salmon Primavera, 201
　in Mom's Garlic Pasta, 210
　in One-Minute Avocado Spread, 26
　in Pasta Chiller, 390
　with peppers, 60
　in Super Summer Quesadillas, 167
　in Tuscan Tomato-Basil Spread, 305
Basil Balsamic Vinaigrette, 106
Beans, dried, 41–46. *See also* Lentils
　chickpeas, 349
　　with curry powder, 179
　　hummus, 42–43, 119, 349, 477, 493
　　roasted, 43
　　Whole Wheat Pita Wedges with Home-
　　　made Hummus, 477, 493
　in Southwestern Sprout Wrap, 85
Beans, green, 46, 223–226
Beef, 47–53, 149, 339
Beef Stir-Fry, 53
Beer, 480
Beets, 54–57, 315
Bell peppers, 58–62
　in All-Occasion Vegetable Platter, 122
　in Aunt Shirley's Three-Bean Salad, 46
　in Barley-Feta Toss, 36
　in Beef Stir-Fry, 53
　in Bok Choy and Rice Noodles, 75
　in Broccoli-Cauliflower Wreath, 121
　in flavored pasta, 325
　in Grilled Salmon Primavera, 201
　in Guilt-Free Grilled Cheese, 137
　in Healthy Hot Pockets, 90
　in Holiday Green Beans, 226
　in Italian Braised Celery, 126
　in Last-Minute Pasta Salad, 331
　in Oriental Chicken Salad, 375
　in pasta sauce, 25
　with quinoa, 383, 386
　in Quinoa Pilaf, 386
　in Super Summer Quesadillas, 167
　in Wheatberries 'n Veggies, 467
Berries. *See* Blackberries; Blueberries; Cranberries;
　　Raspberries; Strawberries

Berry-Good Muffins, 105
Beverages
　with cinnamon, 161
　citrus, 218
　juice
　　cherry, 141
　　cranberry, 170, 171
　　grape, 219, 221
　　orange, 313, 487, 491
　　pomegranate, 361
　with papaya, 319
　slushes
　　cantaloupe, 109
　　chocolate, 159, 493
　　watermelon, 461, 491
　smoothies
　　blueberry, 71, 493
　　cherry, 141
　　grape, 222, 492
　　kiwifruit strawberry, 242
　　peanut butter, 337
　　with seeds, 405
　　strawberry, 435, 487
　　with yogurt, 487
　wine cooler, 479, 482
Birth defects
　asparagus, 16, 18
　beans, 41, 44
　brussels sprouts, 91, 94
　cauliflower, 117, 120
　kiwifruit, 240, 243
　lentils, 245, 246
　lettuce, 249, 252
　oranges, 311, 314
　pasta, 325, 328
　strawberries, 434, 436–437
　wheat germ, 468, 470–471
Blackberries, 63–67, 138
Blackberry Cheese Dip, 138
Blackberry-Peach Crisp, 67, 493
Blindness. *See* Age-related macular degeneration;
　　Cataracts
Bloating, 37, 39, 162, 317. *See also* Lactose intoler-
　　ance
Blueberries, 65, 68–71, 131, 171, 399
Blueberry Breeze, 71, 493
Bok choy, 72–75, 97
Bok Choy and Rice Noodles, 75

Bones
 basil, 37, 39
 bok choy, 72, 74
 broccoli, 76, 78
 brussels sprouts, 91, 93–94
 cabbage, 96-99
 cantaloupe, 107, 110
 carrots, 112, 114–115
 cheese, 132, 134
 cherries, 139
 eggs, 181, 185
 greens, 227, 229
 kale, 235, 238
 milk, 266, 267, 269, 271
 nuts, 286, 290
 okra, 292
 onions, 306
 oranges, 311, 312
 parsley, 321, 322
 pork, 363, 365
 potatoes, 368, 370
 seeds, 404, 406
 shellfish, 409, 410, 412
 soy, 415, 420
 squash, 429, 432
 tea, 443, 447
 wheat germ, 468, 471
 wine, 478, 481
 yogurt, 484, 488
Bowel movements. *See* Regularity
Brain development in infants, 181–183, 196, 200,
  202, 205
Brain function, 181, 183, 185, 478, 480
BRAT diet, 3
Bread
 with figs, 193
 with flax, 204, 206
 with garlic, 209
 whole wheat, 473–477
Breakfast foods. *See also* Cereal
 banana Danish, 32
 cinnamon toast, 161
 french toast, 394
 with mangoes, 257
 muffins
  berry, 105
  with cherries, 141
  cranberry, 172, 493
   with figs, 193
   with flaxseeds, 204
   with wheat germ, 469
 omelettes, 153
 pancakes and waffles
  with apricots, 10, 492
  with blackberries, 64
  with kiwifruit, 242
  with nectarines, 284
  with poached egg, 184
  with raisins, 393
  with sweet potatoes, 440
  with yogurt, 487
 parfait, 399, 492
 with pineapple, 355
 with quinoa, 385
Breakfast menus, 490–494
Brie-Stuffed Figs, 195
Broccoli, 76–80, 98
 in All-Occasion Vegetable Platter, 122
 in Broccoli-Cauliflower Wreath, 121
 in Five-Minute Asian Slaw, 100
 in Oriental Chicken Salad, 375
 in Pasta Primavera Marinara, 62
 in Stressful-Day Stir-Fry, 423
Broccoli-Cauliflower Wreath, 121
Broccoli sprouts, 81–85
Bruschetta, 60
Brussels sprouts, 91–95
Burns, 306, 307

C

Cabbage, 96–100
Callus softening, 356
Cancer
 apples, 1, 3
 apricots, 5, 8
 artichokes, 11, 13
 avocados, 20, 21–22
 bananas, 28, 31
 basil, 37, 39
 beans, 41, 42
 beef, 47, 49, 52
 beets, 54, 55
 bell peppers, 58
 blackberries, 63, 65, 66
 blueberries, 68, 70
 bok choy, 72, 74

Cancer *(Continued)*
  broccoli, 76, 78, 81, 84, 98
  broccoli sprouts, 81, 82, 84
  brussels sprouts, 91, 93
  cabbage, 96, 97–98
  canola oil, 101, 103
  cantaloupe, 107, 110
  carrots, 112, 114
  cauliflower, 117–118
  cheese, 132, 136
  cherries, 139, 140
  chiles, 150
  chives, 152
  corn, 164, 166
  cranberries, 168, 171
  cruciferous vegetables, 78, 79, 81–82
  cucumbers, 173, 174
  curry powder, 177, 178
  fennel, 188
  figs, 192, 194
  flaxseeds, 202, 205
  garlic, 207–208
  ginger, 211, 212
  grapefruit, 215, 216
  grapes, 219
  green beans, 223, 225
  greens, 227, 229
  horseradish, 231, 232
  kale, 235, 236
  kiwifruit, 240, 241
  lentils, 245
  lettuce, 249
  mangoes, 255, 258
  milk, 266
  mint, 272, 273
  mushrooms, 277, 281
  nectarines, 282, 283
  okra, 292, 294
  olive oil, 295, 298
  olives, 300, 301
  onions, 306, 308
  oranges, 311, 312
  papaya, 316, 317
  parsley, 321, 322
  peaches, 332, 334
  peanut butter, 336, 338
  pears, 341, 344
  pineapple, 353, 354, 355–356
  pomegranates, 358, 359
  prunes, 372
  pumpkin, 376, 377
  quinoa, 382, 384
  radishes, 387–389
  raisins, 391, 392
  raspberries, 395–398
  rosemary, 400, 401
  shellfish, 409, 412–413
  soy, 415, 420–421
  spinach, 424, 428
  squash, 429, 431
  strawberries, 434, 436
  sweet potatoes, 438, 439
  tea, 443, 444, 445–446
  tomatoes, 448–449
  watermelon, 457, 458–460
  whole wheat bread, 473, 476
  wine, 478, 480
  yogurt, 484, 485, 488
Canker sores, 484
Canola oil, 101–106, 197, 381
Cantaloupe, 107–111, 357
Cardiovascular function, 219, 221
Carrots, 112–116, 439
  in All-Occasion Vegetable Platter, 122
  in Bok Choy and Rice Noodles, 75
  in Five-Minute Asian Slaw, 100
  in Grandma's Old-World Chicken Soup, 147
  in Healthy Hot Pockets, 90
  in One-Dish Fennel Pork, 191
  in Oriental Chicken Salad, 375
  in Pasta Primavera Marinara, 62
  in Quinoa Pilaf, 386
  in slaw, 113
  in Stressful-Day Stir-Fry, 423
  in Tuna Tucks, 234
Cataracts
  kiwifruit, 240, 241
  onions, 306, 307
  spinach, 424, 425
  tea, 443, 447
Cauliflower, 117–122
Celery, 123–126
  in All-Occasion Vegetable Platter, 122
  in Egg Salad Sandwich, 187
  in Grandma's Old-World Chicken Soup,
    147

in Terrific Turkey Salad Sandwiches, 456
in Waldorf Wrap, 346
in Wheatberries 'n Veggies, 467
Cellular repair, 215–216
Cereal, 127–131. *See also* Breakfast foods
with chocolate chips, 158
with cinnamon, 161
with figs, 193
with nuts, 287
quinoa, 385
with raisins, 393
with raspberries, 398
with seeds, 405
soy, 416
wheatberry, 465
with wheat germ, 469
Cheery Chocolate Slush, 159, 493
Cheese, 132–138
brie, in Brie-Stuffed Figs, 195
calcium quotients, 135
cheddar, in Super Summer Quesadillas, 167
cottage
in Chive Baked Potatoes, 154
in fruit salad, 109
and watermelon, 459
fat-free, in roasted red pepper dip, 60
feta
in Barley-Feta Toss, 36
in Five-Ingredient Cucumber Toss, 176
with green beans, 224
in Mediterranean Salad, 27
in Strawberry-Spinach Salad, 437
in Last-Minute Pasta Salad, 331
in My Mother-in-Law's Lasagna, 330–331
Parmesan
in Baked Brussels Sprouts, 95
in Family-Party Pesto, 299
in Grilled Salmon Primavera, 201
in Lentil-Stuffed Mushrooms, 248
in Mom's Garlic Pasta, 210
in Pasta Primavera Marinara, 62
in Tomato-Basil Summer Salad, 40
ricotta
in Banana Breakfast Danish, 32
in Wild Creamy Mushroom Soup, 281
Chemoprotection, 82
Cherries, 139–142
Cherry Pork Wrap, 142

Chicken, 143–147
with barley, 35
in Chicken Kiwi, 244
in Crunchy Salsa Chicken, 472
with garlic, 209
in Michael's Rosemary Chicken, 403
with mint sauce, 275
in Oriental Chicken Salad, 375
in Sesame Chicken with Whole Wheat Linguine, 408
Chicken Kiwi, 244
Chiles, 148–151
Chile Shrimp and Melon Salad, 151
Chill-a-Melon Soup, 111, 493
Chilly Beet Soup, 57, 494
Chive Baked Potatoes, 154
Chives, 152–154
Chocolate, 155–159
Chocolate Raspberry Thumbprint Cookies, 264–265
Chunky Fresh Applesauce, 4, 491
Cinnamon Acorn Squash, 163
Cinnamon-Raisin French Toast, 394
Circulation, 311
Cleaning fruits and vegetables. *See specific foods*
Colds. *See also* Stuffy nose
bell peppers, 58, 59
cauliflower, 120
chicken, 143, 146
garlic, 208
shellfish, 410
tea, 445
Collard. *See* Greens
Colleen's Famous Gingerbread, 214, 492
Constipation. *See* Regularity
Cooking tips. *See specific foods*
Cookout Citrus Splash, 218
Corn, 164–167, 179
Cozy Quinoa Breakfast, 385
Crab-Stuffed Papaya, 320, 492
Cranberries, 168–172, 264–265, 367, 456
Cranberry Muffins, 172, 493
Cruciferous vegetables, 78, 79, 81–82, 93, 118, 314
See also Bok choy; Broccoli; Brussels sprouts; Cabbage; Cauliflower; Kale; Radishes
Crunchy Salsa Chicken, 472
Cucumber, 173–176, 187, 467

Curry powder, 177–180
Curry Rice Pilaf, 180
Cuts. *See* Wound healing

D

Dehydration. *See* Hydration
Depression, 52, 196, 200
Desserts
   blackberry peach crisp, 67, 493
   with blueberries, 69
   cheese for, 133
   with chocolate, 158
   chocolate-dipped fruit, 158
   chocolate raspberry cookies, 264–265
   with flaxseeds, 204
   frozen yogurt, 485
   gingerbread, 214, 492
   with mangoes, 257, 259
   in menus, 491, 493, 494
   with nectarines, 284
   peach trifle, 335
   piecrust, 381, 469
   prune topping, 373
   pudding
      banana-peanut, 31
      with blackberries, 64
      with cinnamon, 161
      pumpkin custard, 380
      vanilla soy, 422, 494
   pumpkin pie, 376–377, 380–381
   with raspberries, 397
   with yogurt, 485, 487
Diabetes
   apples, 1, 4
   barley, 33, 34
   beans, 41, 44–45
   beets, 54, 55–56
   brown rice, 86, 89
   cereal, 127, 129–131
   curry powder, 177, 178
   kiwifruit, 240, 241
   onions, 306, 310
   peas, 347, 351
   quinoa, 382, 384
   turkey, 453
   wheatberries, 462, 464
   whole wheat bread, 473, 476
   wine, 478, 481

Diarrhea, 3, 4, 11, 14, 108, 484, 485
Dietary Approaches to Stop Hypertension
     (DASH), 124, 269, 288
Digestion
   artichokes, 11
   blueberries, 70
   curry powder, 177, 178
   ginger, 211
   mangoes, 255, 258
   mint, 272, 273
   papaya, 317
   pineapple, 353, 356
   yogurt, 484, 486
A Dilly of a Dip, 489
Dinner menus, 490–494
Dips
   blackberry cheese, 138
   with chives, 153
   with curry powder, 179
   gazpacho, 15
   with olive oil, 296
   with peppers, 60
   with soy, 418
   yogurt and dill, 489
Diverticulosis, 462, 463
Dizziness, 401
Dreamy Vanilla Pudding, 422, 494
Dry hair, 20, 21
Dry nails, 295, 297
Dye, from beets, 55

E

Early Peas in Lettuce Cups, 352
Eggs, 153, 181–187
Egg Salad Sandwich, 187, 491
Energy
   bananas, 28, 29
   beans, 41
   beef, 47
   chicken, 143
   mint, 273
   pasta, 325, 328–329
   peas, 347, 351
   potatoes, 368, 370
   prunes, 372, 374
   raisins, 391, 392
   turkey, 453, 455
   watermelon, 457, 460

Enzyme activity, 358, 359
Escherichia coli. See under bacteria
Estrogen and cancer, 118, 205, 420–421
Exercise performance, 272, 273
Eyes, puffy, 173, 174. *See also* Vision

F

Fajitas, 364
Fall Fruit Salad, 276
Family-Party Pesto, 299
Fatigue. *See* Energy
Fats
    in butter, 154
    in various fish, 197
    in various margarines, 262
    in various milks, 269
    in various oils, 103
    in various pork cuts, 366
    in various spreads, 23
Fennel, 188–191
Fibroids, 424, 428
Figs, 192–195
Fish. *See under* Seafood
Five-Ingredient Cucumber Toss, 176
Five-Minute Asian Slaw, 100, 492
Flatulence. *See* Bloating
Flax Prairie Bread, 206
Flaxseeds and flax oil, 197, 202–206
Food poisoning
    from bagged lettuce, 251
    cinnamon, 160, 162
    horseradish, 231, 232
    rosemary, 400, 401
    from shellfish, 411
Foods *vs.* pills, 115, 208, 441
Fruit, dried, 7, 171, 372–375. *See also* Raisins

G

Gallstones, 311, 312
Garlic, 207–210
    in Basil Balsamic Vinaigrette, 106
    in Beef Stir-Fry, 53
    in Bok Choy and Rice Noodles, 75
    in Chile Shrimp and Melon Salad, 151
    in Garlic Crisp Potatoes, 371, 492
    in Ginger Butternut Soup, 433
    in Grilled Salmon Primavera, 201
    in Healthy Hot Pockets, 90

    in Holiday Green Beans, 226
    in hummus, 42–43, 349, 477
    in Indian-Style Greens, 230
    in Italian Braised Celery, 126
    in Pasta Primavera Marinara, 62
    in Quinoa Pilaf, 386
    in roasted red pepper dip, 60
    in Simple Stir-Fried Broccoli, 80
    in Summertime Okra, 294
    in Super Summer Quesadillas, 167
    in Tapenade, 304
    in Thai Beef Salad, 339
    in Tropical Marinade, 366
Garlic Crisp Potatoes, 371, 492
Gazpacho Dip, 15
Ginger, 53, 142, 211–214, 230, 339, 433, 491
Ginger Butternut Soup, 433, 491
Grains
    barley, 35
    brown rice pita pockets, 90
    cereal, 127–131, 161
    with olives, 303
    quinoa, 382–386, 494
    quinoa pilaf, 386, 494
    tabbouleh with parsley, 323
    wheatberries, 462–467
    wheat germ, 468–472, 476
    whole wheat bread, 473–477
Grandma's Old-World Chicken Soup, 147
Grapefruit, 215–218
Grapes, 219–222, 324, 428
"Gravies." *See* Sauces
Greens, 74, 197, 227–230
    with figs, 193
    in Mediterranean Salad, 27
    in Pomegranate, Clementine, and Kiwi Salad, 362
    spinach, 424–428
Grilled Salmon Primavera, 201, 493
Guilt-Free Grilled Cheese, 137

H

Hair, dry, 20, 21
Hazelnut Asparagus Salad, 19, 492
Healthy eating, cinnamon to promote, 160
Healthy Hot Pockets, 90
Heartburn, 177, 178, 274

Heart disease
  apples, 1
  apricots, 5, 9
  artichokes, 11, 13
  asparagus, 16, 18
  avocados, 20, 21–22
  bananas, 28, 29
  barley, 33–34
  beans, 41, 42–43, 44
  beef, 47–48, 52
  beets, 54, 55
  bell peppers, 58
  blackberries, 63, 65
  blueberries, 68
  broccoli, 76, 78
  brown rice, 86, 88, 89
  brussels sprouts, 91, 93, 94
  cabbage, 96
  canola oil, 101–102, 103
  cauliflower, 117, 120
  cereal, 127–128
  cherries, 139, 140
  chicken, 143, 144–145
  chiles, 148, 150
  chives, 152
  chocolate, 155, 156–157
  cinnamon, 160, 162
  cranberries, 168
  cucumbers, 173
  eggs, 181, 182, 185–186
  fennel, 190
  figs, 192, 194
  flaxseeds, 202, 203, 205
  garlic, 207, 208
  ginger, 211, 212
  grapefruit, 215, 216-217
  grapes, 219, 221
  green beans, 223, 225
  greens, 227, 229
  horseradish, 231, 232
  kale, 235, 236–238
  kiwifruit, 240, 241, 243
  lentils, 245, 247
  lettuce, 249, 252
  mangoes, 255, 258
  margarine, 260–261, 263
  nuts, 286, 288
  olive oil, 295, 297
  olives, 300, 301
  onions, 306, 307
  oranges, 311, 314
  papaya, 316, 318–320
  parsley, 321, 322
  pasta, 325, 328
  peaches, 332
  peanut butter, 336, 338
  pears, 341, 344
  pineapple, 353, 354
  pomegranates, 358, 359
  pork, 363
  prunes, 372, 374
  pumpkin, 376, 377
  quinoa, 382, 384
  raisins, 391
  raspberries, 395, 398
  rosemary, 400
  salmon, 196, 197, 200
  seeds, 404, 406
  shellfish, 409, 410
  soy, 415, 418–419, 420
  squash, 429, 431
  strawberries, 434, 436
  sweet potatoes, 438, 439
  tea, 443, 446
  tomatoes, 448, 449
  turkey, 453
  watermelon, 457, 460
  wheatberries, 462, 464
  wheat germ, 468, 470, 471
  whole wheat bread, 473
  wine, 478, 480
Hearty Purple Cow, 222, 492
Heat tolerance, 249
Hemorrhoids, 462, 463
Herbs. *See also* Spices
  basil, 37–40
  chives, 152–154
  garlic, 207–210
  horseradish, 231–234
  mint, 272–276
  rosemary, 195, 400–403
High blood pressure
  apricots, 5, 9
  bananas, 28
  barley, 33–34
  bok choy, 72, 74
  brussels sprouts, 93

celery, 123, 124
cereal, 127, 128
figs, 192, 194
milk, 266, 269–270
mushrooms, 277, 281
nuts, 286, 288, 290
olive oil, 295, 297
papaya, 316, 318–319
pork, 363, 365
potatoes, 368
pumpkin, 376
salmon, 196, 197, 200
squash, 429, 432
watermelon, 457, 460
yogurt, 484, 488
High cholesterol
    apples, 1, 4
    apricots, 5, 9
    artichokes, 11, 13
    avocados, 20, 21
    barley, 33–34
    beans, 41, 42–43, 44
    beef, 52
    blackberries, 63, 65
    canola oil, 101–102
    cereal, 127–128
    chicken, 143, 144
    chives, 152
    figs, 192, 194
    garlic, 207, 208
    grapefruit, 215, 216–217
    lentils, 245
    margarine, 260–261, 263
    oranges, 311, 312
    parsley, 321, 322
    peanut butter, 336, 338
    pears, 341, 344
    peas, 347
    pork, 363
    prunes, 372, 374
    raspberries, 395, 398
    soy, 415, 418
    tomatoes, 448, 449
    watermelon, 457, 460
    wheat germ, 468, 470
High-risk populations, 186
Hives, 128
Holiday Green Beans, 226
Horseradish, 231–234

Hot flashes, 415, 419–420
Hummus, 42–43, 119, 349, 477, 493
Hydration, 123, 124, 173, 174, 457, 460
Hypertension. *See* High blood pressure
Hypoglycemia, 181, 183

I

Immune function
    apricots, 5, 8
    artichokes, 14
    asparagus, 16, 18
    beef, 47, 49
    bell peppers, 59
    broccoli sprouts, 81
    brussels sprouts, 91
    canola oil, 101, 103
    cantaloupe, 107, 110
    carrots, 112
    cauliflower, 117, 120
    and chemoprotection, 82
    chicken, 143, 146
    chives, 152
    curry powder, 177
    eggs, 181, 184, 185
    garlic, 207, 208
    kiwifruit, 240, 243
    lettuce, 249, 250
    mushrooms, 277, 281
    nectarines, 282, 283
    okra, 292
    oranges, 311
    papaya, 316, 317
    peaches, 332, 334
    pineapple, 353, 354
    pork, 363
    pumpkin, 376, 377
    quinoa, 382, 384
    seeds, 404, 407
    shellfish, 409, 410, 413
    squash, 429, 431–432
    sweet potatoes, 438, 439
    tea, 443, 445, 447
    turkey, 453, 455
    yogurt, 484, 488
Indian-Style Greens, 230
Infants and children. *See* Birth defects; Brain development in infants; Vision development in infants

Infection
    apricots, 5, 8
    basil, 37, 39
    beef, 49
    blueberries, 68, 70
    cranberries, 168, 170
    garlic, 208
    ginger, 211
    onions, 306, 307
    peaches, 334
    pumpkin, 377
    sinusitis, 334
    sweet potatoes, 438, 439
    tea, 447
    turkey, 453
    urinary tract, 68, 70, 168, 170
    wine, 478
    yeast, 5, 8, 438, 439, 484, 485
    yogurt, 484, 485
Inflammation, 37, 39, 188, 190, 211, 212
Insulin sensitivity, 127, 129–131
Irregular heartbeat, 196, 197, 200, 457, 460
Italian Braised Celery, 126, 491

K

Kale, 235–239. *See also* Greens
Kebabs, fruit, 193, 220
Kidney stones, 28, 29
Kiwifruit, 240–244, 362

L

Lactose intolerance, 156, 267
Last-Minute Pasta Salad, 331
Leg cramps, 438, 439
Lentils, 245–248
Lentil-Stuffed Mushrooms, 248
Lettuce, 249–254, 305
Longevity, 155, 156, 473
Lunch menus, 490–494

M

Mangoes, 255–259, 357, 447
Mango Iced Tea, 447, 492
Mango Pops, 259
Margarine, 260–265
Marinade, 213, 257, 366, 397
Mediterranean Radicchio Topping, 305
Mediterranean Salad, 27, 493
Melons, 107–111, 151, 324, 357, 457–461

Memory
    beans, 41, 45
    beef, 49
    blueberries, 68, 70
    eggs, 181, 182–183, 185
    raisins, 391, 392
    spinach, 424, 426–427
    strawberries, 434, 436
Menopausal symptoms, 415, 419–420
Menstrual pain, 196, 200
Menstrual regularity, 196, 200
Menus, 490–494
Mesquite Onion Bloom, 310
Metabolism, 277, 280, 446
Michael's Rosemary Chicken, 403, 491
Milk, 71, 109, 131, 159, 259, 266–271. *See also* Soy
        milk
Minerals. *See specific foods*
Mint, 272–276, 357
Miso. *See* Soy
Mom's Garlic Pasta, 210
Mood
    chiles, 148, 150
    chocolate, 155, 157
    garlic, 207, 210
    pasta, 325, 328
    potatoes, 368, 370
    prunes, 372
    turkey, 453
Morning sickness, 219, 221, 460
Motion sickness, 300
Muffins. *See under* Breakfast foods
Muscle cramps, 13. *See also* Leg Cramps
Mushrooms, 35, 90, 248, 277–281
Mustard. *See* Greens
My Mother-in-Law's Lasagna, 330–331

N

Nachos, 42
Nails, dry, 295, 297
Nausea, 211, 212, 219, 221, 272, 273, 300,
        460
Nectarines, 282–285
"Negative calories," 123
Night blindness, 424, 425, 432
No-Fail Kale, 239, 494
Nutritional data. *See specific foods*
Nuts, 286–291
    hazelnuts, 19

peanut butter, 31, 336–340
peanuts, 7, 100
pecans, 172
pine, 95, 299, 428
in trail mix, 7
walnuts, 4, 32, 163, 197
Nuts Among the Berries, 291, 491

O

Oats, 67, 105, 127–128, 129, 130, 131
Oils, amount and types of fat in, 103. *See also*
　　　　Canola oil; Olive oil
Okra, 292–294
Olive oil, 101, 103, 295–299, 427
Olives, 27, 40, 300–305, 467
One-Dish Fennel Pork, 191
One-Minute Avocado Spread, 23, 26
Onion, 306–310
　　in Aunt Shirley's Three-Bean Salad, 46
　　in Barley-Feta Toss, 36
　　in Bok Choy and Rice Noodles, 75
　　in Ginger Butternut Soup, 433
　　in Grandma's Old-World Chicken Soup, 147
　　in Healthy Hot Pockets, 90
　　in Indian-Style Greens, 230
　　in Quinoa Pilaf, 386
　　in Southwestern Sprout Wrap, 85
　　in Strawberry-Spinach Salad, 437
　　in Stressful-Day Stir-Fry, 423
　　in Super Summer Quesadillas, 167
　　in Terrific Turkey Salad Sandwiches, 456
　　in Thai Beef Salad, 339
　　in Tuna Tucks, 234
Orange juice, 218, 366, 439, 487
Oranges, 311–315, 362, 472
Oranges to Beet the Band, 315
Oriental Chicken Salad, 375
Osteoporosis. *See* Bones
Oven-Roasted Tomatoes, 452
Overeating, 409, 412

P

Pain management, 139, 140, 148, 150, 196, 200
Pancakes. *See under* Breakfast foods
Papaya, 316–320, 408
Parsley, 147, 154, 321–324
Pasta, 325–331. *See also* Pasta sauce
　　with chicken, 145
　　garlic pasta, 210

with greens, 228, 237
lasagna, 330–331
with melon, grapes, and parsley, 324,
　　492
salads, 109, 175, 199, 331, 390
salmon primavera, 201, 493
sesame chicken with linguine, 408
Pasta Chiller, 390
Pasta Primavera Marinara, 62, 493
Pasta sauce
　　with avocado, 25
　　with broccoli, 62, 77, 493
　　with cabbage, 99
　　marinara, 62, 493
Patriotic Breakfast Parfait, 399, 492
Peaches, 67, 332–335
Peach Trifle, 335
Pears, 341–346
Peas, 347–352
Peppers. *See* Bell peppers; Chiles
Perfect Red Salad, 254, 491
Pesticides. *See* Washing produce
Pesto, 275, 299
Piecrust, 381, 469
Pills *vs.* whole food, 115, 208, 441
Pineapple, 259, 353–357
Pizza, 145, 149, 199, 247, 303
Poison ivy, 266
Pomegranate, Clementine, and Kiwi Salad,
　　362
Pomegranates, 358–362
Pork, 142, 191, 363–367, 373
Portions, 329, 421
Potatoes, 154, 191, 247, 368–371. *See also* Sweet
　　potatoes
Premenstrual syndrome
　　bananas, 28, 29
　　cheese, 132, 136
　　milk, 266, 270
　　pasta, 328
Preparation. *See specific foods*
Prunes, 372–375
Pumpkin, 376–381

Q

Quesadillas, 167, 454, 493
Quick Bouillabaisse, 414
Quinoa, 382–386, 494
Quinoa Pilaf, 386, 494

R

Radishes, 387–390
Raisins, 372, 391–394
    in barley pilaf, 35
    in Chunky Fresh Applesauce, 4
    in Curry Rice Pilaf, 180
    in trail mix, 7, 405
Raspberries, 65, 105, 264–265, 291, 395–399
Regularity
    apples, 1, 3-4
    artichokes, 11, 13–14
    barley, 33, 34
    beets, 54, 57
    blackberries, 63, 66
    cereal, 127
    figs, 192, 194
    flaxseeds, 202, 205
    lentils, 245, 247
    lettuce, 249, 253
    nectarines, 282
    pears, 341, 344
    peas, 347, 350
    prunes, 372, 374
    quinoa, 382, 384
    raisins, 391, 392
    raspberries, 395, 398, 399
    strawberries, 434
    wheatberries, 462, 463
    whole wheat bread, 473, 476
Relaxation, 400, 401
Replacements. *See* Substitutions
Rheumatoid arthritis, 101, 103, 196, 200
Rice
    brown, 86–90, 142, 423
    with cranberries, 169
    in Curry Rice Pilaf, 180
    salad, 487
    white, 86, 88, 89, 169, 180
    wild, 169
Rosemary, 195, 400–403

S

Salad dressings
    with apricots, 7
    for barley salad, 36
    basil with canola oil, 106
    on corn, 165
    powdered, on baked potatoes, 369
    soy sauce, walnut oil, and honey, 19
Salads
    barley, 36
    with blueberries, 69
    with bok choy, 73
    with broccoli sprouts, 83
    with cantaloupe, 109
    chicken, 375
    cucumber, tomato, and feta cheese, 176
    egg, 187, 491
    with eggs, 184, 187, 491
    with fennel, 189
    fruit, 276, 355, 357, 405
    with garlic chives, 153
    with grapefruit, 217
    with grapes, 220
    green bean, 224
    ham and watermelon, 459
    hazelnut asparagus, 19, 492
    with lentils, 247
    Mediterranean, 27, 493
    with mint, 275
    with nuts, 287
    with olives, 303
    orange and beet, 315
    with oranges, 313, 315, 362
    pasta, 109, 175, 199, 331, 390
    with pears, 343
    pineapple, 355, 357
    pomegranate, clementine, and kiwi, 362
    with raspberries, 397
    red, 254, 491
    rice and yogurt, 487
    shrimp and melon, 151
    slaw, 99, 100, 113, 389, 492
    with strawberries, 435, 437
    strawberry-spinach, 437
    three-bean, 46, 493
    tomato-basil, 40
    with tomatoes, 40, 176, 450
    turkey, 456, 494
    types of "greens," 250, 252
    wheatberries and veggies, 465, 467, 493
    with wheat germ, 469
Salmon. *See under* Seafood

Salmonella. *See under* Bacteria
Salmon Poached in Red Wine, 483
Salmon with Nectarines, 285
Salsa
    with apricots, 7
    with avocado, 25
    with corn, 165
    in Crunchy Salsa Chicken, 472
    with nectarines, 284
    with potatoes, 369
    in Super Summer Quesadillas, 167
Sandwiches and wraps
    with broccoli sprouts, 83
    cherry pork, 142
    with cucumbers, 175
    egg salad, 187
    fajitas, 364
    grilled cheese, 137
    with lettuce, 251
    with olives, 303
    onion and portobello mushroom, 309
    with peanut butter, 220, 337
    with pineapple, 355
    pita pockets, 90, 234, 427, 474, 492
    quesadillas, 167, 454
    with radishes, 389
    southwestern sprout, 85, 491
    soy burgers, 417–419
    with spinach, 427
    tuna, 199, 234, 492
    turkey salad, 456, 494
    Waldorf, 346
Sauces
    carrot "gravy," 113
    cucumber, 175
    horseradish, 233
    kiwifruit, 242
    to match pasta shape, 327
    mint, 275
    with mushrooms, 279
    papaya, 319
    peanut, 340
    pesto, 275, 299
    pumpkin "gravy," 379
    squash "gravy," 430
    with vegetables, 327
    white, 271
Sauerkraut, 97, 99, 191

Seafood
    with grapefruit juice, 217
    salmon, 102, 196–201, 279, 285, 369, 483
    shellfish, 151, 319, 320, 409–414, 492
    sushi, 199, 411
    tuna, 199, 234, 492
Seeds, 404–408
    fennel, 188, 189, 190
    flaxseeds, 197, 202–206
    pomegranate, 358–362
    toasting, 406
Serving sizes, 329, 421
Shellfish. *See under* Seafood
Shopping and serving tips. *See specific foods*
Simple Stir-Fried Broccoli, 80
Simply Sweet Potatoes, 265
Sinusitis, 334
Skin, 52
    artichokes for, 13
    cantaloupe for, 107, 110
    jaundice, 115
    oranges for, 115
    squash for, 431, 432
    sunburn, 431, 432
    wrinkles, 68, 311, 312, 400–401
Smelling salts, 401
Smoking, 58–59, 82, 114
"S'Mores Yogurt," 487
Snacks
    with apricots, 7, 405
    with beans, 42, 43, 477, 493
    with chocolate, 158
    with curry powder, 179
    with fish, 199
    ice pops, 259, 459
    in menus, 491, 492, 493, 494
    with nuts, 287
    with peanut butter, 158, 337
    pita wedges with hummus, 477, 493
    with seeds, 7, 405
    with sweet potatoes, 440
    trail mix, 7, 405
    with wheatberries, 465
Snow peas, 348–350. *See also* Peas
Soups
    beet, 57, 494
    with bok choy, 73
    bouillabaisse, 414

Soups *(Continued)*
  with broccoli sprouts, 83
  cantaloupe, 111, 493
  with cauliflower, 119
  with celery, 125
  chicken, 146, 147
  with chiles, 149
  with fish, 199
  with ginger, 213, 433, 491
  ginger butternut, 433, 491
  with kale, 237
  mushroom, 281, 492
  with okra, 293
  onion, 309
  with pumpkin, 379
  with quinoa, 383
  with spinach, 427
  with squash, 430
  with wheatberries, 465
Southwestern Sprout Wrap, 85, 491
Soy, 131, 291, 415–423
Soy milk, 131, 291
Sparkling Red Wine Cooler, 482
Spices. *See also* Herbs
  cinnamon, 160–163
  curry powder, 177–180
  ginger, 211–214
Spicy Peanut Sauce, 340
Spicy Pumpkin Custard/Pie Filling, 380
Spinach, 184, 325, 424–428, 437. *See also* Greens
Spinach Pignoli, 428, 493
Spreads
  with avocado, 23, 26
  with cranberry sauce, 169
  with garlic, 209
  with goat cheese, 133
  with horseradish, 233
  hummus, 42–43, 119, 349, 477, 493
  with prunes, 373
  with raspberry, 397
  tapenade, 303, 304
  tomato-basil, 305
Sprouts, broccoli, 81–85
Squash, 161, 163, 429–433
Stir fry
  beef, 53
  with bok choy, 73, 75
  broccoli, 80

cabbage, 99
  with canola oil, 104
  with ginger, 213
  with okra, 293
  with radishes, 389
  with snow peas, 349
  tofu and vegetable, 423, 492
Stomachache. *See* Digestion
Storage tips. *See specific foods*
Strawberries, 65, 156, 434–437
  in Chill-a-Melon Soup, 111
  in Peach Trifle, 335
  in smoothies, 242
  in Tropical Fruit Salad, 357
Strawberry-Spinach Salad, 437
Stressful-Day Stir-Fry, 423, 492
Stroke
  apples, 1, 3
  apricots, 5, 9
  bananas, 28, 29
  brussels sprouts, 91, 93
  cabbage, 96
  canola oil, 101, 103
  cauliflower, 117, 118, 120
  chiles, 150
  eggs, 181, 182, 185, 186
  figs, 192, 194
  ginger, 211, 212
  grapefruit, 215, 216
  kiwifruit, 240, 241
  nuts, 286, 288
  onions, 306, 307
  oranges, 311, 314
  pumpkin, 376
  quinoa, 382, 384
  salmon, 196, 197, 200
  squash, 429, 432
  tea, 443, 446
  watermelon, 457, 460
  wheat germ, 468, 470
  wine, 478
Stuffy nose, 148, 150, 177, 213, 231, 232. *See also* Colds
Substitutions
  canola oil for butter or shortening, 104
  flaxseeds for eggs, 203
  flaxseeds for oil, 204
  mangoes for peaches, 257

parsley for basil, 323
prune puree for butter or oil, 373
raisins for chocolate chips, 393
sweet potatoes for white potatoes, 440
turkey for chicken or beef, 454
yogurt for mayonnaise or sour cream, 487
Sugar Baby Carrots, 116
Summertime Okra, 294
Super Summer Pasta, 324, 492
Super Summer Quesadillas, 167, 493
Sweet potatoes, 147, 265, 438–442
Sweet Potato Fries, 442, 491

T

Tacos, 145
Tahini, 407
Tapenade, 303, 304
Tea, 443–447
    basil, 39
    ginger, 212
    how to brew, 446
    iced, 444, 446, 447
    mango, 447
    mint, 275
Teeth, 132, 136, 311, 312, 443, 447
Tempeh. *See* Soy
Terrific Turkey Salad Sandwiches, 456, 494
Thai Beef Salad, 339
Tofu. *See* Soy
Tomato-Basil Summer Salad, 40
Tomatoes, 448–452
    in Artichoke Appetizer with Fresh Gazpacho
        Dip, 15
    in Barley-Feta Toss, 36
    in Five-Ingredient Cucumber Toss, 176
    in flavored pasta, 325
    in Italian Braised Celery, 126
    in Mom's Garlic Pasta, 210
    in My Mother-in-Law's Lasagna, 330–331
    in pasta sauce, 25
    in Quick Bouillabaisse, 414
    in Southwestern Sprout Wrap, 85
    in Summertime Okra, 294
    in Tomato-Basil Summer Salad, 40
    in Tuscan Tomato-Basil Spread, 305
Trail mix, 7, 405
Tropical Fruit Salad, 357
Tropical Marinade, 366

Tuna Tucks, 234, 492
Turkey, 346, 453–456
Turnip. *See* Greens
Tuscan Tomato-Basil Spread, 305

U

Ulcers
    basil, 37, 39
    chiles, 148, 150
    cinnamon, 160, 162
    tea, 443, 447
Upset stomach. *See* Digestion
Urinary tract infection, 68, 70, 168,
        170

V

Vegetable side dishes
    with cauliflower, 119
    garlic crisp potatoes, 371, 492
    green beans, 226
    Indian-style greens, 230
    kale, 239, 494
    okra, 294
    oven-roasted tomatoes, 452
    spiced sweet potatoes, 265
    spinach pignoli, 428, 493
    sweet potato fries, 442, 491
"Veggie burgers," 417–419
Vibrio vulnificus. See under Bacteria
Vision. *See also* Age-related macular degeneration;
            Cataracts
    bell peppers, 58, 59, 61
    broccoli, 76, 79
    cabbage, 96
    cantaloupe, 107, 110
    carrots, 112
    corn, 164, 166
    eggs, 181
    greens, 227, 229
    kale, 235–236
    kiwifruit, 240, 241, 243
    mangoes, 255, 258
    nectarines, 282, 283
    onions, 306, 307
    papaya, 316, 317
    peaches, 332
    pumpkin, 376, 377–379
    spinach, 424–425

Vision *(Continued)*
squash, 429, 431, 432
tea, 443, 447
Vision development in infants, 196, 200, 202, 205
Vitamins. *See specific foods*

W

Waffles. *See under* Breakfast foods
Waldorf Wrap, 346
Washing produce, 2, 83, 108, 175, 228, 251, 426
Watermelon, 151, 457–461
Watermelon Slush, 461, 491
Weight control
artichokes, 11, 14
avocados, 20, 22–23
beans, 41
blackberries, 63, 66
celery, 123
chicken, 143, 146
chives, 152
cucumbers, 173, 174
fennel, 188, 190
figs, 192, 194
garlic, 207, 210
ginger, 211, 212–213
green beans, 223, 225
milk, 266, 270–271
mushrooms, 277, 279
nuts, 286, 290
peanut butter, 336, 338
radishes, 387, 389–390
rosemary, 400, 401
shellfish, 409, 412
tea, 443, 446
wheatberries, 462, 465
yogurt, 484, 488
Wheatberries, 462–467
Wheatberries 'n Veggies, 467, 493

Wheatberry Breakfast, 466
Wheat bread, 473–477
Wheat germ, 468–472, 476
Whole Wheat Pita Wedges with Homemade
Hummus, 477, 493
Wild Creamy Mushroom Soup, 281, 492
Wine, 478–483
Wound healing
bok choy, 72, 74
horseradish, 231, 232
lettuce, 249, 253
oranges, 311, 312
papaya, 316, 317
peaches, 332, 334
potatoes, 368, 370
strawberries, 434, 436
Wraps. *See* Sandwiches and wraps
Wrinkles, 68, 311, 400–401, 412

Y

Yams, 441
Yeast infection, 5, 8, 438, 439, 484, 485
Yogurt, 132, 484–489
in Amazing Apricot Waffles, 10
in Banana-Peanut "Pudding," 31
in Blackberry Cheese Dip, 138
in Blueberry Breeze, 71
with cantaloupe, 109
in Chile Shrimp and Melon Salad, 151
in Chill-a-Melon Soup, 111
in Chilly Beet Soup, 57
in Chive Baked Potatoes, 154
in Hearty Purple Cow, 222
in Patriotic Breakfast Parfait, 399
with pineapple, 355
in Sesame Chicken with Whole Wheat Linguine, 408
in Tuna Tucks, 234